EXERCISE MANAGEMENT

Concepts and Professional Practice

LAUREL T. MACKINNON

CARRIE B. RITCHIE

SUE L. HOOPER

PETER J. ABERNETHY

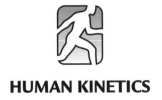

HUMAN KINETICS

Library of Congress Cataloging-in-Publication Data

Exercise management : concepts and professional practice / Laurel T.
Mackinnon ... [et al.].
        p. ; cm.
Includes bibliographical references and index.
  ISBN 0-7360-0023-2 (hard cover)
  1. Exercise therapy--Mangement. 2. Physical educaton and
training--Management.
  [DNLM: 1. Physical Education and Training. 2. Exericse Therapy. 3.
Physical Fitness. 4. Professional Practice. QT 255 E9555 2003] I.
Mackinnon, Laurel T., 1953-
  RM725 .E933 2003
  615.82 MAC   2002009621
ISBN 0-7360-0023-2

Copyright © 2003 by Laurel T. Mackinnon, Carrie B. Ritchie, Sue L. Hooper, and Peter J. Abernethy

The Web addresses cited in this text were current as of August 12, 2002, unless otherwise noted.

Acquisitions Editor: Michael S. Barhke, PhD; **Developmental Editor:** Jennifer L. Walker; **Assistant Editor:** Sandra Merz Bott; **Copyeditor:** Patricia L. MacDonald; **Proofreader:** Pamela Johnson; **Indexer:** L. Pilar Wyman, Wyman Indexing; **Permission Manager:** Dalene Reeder; **Graphic Designer:** Robert Reuther; **Graphic Artist:** Dawn Sills; **Photo Manager:** Leslie A. Woodrum; **Cover Designer:** Jack W. Davis; **Art Manager:** Kelly Hendren; **Illustrators:** Tom Roberts; Keith Blomberg; **Printer:** Sheridan Books

Printed in the United States of America   1 2 3 4 5 6 7 8 9 10

Human Kinetics
Web site: www.HumanKinetics.com

United States: Human Kinetics
P.O. Box 5076
Champaign, IL 61825-5076
800-747-4457
e-mail: humank@hkusa.com

Canada: Human Kinetics
475 Devonshire Road Unit 100
Windsor, ON N8Y 2L5
800-465-7301 (in Canada only)
e-mail: orders@hkcanada.com

Europe: Human Kinetics
107 Bradford Road
Stanningley
Leeds LS28 6AT, United Kingdom
+44 (0) 113 255 5665
e-mail: hk@hkeurope.com

Australia: Human Kinetics
57A Price Avenue
Lower Mitcham, South Australia 5062
08 8277 1555
e-mail: liahka@senet.com.au

New Zealand: Human Kinetics
P.O. Box 105-231, Auckland Central
09-523-3462
e-mail: hkp@ihug.co.nz

To our families

and

To those practitioners, scientists and academics
working to promote and expand our understanding
of the role of physical activity in health, fitness and sport.

CONTENTS

PREFACE

Exercise management is a dynamic profession in which practitioners design, deliver, promote and evaluate physical activity programs for the widest possible audience. It blends a strong foundation in kinesiological or exercise sciences (exercise physiology, exercise and sport psychology, motor development and control, and biomechanics) with business principles, such as business planning, marketing and professional leadership—hence the term exercise *management*.

This dual approach, combining exercise science with business management principles, gives the exercise manager unique skills to develop and manage optimal physical activity programs for all people, whether exercising alone, in a group or in a community setting. Exercise managers are found in a wide variety of settings, from clinics for children with movement disorders, to exercise rehabilitation programs for cardiac patients, to commercial or community-based activity programs for healthy adults and, of course, in organised sport. Regardless of the setting, the hallmark of a successful exercise manager is the effectiveness of his or her interaction with the stakeholders in physical activity—individual clients, the local community, government and private organisations, professional peers, other health professionals and colleagues within an exercise management practice.

Our Mission

Our mission in developing and writing this text is to provide a solid introductory foundation that challenges students to develop the professional skills to design physical activity programs that enhance the health and well-being of all clients, regardless of the particular exercise management setting. Physical activity has the potential to enhance the health, well-being and physical performance of virtually all people, regardless of age, disease or disability. Since the 1996 release of the landmark *Physical Activity and Health: A Report of the* [U.S.] *Surgeon General,* many government and community health organisations throughout the world now advocate that all individuals—young or old, healthy or infirm—maintain a physically active lifestyle.

How to Use This Book

Because of the inherent diversity of the exercise management profession, this book's design and purpose are twofold. First, it serves as a comprehensive text to introduce undergraduate students to the broad application of professional exercise management principles in diverse physical activity settings. Second, we have designed the text with other health professionals in mind, specifically those who either work with exercise managers or who are involved in the design of physical activity programs in the clinical setting.

The book has four main sections, each addressing a broad topic relating to the practice of exercise management. In section 1, we define the field of exercise management and discuss important professional issues within the broader context of the health benefits of physical activity and for promoting physical activity among the wider community. Section 2 discusses the basic principles of exercise prescription and programming for healthy individuals, including tools for pre-program screening and fitness assessment and behavioural interventions to facilitate adoption and maintenance of regular physical activity. In section 3, we apply these basic principles of exercise prescription and programming to groups with special needs, such as children, the elderly, athletes, and people with diseases or conditions affecting physical capacity, such as cardiovascular, respiratory, metabolic, neurological and musculoskeletal impairments. Finally, because successful professional practice requires sound technical *and* business skills, the application of business principles and human resource management in exercise management settings is introduced in section 4.

We also wish to note that this book draws from best practice both overseas (primarily North America, where many initiatives originate) and in Australia and New Zealand. Because the practice of exercise management is defined by diverse contextual and cultural factors, we invite instructors, students and other readers to supplement this text with local examples and recent research reports to best illustrate the principles presented.

Features of the Book

Glossary—At the end of each chapter is a compilation of key terms used within that chapter along with their abbreviations and definitions. The glossary at the end of the book contains all of the chapter glossary terms as well as additional key terms.

Case studies—Within most chapters are case studies. Students can use these case studies to apply their knowledge in realistic exercise management settings. Some of the case studies are based on real people or situations we have encountered in the practice of exercise management. For the case studies, we have included key issues to provide some direction to students. We have intentionally avoided solving the cases because, as students will come to realise, there is rarely only *one* way to develop and deliver a physical activity program. We think that providing only one solution could inhibit students from finding their own creative solutions. In our teaching at university level, we have used these and other case studies in many ways: student assignments, small group tutorials, role-playing and examination questions.

Student activities and study questions—At the end of each chapter are student activities and study questions that require the student to independently seek additional information beyond that presented in the book. For some activities, students will need to visit various exercise management sites to gain first-hand appreciation of the scope of professional practice.

References—To make the text more user friendly, we have generally avoided citing references within the text. Instead, we cite specific references only to support or illustrate a particular point or when referring to a particular report or research paper.

Suggested readings—At the end of the book are suggested readings for each section for those interested in pursuing particular topics at a more advanced level.

Laurel T. Mackinnon
Carrie B. Ritchie
Sue L. Hooper
Peter J. Abernethy

Brisbane, Australia, January, 2002

ACKNOWLEDGEMENTS

. . . .

We gratefully acknowledge the following people who assisted in the preparation of this book by providing ideas for case studies, "day in the life" scenarios in chapter 1, relevant references or information, or critical review of parts of the book: Tom Briffa, Rachelle Foreman, David Jenkins, Vince Kelly, Sophia Ljaskevic, Graeme Maw, Chris Nunn, Victor Pendleton, Sharon Bishop Sibthorpe, Stewart Trost, and Sean Tweedy.

We wish to thank Deb Noon for her expert assistance in preparation of tables and figures.

We also wish to acknowledge the patience and guidance of editors and other staff at Human Kinetics, especially Rainer Martens, Mike Bahrke, Jennifer Walker, and Sandra Merz Bott.

THE PROFESSION OF EXERCISE MANAGEMENT: PROMOTING PHYSICAL ACTIVITY IN THE COMMUNITY

Physical inactivity is acknowledged as a health risk in most developed countries, contributing to a number of diseases or conditions including cardiovascular diseases (heart disease, stroke, peripheral vascular disease), obesity, hypertension, type 2 (non-insulin-dependent) diabetes, osteoporosis and certain types of cancer. Regular moderate physical activity has potential to reduce the burden of disease by helping to prevent these conditions. In addition, regular moderate physical activity plays an important role in the management of other diseases or conditions such as cardiac event recovery, neurological and musculoskeletal disorders, and anxiety and depression. Regular physical activity also provides many psychological health benefits such as enhanced self-esteem and self-efficacy. Consequently, many developed and developing countries have initiated strategies to encourage their populations to become more physically active as a means of improving health, quality of life, and to contain ever-increasing health care costs.

Section 1 contains three chapters aimed at introducing and explaining the field of exercise management. Chapter 1 introduces the exercise management profession, defining the profession, and discussing essential skills and training needed by the exercise manager, as well as professional ethics and organisations representing the interests of exercise managers throughout the world. Chapter 2 introduces and examines the myriad health benefits of physical activity and current rates of participation in physical activity in developed countries. This is followed by a presentation of current recommendations for the amount of physical activity needed to realise these health benefits. Although the health benefits of regular physical activity are well-documented, there remains an alarmingly high proportion of the population in developed countries that is not sufficiently active to positively influence health, presenting a significant challenge to those working in the fields of health promotion and exercise management. Chapter 3 discusses how national and community efforts are trying to meet the challenge of encouraging wider participation in regular physical activity.

CHAPTER 1

- - - - - - - - - - -

The Profession of Exercise Management

As described in the preface, **exercise management** is a dynamic **profession** involved in the design, delivery, promotion and evaluation of **physical activity** programs for the widest possible audience, including elite athletes, healthy individuals of all ages and people with disease or impairment. Exercise management principles are used in any setting in which physical activity, **exercise** or sports are performed. Regardless of the particular setting, a common feature of exercise management is the manager's consistent focus on enhancing the physical capacity and well-being of all clients using sound management and leadership principles.

The **Australian Association for Exercise and Sports Science (AAESS)**, a professional association representing exercise managers, defines exercise and sport science as

> A multidisciplinary field concerned with the understanding and enhancement of human movement in the broadest sense, including general physical activity pursuits such as goal oriented fitness regimens and recreational sport as well as elite sport and the area of performance enhancement. It includes the knowledge, methods and applications of subdisciplines (i.e., exercise physiology, biomechanics, motor control and motor development, exercise and sport psychology) as well as how they interact. (AAESS Web site)

Settings Where Exercise Management Professionals Are Employed

The profession of exercise management is diverse, and professionals may be found working in many settings. While the settings may differ, all exercise managers work with a common purpose: to develop, deliver and manage the most appropriate physical activity programs for the client(s), whether the client is an individual, small group or large community. Services provided by exercise managers include (but are not limited to)

- ▶ assessment of **physical fitness** for sport, recreation or employment;
- ▶ exercise counselling, prescription and programming for individuals and small or large groups;
- ▶ movement and exercise rehabilitation for those with, or at risk of, disease or impairment;

▶ design and delivery of exercise training programs to enhance sport performance;

▶ applied, basic and clinical research relating to physical activity, exercise and sport;

▶ promotion of healthy lifestyles, including physical activity, in the wider community; and

▶ evaluation of individual or group physical activity programs and efforts to promote physical activity among the wider community.

Exercise managers are employed in an ever-increasing variety of settings, including corporate and commercial health and fitness centres, hospitals, aged care facilities and rehabilitation clinics, private consultancies, government and non-government health promotion agencies, sports academies/institutes and community or professional sports clubs, and public and private educational or other community organisations. Exercise management requires knowledge and skills gained in an undergraduate degree in human movement studies/science or exercise science, coupled with extensive practical experience in at least one aspect of professional practice. Advanced study, through a research or coursework postgraduate degree, is often recommended for those working with special groups such as elite athletes or clients with disease or impairment. As with many professions in this fast-changing world, some exercise management employment opportunities did not exist a few years ago, and new ones will be created in the coming years. The depth and variety of exercise management settings are best illustrated by describing a typical day in the lives of exercise managers working in different settings.[1]

Sport Science Consultant

I am a private consultant specialising in strength and conditioning for sport. My clients are varied, from promising young athletes in individual sports to professional teams. I have an undergraduate degree with honours in exercise science and practical experience working with elite and professional athletes.

The first job of the day starts at 7:00 A.M. with an individual conditioning session for a state-level tennis player. In this session, we focus on her speed and agility because she was lacking speed when coming forward to the net in her last match.

At 9:00 A.M., I administer a battery of tests to a young AFL (Australian Football League) player who has been invited to the AFL national draft camp at the AIS (Australian Institute of Sport). The athlete performs tests of speed (20-m sprints), agility, power (vertical jumps), strength (bench presses), anaerobic power capacity and aerobic endurance (shuttle runs); anthropometric measures (body mass, skinfolds) are also taken.

In the afternoon, I examine the AFL player's test results and compare them with results from the previous year's draft camp. These comparisons are used to identify any fitness components that the player needs to improve. Once identified, these weaker areas are incorporated into a program to help the athlete prepare for the draft camp in 2 months. This process takes about 3 h.

In the early evening, I run a conditioning session for a squad of elite junior tennis players. The session will vary depending on the phase of the competitive season but will always include some focus on agility, footwork and movement patterns.

Finally, I attend a strength and power session in the gym with a squad of rugby athletes. This session includes a wide variety of resistance exercise, including Olympic lifts and other methods to maximise power development.

Throughout the day, I am aware of the need to tailor strength and conditioning training to the athletes' specific needs to help them improve performance in their sports.

High-Performance Manager in a State Institute of Sport

In my job I provide sport science services for high-performance athletes at the state and national level. I work closely with the athletes, coaches and other support personnel (doctors, dietitians, physiotherapists) to help optimise the athletes' training and performance. I have an undergraduate degree in exercise science and a doctorate in exercise physiology; my research background is especially useful since much of my job involves data collection and analysis to advise the coaches on optimal training methods to enhance the athletes' performances.

The day begins early (5:30 A.M.) at the pool. It is "skinfold day"—one of our regularly scheduled ses-

---

[1]These are actual statements obtained from exercise managers working in the different contexts described. They were each asked to provide a statement about a typical day at work.

sions to assess body composition, which tend to increase in frequency as competition approaches. While the swimmers train, I compile the data so that I can discuss the numbers with the swimmers and coach at the end of the session and refer any swimmers needing or requesting dietary advice.

Back at my office, I eat breakfast while catching up with the world electronically, reading relevant literature and perusing Web sites relating to swimming and exercise science. I next start to analyse yesterday's data collected on elite rowers, compiling these into a report for the coach. Our lab has recently been discussing a new perspective on lactate curves related to rowing, and I wanted to take some extra time to compare the data analysed the usual way with our proposed new analysis. As soon as I finish, I fax the data to the coach, who is eager for the results; he will modify training over the next few days to reflect what the data showed.

After lunch, I meet with a postgraduate student who will be conducting his research with us by planning his testing program within the athletes' training schedule. I then return to the pool to conduct more testing with the swimmers, who were to complete a set of "quality" sprints. This type of testing is part of a long-term periodised program, and we monitor heart rates, blood lactate and swimming mechanics (technique). I also schedule a session for the following week in which I will add video analysis to the physiological measures as part of our regular testing program. To me, it is vital to be able to integrate measures of fitness, technique and psychological readiness to really help these athletes improve performance.

Exercise Cardiac Rehabilitation Manager

I work in a hospital **exercise cardiac rehabilitation** clinic. We provide exercise advice and programs for both in-patients (before discharge from hospital) and out-patients (after discharge). Our patients all have some form of heart disease or are at high risk of developing heart disease; some have recently had heart surgery. I have a bachelor's degree in exercise science and a master's degree in clinical exercise science, both of which included practical work experience with exercise cardiac rehabilitation programs. During my postgraduate study, I also worked as a cardiac technician, assisting a cardiologist administer exercise stress tests.

The working day starts at 7:30 A.M. when I meet 12 patients attending our maintenance activity program at the outdoor oval next to the hospital. These patients have some type of heart disease or experienced a cardiac event at least several months ago but have been exercising regularly since then. Today the group plays a modified game of soccer that involves no running. Before the game begins, I measure their resting heart rates and blood pressures and lead them in a 15-min warm-up. We will repeat this as a cool-down at the end of the 35-min game.

After the game, I return to the centre's gym to lead two out-patient exercise sessions. I measure resting and exercise heart rates and blood pressures for all patients to ensure these remain within the recommended levels. I also help two patients decide how much to increase the resistance on the weight machines because their muscular strength has improved over the past month. At 10:45 A.M., after morning tea with these out-patients, I attend a group discussion for patients led by the hospital pharmacist in which the various medications used by cardiac patients are discussed. Between the two morning exercise sessions, I also phone recently discharged patients to discuss the best out-patient programs for them to attend.

The afternoon is filled with assessment of two new patients—one is 2 weeks post-angioplasty and the other is 3 weeks post-myocardial infarction (heart attack). I have already talked with their cardiologists about their histories and current medications. The patients will complete questionnaires on health status, quality of life, physical activity habits, and leisure and work activities; these allow us to individualise their exercise programs to best suit their interests and needs. I then supervise submaximal fitness testing of these patients on a cycle ergometer and assess their body composition and muscular flexibility.

The last task of the day is to consult with the hospital's social worker to discuss a new patient and his spouse, whom I have referred for counselling. I find it especially rewarding to work with a variety of health professionals to help patients change their lifestyles and health in a positive way.

Clinical Musculoskeletal Exercise Rehabilitation Consultant

The work is varied in my practice as a clinical **musculoskeletal exercise rehabilitation** consultant. I work with individual clients with particular diseases or impairments, and I also provide public and patient educational programs. I work closely with a small private hospital, but I also see clients in their homes. I have a bachelor's degree in exercise science, which included practical experience working with the local Diabetes Association to develop exercise and public education programs for people with diabetes.

My day starts at 7:30 A.M. when I meet at the clinic a 39-year-old man with chronic back pain who has been referred from a physiotherapist. Although he has worked for several years in a job requiring manual handling (e.g., lifting and moving heavy objects), his current problem had a sudden onset, suggesting some type of acute injury. When I assessed him previously, it was clear that he had poor strength in the pelvic and lower back region. It is also obvious that he is apprehensive about using these muscles because of the pain, and this affects his ability to work and enjoy a normal lifestyle. In today's session we focus on core stability exercises to improve his strength in this area.

Between 8:30 and 9:30 A.M., I discuss over the phone the treatment details of clients referred by physiotherapists and chiropractors, and I complete relevant Work Cover forms.

At 9:30 A.M., I meet for the first time with another client with low back pain. This session is spent assessing his range of motion and readiness to exercise and discussing his expectations and goals for an exercise program.

From 12 noon to 2:00 P.M., I deliver an information seminar on exercise and type 2 diabetes as part of a public education program through the hospital. I discuss the benefits of physical activity in managing type 2 diabetes, precautions for diabetics who exercise, and safe ways for people with diabetes to become more physically active.

At 3:30 P.M., I meet with an 11-year-old client at her home to develop a program of sensible weight loss and physical fitness. During the meeting I realise that, in addition to simple weight loss, she hopes to improve her coordination and basic body awareness. Together we develop a home-based fitness program of games and drills, emphasising continual movement and enjoyment, that she can do in the privacy of her backyard.

At 5:00 P.M., I meet at the home of a 13-year-old boy with impaired muscle development and motor function. His goals are to improve muscular strength and coordination. We develop a program of activities to improve proprioception and coordination (using the Swiss Ball) and to teach basic weightlifting technique in preparation for a future gym-based program that he desires. Because of his limited muscular strength and endurance, the initial program comprises brief low-intensity exercises, with an eye to gradual progress.

At 6:30 P.M., I meet with a 45-year-old woman with type 1 diabetes and osteoarthritis in her feet. I demonstrate some recommended exercises using resistive rubber bands (Thera-Band®). The aim of her program is to gently increase energy expenditure while avoiding hypoglycaemia and foot pain.

Personal Trainer

As a **personal trainer** and health consultant, I typically work when everyone else does not—my peak working times are between 5:30 and 9:30 A.M. and then again from 4:30 to 7:30 P.M. Each day is different, depending on my clients' interests. As a small business owner, I also spend some of each day on paperwork and business planning. My background includes an undergraduate degree in human movement studies and education, in which I prepared for a career as a health and physical education teacher, followed by an honours degree in exercise physiology. I have previously worked for the public service, developing and managing a fitness facility for a local government council.

My typical day starts at 5:30 A.M. when I meet my first client at the local heated pool. She was not a strong swimmer to start, and we have been focusing on stroke technique and fitness. She swims a 300-m time trial to assess her progress—25-s improvement in the past 6 weeks; she is pleased. In the rest of the 1.8 km session, we focus on high elbow lift and the pull through the water.

My next session begins at 7:15 A.M. at the home of a client who is recovering from a back injury. She has been diligent in her home-based program, to which we are starting to add some variety. Today we walk briskly for 40 min, followed by core stability exercises for the lower back and a good stretch.

I meet my next client at 8:30 A.M. for a cycle session. She is new to road cycling and is learning to maintain pedal revolutions while changing gears. Today we test one of two new routes, timing the ride as a baseline to measure improvement over the next 6 weeks.

Between 9:30 A.M. and 4:00 P.M., I attend to billing and accounts, write programs for this week's clients and make some phone calls to clients. Since I also employ three trainers, I discuss with them via phone or e-mail their current clients' progress and any problems. I also eat lunch and take a nap to be ready for the evening sessions.

At 4:30 P.M., I meet with a male client, a rock climber, who is working on improving his strength and physical fitness for climbing. We train together once each week, and he completes on his own three other sessions each week that we have developed together to meet his specific goals. Today we are doing a gym session made up of specific exercises to strengthen the upper body muscles he needs for rock climbing.

At 5:30 P.M., I meet with my final client of the day, who is training for the Noosa Triathlon in 4 months' time. Today he completes a 10 km time trial, trying to maintain a 4:45 per km target pace; this pace is a bit too fast for me to run, so I ride alongside on my bike, giving him encouragement and split times for each km. After a cool-down, we discuss the next 6 weeks of the program, which is aimed at improving his pace during the run phase of the triathlon.

Health Promotion Officer

I work with a non-government, non-profit organisation. My main job is to develop a community physical activity program that can be delivered locally but coordinated at a state level. To develop a program that is responsive to the needs of the community throughout the state, I meet and liaise with people employed in health care and community activities. In addition, I work directly with members of the public who are involved in our community walking program. I have an undergraduate degree in exercise science and a master's degree in clinical exercise science, in which I specialised in working in clinical exercise settings with older, healthy people and with cardiac and cancer patients.

My typical day starts with attending to recent phone and e-mail messages from our current group leaders and participants and with updating our current database on the program. I then have morning tea with my staff (e.g., volunteers and project officers) to discuss the program's progress and ways to address any problems that may have arisen in the past few days.

The rest of the morning is spent developing the content of resources for our program, such as booklets, newsletters, posters, advertising in the print and electronic media, and our Web site. I also spend time on development of our merchandise, such as T-shirts and water bottles. All of these activities educate the public about the health benefits of walking and promote our community programs.

Over lunch, I read through a draft of an honours thesis by a student evaluating our program as part of her research. After lunch, I attend a meeting of representatives from a wide variety of health and community groups, **stakeholders** in our physical activity programs. We discuss the best ways to promote physical activity in general, and our programs in particular, among the wider community, especially in the smaller regional and remote areas.

At the time of writing this, I am also involved in a state-wide taskforce on physical activity. We are holding a series of 23 regional consultation forums and focus groups to develop a state-wide policy and framework to increase participation in physical activity. I spend some of each day involved in the planning of the forums (which I attend) and liaising with other stakeholders in the process (government, sport and community groups).

As can be seen in these examples, exercise management is very much a "hands on" profession, involving direct work with individual clients and groups with various needs. Broad training across the subdisciplines of exercise science and health promotion provides the exercise manager with the knowledge and technical skills to tailor programs to meet these diverse needs.

Skills and Personal Attributes of the Exercise Manager

Exercise management is a multidisciplinary field requiring knowledge and skills from a number of subdisciplines; these are usually incorporated into the undergraduate degree in exercise science or human movement studies. The field of exercise management comprises a knowledge base from the four subdisciplines of exercise science—exercise physiology, motor learning and control, biomechanics, and sport and exercise psychology. To this base is added further study and practical experience in technical skills (**pre-activity screening**, **fitness assessment**, exercise leadership and **exercise prescription and programming**). Effective program development (How do we develop an effective program? How do we assess the effectiveness of a program?) requires problem solving, communication and evaluation skills. In addition, exercise managers providing physical activity services aim to run a successful business and need basic business skills, such as business planning, marketing, professional leadership, human resource management and effective communication. The relationship between these skills and knowledge is depicted in figure 1.1.

Exercise physiology provides much of the knowledge base for exercise management. It is too simplistic to think of the discipline and professional practice as simply "applied exercise physiology". This is illustrated by the following simple example.

An overweight man on medication for hypertension is referred to a community fitness program by his doctor in the belief that regular physical activity may help in the management of his blood pressure.

Knowledge from several disciplines needs to be considered to safely and effectively prescribe exercise for this client:

▶ Regulation of blood pressure and physiological responses to exercise in hypertensive individuals (systemic physiology, exercise physiology)

▶ Regulation of body weight and fat metabolism and effectiveness of exercise in weight loss (physiology, biochemistry, nutrition, exercise physiology)

▶ Effects of blood pressure medication on exercise capacity and prescription (pharmacology)

▶ Technical skills in fitness assessment and exercise leadership (exercise physiology, exercise prescription and programming)

▶ Effects of excess body mass on mechanical forces stressing the body during exercise and risk of musculoskeletal injury (biomechanics, sports medicine)

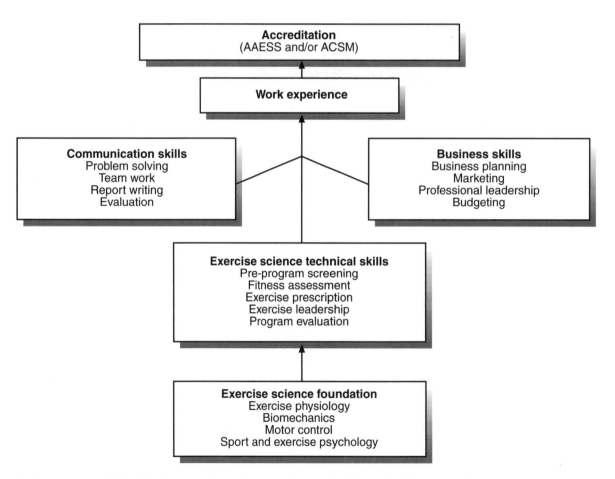

FIGURE 1.1   Relationship between the various professional skills needed by an exercise manager.

▶ Factors influencing adherence to an exercise program (exercise and health psychology)

▶ Factors influencing health behaviour changes (health psychology)

▶ Oral and written communication and individual counselling skills (pedagogy, communication, psychology)

▶ Models of physical activity skill acquisition (pedagogy, motor learning and control)

It can be seen from this example that the exercise manager must take a holistic view of the individual client to effectively prescribe exercise that meets the client's goals and objectives. By holistic, we mean considering the client from all perspectives. That is, an exercise prescription will only be successful if it also incorporates and integrates all the key issues relating to the individual client (or group, discussed later). While one type of exercise may seem appropriate from the physiological perspective, an exercise program is doomed to fail if it does not also incorporate the client's perceived and actual needs, goals, preferences, previous experience, skill level, health risks and readiness to change health behaviour (these topics are discussed in more detail in section 2).

Technical Skills in Exercise Management

In addition to expertise in exercise science and more general skills (communication, problem solving, business planning) listed previously, exercise management requires a broad range of technical competence. The basic technical skills required by exercise managers include the following:

▶ Health risk screening—Identifying clients at risk of or with disease for whom vigorous exercise may be problematic and who need referral to a physician before beginning an exercise program.

▶ Assessment of physical fitness and interpretation of data—Measuring the client's fitness level and using these data as a basis for exercise prescription.

▶ Exercise prescription and programming—Writing an exercise prescription to meet the needs of individual or group clients.

▶ Exercise leadership—Demonstrating and teaching physical activity skills to clients.

These basic technical skills are discussed in greater detail in section 2. In addition to these basic

skills, further technical skills may be needed to work with a particular individual client or group. For example, a sport scientist employed to enhance performance of a group of athletes would use a variety of sport-specific assessment tools; in a musculoskeletal rehabilitation clinic, the exercise manager would apply a number of tests to assess patient progress during recovery.

Evaluation Skills in Exercise Management

Evaluation is a critical, but sometimes overlooked, function of exercise managers. Evaluation can be defined as a process of asking meaningful questions and collecting relevant data to be used in developing the most appropriate program for a given individual, group or community. Evaluation is an ongoing process in which the data collected are used for program planning, development, delivery and modification. In the exercise management context, the process of evaluation can be applied to individuals (e.g., using client goals and fitness assessment data to develop the exercise prescription) as well as to programs (e.g., determining program goals in advance and then later deciding if these goals have been met).

The general goals of evaluation in exercise management are to

▶ determine program effectiveness;

▶ identify and assess program achievements and outcomes;

▶ identify program shortcomings and, thus, the need and opportunities for improvement;

▶ assess program quality; and

▶ provide data and make recommendations for future directions.

In addition to the exercise science technical skills described previously, the successful exercise manager needs a variety of evaluation skills. Evaluation skills include the ability to manage information, to systematically collect and analyse quantitative and qualitative data, to effectively communicate the findings to individuals and groups, and to incorporate this information in future planning (lateral thinking and problem-solving skills).

The topic of evaluation is discussed further throughout this book, in particular as applied to community programs (chapter 3), as applied to individual exercise prescription (chapters 4-7) and as part of business planning (chapters 12-13).

Business Skills in Exercise Management

Exercise managers also need a variety of business skills in addition to the exercise science technical and evaluation skills described in the previous section. Many exercise managers own their own businesses as sole proprietors (self-employed) or business partners (with one or more co-owners) or head larger businesses that employ many staff. Other exercise managers work in supervisory or management roles within organisations, such as governmental agencies, hospitals, professional sports teams, private practice or large companies. Basic business skills needed by the exercise manager include the following:

- ▶ Business planning—A process to identify the program's or organisation's mission and goals and then implement an effective strategy to achieve these goals.

- ▶ Professional leadership—The ability to inspire and guide others to work toward a common goal.

- ▶ Effective oral and written communication— The ability to clearly articulate to staff, clients and other stakeholders the business' mission, purpose, strategies and effectiveness.

- ▶ Marketing—The promotion of the business to attract and retain clients.

- ▶ Financial planning and management—The ongoing management of income and expenditure, essential to maintaining the viability of a business.

The extent to which exercise managers need to develop expertise in these particular skills depends on the type of business and the role the exercise manager plays in the business. For example, a sole proprietor will need to develop planning, marketing and financial skills, whereas an exercise manager supervising other staff in a larger organisation may need to develop skills in professional leadership. These topics are discussed in further detail in section 4.

Application of Skills at Different Levels

It can be seen from the preceding discussion that the exercise manager uses technical, evaluation and business skills at different levels, which can be broadly divided into the individual level and program level. Individual-level applications include mainly the technical and evaluation skills applied directly to individual clients, such as pre-exercise screening, physical fitness assessment, exercise prescription and exercise leadership. In the "typical day" examples described previously, these skills formed a substantial part of the working day of nearly all of the exercise managers, with the exception of the health promotion officer. Program-level applications include more of the business, evaluation and communication skills needed to develop and administer effective physical activity programs. These incorporate business planning, marketing, professional leadership, managing staff, budgets, report writing and evaluation. These functions were mentioned in the "typical day" examples of the high-performance manager, exercise cardiac rehabilitation manager, personal trainer and health promotion officer.

Other Skills

As already mentioned, exercise managers work with more than individual clients; they sometimes work with small or large groups or even an entire community. As a result, the exercise manager may also need to acquire skills in health promotion, research design and statistics, and communication to small and large groups. To build on the previous example, the exercise manager working in community health promotion may be involved in developing recommendations for physical activity interventions for people with high blood pressure. This might involve consultation with other health professionals, health insurers and government, followed by development of effective ways to communicate these recommendations to everyone in the community, such as through brochures available at health centres, doctors' surgeries and pharmacies or public health messages in print and electronic media.

Finally, the exercise manager is often part of a multidisciplinary team that includes professionals from different backgrounds. For example, most cardiac rehabilitation programs involve collaboration among physicians (usually general practitioners and cardiologists), nurses, physiotherapists, occupational therapists, dietitians, psychologists and exercise managers, each contributing distinctive skills and expertise to promote recovery in cardiac patients. Another example might be the elite sport setting, in which the coaches, trainers, physiotherapists, dietitians, masseurs, sport physicians, sport psychologists and sport scientists (exercise managers) work together to optimise an athlete's performance. Thus, teamwork, the ability to work effectively with other professionals toward a common goal, is another essential skill in exercise management.

Professionalism

A profession can be defined as an occupation requiring advanced knowledge in a specialised area. A professional, then, is a practitioner of a particular profession, that is, one who can demonstrate specialised and unique training, knowledge and skills. In some instances, state or national laws strictly define a profession and who may practice that profession. The profession of exercise management has not yet been defined by state or federal law. Exercise management can be described as a profession in which practitioners design, deliver, promote and evaluate physical activity programs for the widest possible audience—from elite athletes to healthy individuals to people with disease or impairment affecting their ability to move.

The term *professionalism* is often used to describe an expected level of professional behaviour, that is, how a professional behaves in the professional context. Professionalism entails a wide range of issues including requisite knowledge and skills; technical competence; interaction with clients, peers and the public; and honest and ethical behaviour. Clients or the public usually have expectations of professional behaviour that may be generalised across professions. For example, honesty and ethical behaviour in dealing with clients are expected of all professionals. Acceptable (and unacceptable) professional behaviour may be delineated by the organisation governing that profession. This usually takes the form of a code of ethics to which all members of that profession are expected to adhere. In some professions, disciplinary action (including withdrawal of professional accreditation) may be taken if the profession's code of conduct is violated. Figure 1.2 gives the Australian Association for Exercise and Sports Science (AAESS) Code of Ethics.

Of importance to the exercise manager are issues such as technical competence, ethical treatment of clients and the public, interaction with peers and **confidentiality**. Technical competence is the ability to perform basic services such as health risk screening, fitness testing, interpretation of test results, and safe and effective exercise prescription and programming. A breach of technical competence

would be failure to give adequate safety instructions to a client as part of the exercise prescription. Technical competence is essential for maintaining high professional standards and for avoiding undesirable events; the example just given could result in injury to the client. Ethical treatment of clients and the public requires open and honest communication. Clearly indicating fee structures and services to be provided and then delivering the services as promised are good examples. Confidentiality is an important part of ethical interaction with clients. It is expected that the exercise manager will treat as confidential and privileged all personal information about individual clients. A breach of confidentiality would occur if the exercise manager discussed a client's health status with another client. Professional behaviour also extends to interactions between practitioners within the profession. Colleagues expect to be treated honestly and ethically by each other, even when they may be competitors in the same type of business. A high standard of professional behaviour by all practitioners enhances the standing of that profession in the eyes of clients, the public and other stakeholders (e.g., health insurers, government).

Professional Organisations Representing Exercise Managers

There are a number of professional organisations in Australia and overseas in which physical activity, exercise or sport is a primary focus. The four most relevant organisations to exercise managers in Australia (although by no means the only ones) are the Australian Association for Exercise and Sports Science (AAESS), **Sports Medicine Australia (SMA)**, the **American College of Sports Medicine (ACSM)** and the International Council of Sport Science and Physical Education (ICSSPE).

Australian Association for Exercise and Sports Science (AAESS)

The AAESS was founded in 1991 to represent the professional needs of exercise and sport scientists in Australia (i.e., exercise managers working in exercise and sport science settings). The mission of the AAESS is "to represent exercise and sports science professionals in Australia as the leading recognised providers of knowledge concerning physical activity, performance and health/wellness" (AAESS Strategic Plan 2001, AAESS Web site).

PREAMBLE

Notwithstanding all other goals of the AAESS, the responsibility of members for the welfare, health and safety of their clients and the community at large shall at all times be paramount. To the end, members should abide by this code of ethics in deciding the standards by which they determine the propriety of their conduct and their relationships with colleagues, with allied professionals, with the public and with all persons with whom a professional relationship has been established. These dimensions of conduct should be addressed by members:

1. **Best practice.** Members should maintain high professional standards of client service:
   a. Service should be based on the best scientific information and professional practice currently available.
   b. Members should be committed to, and involved in, furthering their knowledge, skills and competencies through continuing education.
2. **Client care.** Clients should not be subjected to undue risk before, during and after exercise prescribed by members:
   a. Members should ensure that clients are aware of the risks associated with exercise through the process of informed consent and aware of their rights to withdraw from such interaction without penalty (at any time).
   b. Members should provide instruction and education that minimises the risk of injury and maximises the benefits from their interaction.
   c. Members should ensure that, in the case of injury, treatment and appropriate care are available to clients.
   d. Members should ensure that, in the conduct of experimentation, procedures conform to the principles enunciated by
      i. the NH & MRC (National Health and Medical Research Council) and
      ii. those of the administering institution.
3. **Personal and professional integrity.** The Association has a responsibility to protect the public from members who do not demonstrate professional competence or who behave in an unethical manner.

Individual members should strive to enhance the effectiveness of and the standing of the AAESS as well as respect the confidential nature of their relationships with clients.

FIGURE 1.2   Code of Ethics of the Australian Association for Exercise and Sports Science.

The objectives of the AAESS are to

▶ further the professions of exercise and sport science;

▶ develop and promote career opportunities for members;

▶ promote ethical and honourable practice by members;

▶ promote, progress and improve education and communication in the exercise and sport science professions; and

▶ formulate, implement and manage procedures for registration of exercise and sport scientists.

A complete listing of objectives of the AAESS may be found on their Web site listed at the end of this chapter.

There are four categories of membership in the AAESS—full, adjunct, student and accredited. Full membership requires a 3- or 4-year degree in exercise or sport science or human movement studies. The degree must include study within the four fundamental exercise science subdisciplines (exercise physiology, motor control, biomechanics, sport and exercise psychology), although it is possible to meet this latter requirement by prior learning competencies through tertiary training or work experience. AAESS members may use the post-nominal

MAAESS in professional practice (e.g., on business cards, for marketing purposes). Student members are those studying in courses that eventually lead to membership in the AAESS. Adjunct membership is open to graduates of other degrees with postgraduate qualifications in exercise or sport science. Accreditation is discussed in more detail later in the chapter.

The AAESS recognises the diversity of settings in which exercise and sport scientists are employed and has developed a recommended salary scale to reflect the skills and expertise of its members. In addition, AAESS members may obtain professional indemnity and public liability insurance. The AAESS has been an active advocate for programs to enhance wider participation in physical activity across the entire population and for recognition of the exercise and sport scientist as a professional with requisite expertise in physical activity and sport. Important recent achievements include the recognition by some private health insurers of AAESS-accredited members as providers of health services and the development of a national network of university, clinic and health insurance participants to provide data in support of the effectiveness of exercise rehabilitation and to provide the basis for evidence-based practice.

Besides the national body of the AAESS, there are state and regional branches in Queensland, New South Wales, Victoria, South Australia and West Australia. These groups meet regularly to discuss relevant professional issues and to provide continuing professional education. Further information about membership, accreditation, recommended salary scale, state branches and the Association's activities may be found on their Web site listed at the end of this chapter.

Sports Medicine Australia (SMA)

SMA is a non-profit professional and community educational organisation made up of a variety of professional groups with a common interest in sports medicine and sport science. These groups include professional associations representing the following fields (professional associations listed in parentheses):

▶ Medicine (Australian College of Sports Physicians, Sports Doctors Australia)

▶ Exercise and sport science (AAESS)

▶ Physiotherapy (Australian Physiotherapy Association National Sports Physiotherapy Group)

▶ Dietetics (Sports Dietitians Australia)

▶ Podiatry (Australian Association of Sports Podiatry)

▶ Psychology (Australian Psychology Association College of Sport Psychology)

SMA provides important educational and community services locally and nationally. Community services include medical coverage of sporting events for school and community sports, educational programs in sports first aid and sports training, injury surveillance and prevention, and publication of policy statements and educational brochures for professional practitioners and the public. SMA also provides an important referral and communication network to link the various professional groups, governmental agencies and the community. Recently, SMA has become actively involved in government and community initiatives to promote physical activity across the wider population (e.g., Active Australia, discussed in chapter 3.

The annual SMA conference incorporates scientific and clinical sessions from each of the various disciplines just listed. This offers unique interaction between scientists, practitioners and clinicians with interests across the diverse fields within sports medicine and science. Further information about SMA and its discipline organisations may be found at the Web site listed at the end of this chapter.

American College of Sports Medicine (ACSM)

Founded in 1954, the ACSM is the largest sports medicine and exercise science association in the world, with nearly 18,000 members from more than 75 countries in addition to the United States and Canada. ACSM's mission is "to promote and integrate scientific research, education and practice in the areas of sports medicine and exercise science to maintain and enhance physical performance, fitness and health and quality of life" (ACSM Web site). There are three general interest areas:

▶ Medicine (general practice, sports medicine, cardiology, orthopaedics, other clinical specialities)

▶ Basic and applied science (exercise physiology, biomechanics, sport psychology, motor control, health promotion, epidemiology)

▶ Education and allied health (nursing, physical education, occupational and physical therapy, sports training)

The ACSM annual conference in the United States attracts more than 5,000 delegates. This conference provides an ideal setting for interaction and collaboration between members of the various disciplines of sports medicine and exercise science from around the world. In addition, the ACSM sponsors or endorses more than 165 other conferences and workshops each year that provide continuing education credits required for professional licensure or accreditation.

In addition to its strong research and educational role, the ACSM has been an active and prominent force in increasing recognition by governments and health professions of the importance of physical activity to health, in particular through the release of the landmark 1996 **U.S. Surgeon General's report on physical activity and health** (discussed more fully in chapter 2). The ACSM was the first organisation to certify professionals working in the exercise sciences; it has been instrumental in gaining recognition for the exercise scientist as an important contributor to the clinical management of many illnesses such as cardiac and pulmonary disease. The many ACSM publications are standard references for anyone working in health and fitness or clinical exercise settings. In addition, as discussed in much of this book, the ACSM Position Statements on various topics, especially those relating to exercise prescription for healthy adults and the elderly, have become benchmarks for **best practice** in exercise prescription and programming.

International Council of Sport Science and Physical Education (ICSSPE)

The ICSSPE was founded in 1958 in Paris initially to improve links between the fields of sport, sport sciences and physical education. ICSSPE's main objectives are to encourage international cooperation in the sport sciences; to promote scientific research on physical activity, sport and physical education; and to make available such scientific knowledge to organisations devoted to sport and physical activity. The ICSSPE is currently focusing on its role as a facilitator of links between key organisations, such as the World Health Organization (WHO), the International Olympic Committee (IOC), United Nations (through UNESCO) and other groups, to enhance accessibility of information and resources on sport and physical activity, especially in developing countries. Roughly 200 organisations from approximately 60 countries are members of the ICSSPE. The prestigious Sport Science Award of the IOC President, presented in recognition of outstanding scientific work in the areas of sport and exercise science, was initiated by the ICSSPE.

Other Professional Organisations in Australia and Overseas

Countless other professional organisations may interest the exercise manager, depending on the particular specialist area of practice. Some of these organisations attract professionals from a wide variety of fields; for example, the Australian Cardiac Rehabilitation Association (ACRA) draws its membership from health professionals (e.g., doctors, nurses, exercise managers, dietitians, physiotherapists, occupational therapists, social workers, psychologists) working to enhance health and quality of life in cardiac patients. Similarly, the Australian Health Promotion Association attracts professionals working to promote healthy lifestyles among the wider community; physical activity would be one of many focus areas for this organisation. There are also professional associations representing particular aspects of exercise science, such as the National Strength and Conditioning Association, which attracts coaches, trainers, athletes, exercise managers, sport scientists and fitness consultants, all using the application of resistance training to enhance physical fitness and sport performance. Some international associations with a more specialised focus that may be of interest to the exercise manager include the International Society for the Advancement of Kinanthropometry (body composition analysis), International Society of Sport Psychology, International Society for the Study of Obesity, International Sports Medicine Federation, International Federation of Adapted Physical Activity, and International Research Group on Biochemistry of Exercise; Web sites for some of these organisations are listed at the end of this chapter. It is not unusual for exercise managers (or any professional) to belong to several professional associations at the same time because each organisation provides a unique perspective and opportunity to advance skills, knowledge and career opportunities in the professional practice of exercise management.

Professional Accreditation

Accreditation or certification refers to criteria that practitioners are expected to have to provide certain professional services. These criteria, which are established by a professional organisation, may include a minimum educational level (e.g., a specific tertiary degree) and additional work-related experience outside of formal education. In some professions, certification may also require demonstration of technical competence, successful completion of continuing education courses or passing a standardised examination.

Accreditation or certification serves several functions, ensuring that

▶ practitioners have achieved a specified level of training, education and skill;

▶ clients can expect a certain level of care;

▶ professional practice will incorporate the most recent advances in the profession (best practice); and

▶ practitioners have a forum in which to communicate with each other.

Certification is an important means of quality control to ensure consistency and the highest standard of professional care. It can also serve as a means to educate and promote the image of the profession within the public sphere.

At present, the two most relevant organisations accrediting exercise managers in Australia are the American College of Sports Medicine (ACSM) and the Australian Association for Exercise and Sports Science (AAESS).

American College of Sports Medicine Professional Certification

The first exercise science organisation to certify its professional members was the ACSM. Certification began in 1974 during the early development of exercise cardiac rehabilitation programs. The ACSM viewed the certification process as a means to establish safe and scientifically based exercise services as part of the clinical management of cardiac patients. Over the past 25-plus years, ACSM certifications have expanded to include professionals providing health and fitness services for apparently healthy and low-risk clients and professionals working in other areas of exercise rehabilitation (e.g., clinical exercise physiology, first registration examinations in 2000). There are, at present, two "tracks" of ACSM certification—the Health and Fitness Track and the Clinical Track (ACSM 2000). Within each track are different levels according to education and work experience. Each certification requires a minimum level of education, work experience and other certifications (e.g., lower-level certification within a given track; see table 1.1). Knowledge, skills and abilities (KSAs) are clearly indicated for each certification level and are assessed by a written, and sometimes practical, examination.

The Clinical Track is designed for professionals working with individuals at risk of, or with, known diseases as well as apparently healthy individuals; these professionals work primarily, but not exclusively, in exercise cardiac rehabilitation clinical programs. The Health and Fitness Track is designed for professionals providing leadership in fitness assessment, exercise prescription and program development for apparently healthy individuals and those with controlled diseases; these professionals work primarily in corporate, community and commercial physical activity settings. Levels of certification are listed in table 1.1.

The ACSM certification programs are continually updated to incorporate recent advances in research and professional care. In 2000, in response to recent expansion of the clinical use of exercise-related services for the treatment of diseases and conditions other than cardiopulmonary diseases, the ACSM introduced a new certification level, the Registered Clinical Exercise Physiologist (RCEP). The RCEP is envisioned as a complement to the ACSM Exercise Specialist (ES) certification (ACSM Web site). The RCEP is an allied health professional working in the "application of exercise and physical activity for those with clinical and pathological situations where it has been shown to provide therapeutic or functional benefit" (see figure 1.3). Patients include, but are not limited to, those with cardiopulmonary, musculoskeletal/orthopaedic, neuromuscular, metabolic, immunologic and inflammatory diseases or conditions and the elderly, children and pregnant women. The RCEP is designed to be broad based, in recognition of the diverse issues relating to exercise management of patients with major diseases other than cardiovascular or pulmonary. This is in contrast, and complementary, to the Exercise Specialist certification, which has historically reflected a more detailed level of knowledge and competency in exercise rehabilitation specifically for cardiovascular and pulmonary diseases.

Further information about the ACSM and its certification procedures can be obtained at the Web site listed at the end of this chapter. It is not necessary to take ACSM certification examinations in the United States; some examinations are administered outside of the country.

Australian Association for Exercise and Sports Science Accreditation

In recognition of the varied settings in which exercise managers are employed and the need for specialist skills and competencies, the AAESS has developed accreditation in two streams—sport science and exercise science. The latter is subdivided into

TABLE 1.1—ACSM Certification Levels

CLINICAL TRACK

Certification	Major professional responsibilities	Minimum requirements
Program Director[SM] (PD)	Develops, directs, evaluates safe and effective clinical exercise programs	Advanced degree or equivalent + 2 yr clinical experience + >1 yr relevant experience in administrative authority + current certification in Basic Life Support + recommendation from current PD
Exercise Specialist™ (ES)	Performs graded exercise testing (with clinical staff), exercise prescription and leadership, and education of clinical patients	Bachelor's degree or 2-yr degree + 2 yr experience in clinical exercise science + >600 h practical experience + current CPR certification

HEALTH AND FITNESS TRACK

Certification	Major professional responsibilities	Minimum requirements
Health/Fitness Director™ (HFD)	Administers exercise programs in community, corporate, commercial settings	2-yr, bachelor's or advanced degree + >2 yr/ 4000 h experience as fitness manager or HFI + 2 yr/4,000 h experience as fitness manager and current CPR certification
Health/Fitness Instructor[SM] (HFI)	Assesses, designs, supervises and implements individual and group programs for the apparently healthy and those with controlled disease	2-yr bachelor's or advanced degree or completion of >2 yr of bachelor's program or >900 h experience in fitness setting and current CPR certification
Exercise Leader™ (EL)	Demonstrates and leads safe and effective individual and group programs for apparently healthy and those with controlled disease	Fitness certification from recognised organisation or degree or enrollment in tertiary program or 300 h experience in group exercise leadership and current CPR certification

Within each Track, the certification levels are listed from highest (top of table) to lowest. Degrees listed in "Minimum requirements" are in relevant health and/or exercise science related areas. Similarly, experience is needed in work or practical sites delivering relevant exercise or physical activity programs to the relevant client-base. CPR = cardiopulmonary resuscitation.

Compiled from American College of Sports Medicine, 2000, *ACSM's guidelines for exercise testing and prescription,* 6th ed. (Philadelphia: Lippincott Williams & Wilkins), 322-328.

specific specialties of exercise physiology, cardiorespiratory rehabilitation and musculoskeletal rehabilitation (see table 1.2).

The AAESS-accredited Sports Scientist provides sport science services to individual athletes and groups of athletes. Sport scientists are employed by academies or institutes of sport, elite and community sports organisations and in private consultancies. Their services include assessment of performance and development of training programs to optimise sport performance. The subfields within the Sports Science accreditation are sports physiology, sports biomechanics, sport psychology and sports motor control. The purpose of AAESS accreditation is to ensure a high standard of technical and ethical conduct by sport scientists. To become accredited, the sport scientist must demonstrate technical competence in administering and inter-

MAJOR PROFESSIONAL RESPONSIBILITIES

Application of exercise and physical activity for those with clinical and pathological conditions where it has been shown that exercise/physical activity has therapeutic or functional benefit

MINIMUM REQUIREMENTS

Graduate degree in exercise-science-related field[a]

Pass RCEP registry exam (4 h) in eight competency domains

>1,200 h supervised clinical experience

Relevant clinical experience within RCEP's scope of practice

---

[a]Until December 31, 2002, a person with a bachelor's degree plus 10,000 h of clinical experience may sit the registry exam.

Compiled from ACSM Web site **www.acsm.org**.

FIGURE 1.3   ACSM's Registered Clinical Exercise Physiologist (RCEP).

TABLE 1.2—AAESS Accreditation Levels

Certification	Major professional responsibilities	Minimum requirements
Sports Science—specialisations detailed below	Provides sport science services to assess or train athletes; provides research expertise in sport sciences to sports organisations	Full member of AAESS + >500 h work experience (175 h outside of training institution) + professional indemnity insurance + current CPR + demonstrated selected technical skills in sports science
Specialisation in Sports Science*	Provides specialised sport science expertise to assess and/or train athletes, or to work as research consultant to sports organisations	Accredited Sports Scientist + >100 h advanced or postgraduate study in subdiscipline + >1000 h additional experience in specialisation + regular publication and presentation in specialisation
Exercise Physiology	Provides services for pre-program health risk screening, fitness assessment and exercise prescription and programming for apparently healthy individuals	Full member of AAESS + documented evidence of relevant knowledge, skills and competencies as designated by AAESS + >300 h experience + current CPR
(Exercise) Cardiorespiratory Rehabilitation	Provides services for exercise prescription and programming for individuals at risk of or with known cardiorespiratory diseases	Accredited Exercise Physiologist + documented evidence of knowledge, skills and competencies as designated by AAESS + work experience + current CPR
(Exercise) Musculoskeletal Rehabilitation	Provides services for exercise prescription and programming for individuals with musculoskeletal disease or impairment	Accredited Exercise Physiologist + documented evidence of knowledge, skills and competencies as designated by AAESS + work experience + current CPR

An individual may hold simultaneous accreditations in any areas, provided accreditation requirements have been met.

*Sports science specialisation areas are sports physiology, sports biomechanics, sports motor control and sport psychology (accreditation as sport psychologist by Australian Psychology Association).

Abbreviation: CPR = cardiopulmonary resuscitation certification

Compiled from AAESS Web site at **www.aaess.com.au**.

preting standard tools for assessment of sport performance, competence in developing appropriate training interventions for the athlete, and anthropometric testing skills equivalent to Level 1 accreditation of the International Society for the Advancement of Kinanthropometry (ISAK). In addition, a minimum of 500 h of professional practice experience is needed for accreditation. Specialisation within one of the subfields requires additional professional experience in that subfield.

The AAESS-accredited Exercise Physiologist performs fitness assessment and provides exercise prescription for apparently healthy and low-risk clients (i.e., clients who do not require clinical programs such as rehabilitation). Exercise physiologists are employed in many settings, in particular in community, corporate and commercial physical activity programs and in private consultancies (e.g., personal training). Accreditation requires demonstration of knowledge, skills and competencies in health risk screening, physical fitness testing, nutrition, exercise leadership and prescription, and body composition assessment. A minimum 300 h practical work experience, including technical experience in fitness assessment and exercise leadership and prescription, is also needed for accreditation.

The AAESS-accredited rehabilitation specialists use physical activity to aid in the restoration or maintenance of physical functional capacity in patients with diseases or impairments of the cardiac and pulmonary (Cardiorespiratory Rehabilitation) and musculoskeletal (Musculoskeletal Rehabilitation) systems. These two specialties are accredited separately. Accredited specialists are usually employed in clinical exercise programs, in particular hospital-based programs offering rehabilitation to patients with cardiac, pulmonary, neurological and musculoskeletal conditions. Rehabilitation accreditation requires prior or concomitant accreditation as an exercise physiologist along with additional specialist knowledge, skills and competencies in exercise assessment and prescription for individuals with cardiovascular and pulmonary diseases or musculoskeletal impairments.

The requirements for accreditation are summarised in table 1.2. Details and application forms may be obtained from the AAESS secretariat or on-line through the organisation's Web site listed at the end of this chapter.

Summary

Exercise management is a dynamic profession involved in the design, delivery, promotion and evaluation of physical activity programs for the widest possible audience. The exercise manager's unique expertise and skills in exercise science, exercise prescription and program evaluation are employed in diverse settings, from elite sport to clinical rehabilitation to community health promotion to corporate and community health and fitness. Several Australian and international professional organisations have a core interest in exercise science and represent the professional interests of exercise managers; some of these provide professional accreditation in specific specialty areas. The central and possibly most attractive feature of exercise management is that physical activity can be used to enhance the health, well-being and physical function of a wide variety of clients.

Selected Glossary Terms

American College of Sports Medicine (ACSM)—The largest sports medicine and exercise science professional organisation in the world, dedicated to promoting and integrating scientific research, education and practice in sports medicine and exercise science; founded in 1954.

Australian Association for Exercise and Sports Science (AAESS)—The professional body representing exercise and sport science professionals in Australia; founded in 1991.

best practice—The use of advanced methods and technology, usually backed by research and recommendations by professional organisations, to provide the highest quality of professional service or care.

cardiac rehabilitation—A multifaceted secondary prevention program to help patients return to an active and satisfying life after some type of cardiac event; includes interventions to facilitate weight loss, smoking cessation, blood lipid and blood pressure management, effective use of prescribed medication and physical activity.

confidentiality—Maintaining privacy regarding all personal and health information obtained from a client during, for example, health risk screening, physical fitness testing and exercise programming.

exercise—A subcategory of physical activity that is planned and structured with the intention of improving or maintaining physical fitness.

exercise management—A profession involved in the application of exercise science and business knowledge and principles to the design, delivery, promotion and evaluation of physical activity programs for the widest possible audience.

exercise prescription and programming—Developing an exercise program for a client (or group of clients) designed to meets the client's health, fitness, performance, and other goals and needs.

exercise cardiac rehabilitation—The inclusion of exercise in a multifaceted program to help restore the patient's functional capacity and health.

fitness assessment—Use of standardised tests to measure various components of physical fitness (refer to physical fitness).

musculoskeletal exercise rehabilitation—Exercise programs designed for individuals with musculoskeletal disorders, such as arthritis, injury or low back pain, to help restore physical function and fitness and, if possible, prevent future injury.

personal trainer—An exercise professional who works with individual clients to develop and maintain an ongoing, individualised exercise program; the personal trainer may also exercise with the client.

physical activity—(According to the U.S. Surgeon General) Bodily movement produced by contraction of skeletal muscle that increases energy expenditure above the basal level.

physical fitness—Ability to perform physical tasks without undue fatigue; components include cardiorespiratory endurance, muscular strength and endurance, muscle flexibility, agility, balance and body composition.

pre-activity screening—Use of questionnaires and/or health information to assess an individual's health risk factors to optimise safety and effectiveness of fitness assessment and physical activity prescription.

profession (professional, professionalism)—Occupation requiring advanced knowledge in a specialised area; a professional is a practitioner of a particular profession; professionalism is an expected level of professional behaviour.

Sports Medicine Australia (SMA)—A professional and community educational organisation in Australia made up of several professional groups with a common interest in sports medicine and sport science.

stakeholders—Individuals, groups or organisations directly involved in, or potentially affected by, a program, policy or law; the individual or group is said to have a "stake", or strong interest, in the outcome of the program or policy.

U.S. Surgeon General's report on physical activity and health—A landmark report, published in 1996, that summarised research to date showing a strong relationship between moderate physical activity and health and that called for further promotion of a physically active lifestyle for all Americans.

Student Activities and Study Questions

1. Visit sites in which exercise managers are employed. Try to find a wide variety of sites (e.g., sport-related, clinic-based, community-focused). Visit at least one site and preferably more than one; if the latter, choose sites with different objectives. Observe the types of activities performed by the exercise manager(s) at these sites. If visiting more than one site, compare their different exercise management activities.

2. Talk with at least one, and preferably more, professional employed in the field of exercise management. What are the most satisfying aspects of the job? What skills does he think are essential to successfully work in the field of exercise management? What future developments does he see for the field of exercise management?

3. Study the AAESS Code of Ethics in figure 1.2. What, specifically, is meant by "best practice"? What (in your own words) are the duties of the AAESS member toward client care?

4. What local or regional professional organisation represents exercise managers where you live or study? Is this organisation associated with a national or international organisation? What are the objectives of the local organisation? Inquire about the meetings and events hosted by this organisation; try to attend at least one. How can you, as a student, become involved in this organisation?

5. Look in the telephone directory for your local area. Under what headings do you find services related to exercise management? How do these service providers identify themselves (e.g., What do they call themselves? How do they try to make their businesses stand out?)?

6. Visit the Web site of the AAESS or ACSM (or another relevant professional organisation in your region). What certifications do you think you should achieve in the next 5 years? Ten years? How can you start planning for this now?

Web Site Addresses of Some Professional Organisations Relevant to Exercise Management

Organisation	Web site address
American College of Sports Medicine (ACSM)	www.acsm.org
Australian Association for Exercise and Sports Science (AAESS)	www.aaess.com.au
Australian Cardiac Rehabilitation Association (ACRA)	www.acra.net.au
Australian Council for Health, Physical Education and Recreation (ACHPER)	www.achper.org.au
Australian Health Promotion Association (AHPA)	www.healthpromotion.org.au
International Council of Sport Science and Physical Education (ICSSPE)	www.icsspe.org
International Federation of Sports Medicine (FIMS)	www.fims.org
International Society for the Advancement of Kinanthropometry (ISAK)	http://freshedu.aut.ac.nz/ISAK/
National Strength and Conditioning Association (NSCA)	www.nsca-lift.org
Sports Medicine Australia (SMA)	www.ausport.gov.au/sma

CHAPTER 2

Health Benefits and Recommended Amount of Physical Activity

It is now widely accepted that regular physical activity is an important part of a healthy lifestyle. Regular physical activity lessens the risk of a number of major diseases and helps in the management of many others. For example, physical activity plays an important role in the treatment and management of diseases or conditions such as arthritis, pulmonary disease, neuromuscular impairments and depression, and it retards muscle wasting in conditions such as AIDS or spinal cord injuries (see table 2.1). Regular physical activity can also play a major role in helping to maintain physical **functional capacity** and independence in older individuals and those with physical impairments. Increasing the number of Australians and citizens worldwide who participate in regular physical activity may reduce the burden of disease and injury management as well as decrease health care costs associated with premature death, disease, physical impairment and aging currently assumed by health care institutions and governmental bodies.

The overwhelming evidence supporting the importance of physical activity to health has prompted worldwide efforts to increase the number of people who are regularly physically active. Although no one now disputes the importance of physical activity to disease prevention and health, there still remains considerable debate over how to enhance participation in regular physical activity sufficiently enough to affect the health of entire populations. In other words, most people know that physical activity is important, but few in developed countries are sufficiently active to achieve these health benefits. There are a number of reasons for this insufficiency, including misconceptions by the public about how best to become physically active. The challenge for exercise managers is to develop ways to activate entire populations so that regular physical activity becomes an accepted lifetime habit. This chapter discusses the scientific evidence underlying the relationship between physical activity and health and presents the most recent recommendations for physical activity.

TABLE 2.1—Conditions or Impairments in Which Physical Activity Is Beneficial in Treatment or Prevention of Further Disease Progression (Secondary Prevention)

Condition	Major benefits of physical activity for condition
Coronary heart disease, including after myocardial infarction, bypass surgery or angioplasty	Lowers risk of death from subsequent cardiac event (e.g., reinfarction) Strengthens heart Reduces work of heart by lowering resting and exercise blood pressure and heart rate Assists in control of blood glucose and lipids
Stroke	Assists in regaining muscle function, balance and coordination Reduces resting and exercise blood pressure
Mild-moderate hypertension	Reduces resting and exercise blood pressure and heart rate
Type 2 diabetes	Improves insulin resistance and glucose control Assists in weight loss
Obesity	Reduces body mass and abdominal fat deposition Increases lean body mass and basal metabolic rate
Peripheral vascular disease	Improves exercise tolerance and functional capacity
Arthritis	Maintains joint range of motion, mobility, muscular strength and functional capacity
Low back pain	Improves muscular strength and endurance
Cancer	Maintains muscular strength and functional capacity Lessens nausea and weakness associated with treatment Attenuates increase in weight during treatment for breast cancer
HIV/AIDS	Prevents or attenuates loss of lean body mass
Asthma	Raises threshold at which exercise-induced asthma occurs
Neuromuscular and musculoskeletal impairments	Maintains or improves muscular strength, endurance and flexibility and functional capacity
Aging	Prevents or attenuates loss of bone mass, muscle mass, muscular strength, balance, joint range of motion and functional capacity Attenuates age-related increases in blood pressure, lipids and glucose intolerance

Physical Activity and Health

The exercise management professional should have a clear understanding of the relationship between physical activity and health. Any safe and effective exercise prescription, whether designed for an individual or group, must be shaped by the most recent research on how physical activity enhances health. For example, the 1996 U.S. Surgeon General's report on physical activity and h1ealth provides concrete recommendations regarding the amount and types of physical activity based on a thorough literature review of the relationship between health and physical activity. A more specific example is the prescription of exercise for a client with a particular health concern, say, hypertension; the exercise manager must be familiar with the research literature that shows a clear link between regular physical activity and blood pressure management. Additionally, the exercise management professional, in seeking referrals from other health professionals or rebates from health insurers, must be able to clearly identify the health benefits of physical activity for particular clients or for specific conditions. Finally, the exercise management profession often acts as an advocate, offering expert advice to government or non-government agencies about issues related to physical activity. Thus, being well versed in the links between physical activity and health is in the best interest of both the exercise management profession and the individual practitioners.

Physical Activity, Mortality and Morbidity

It is a frightening, but all too true, statistic: Physically inactive people are at increased risk of dying prematurely compared with active people of similar background. Epidemiological studies in developed countries, such as Australia, the United States and the United Kingdom, indicate that physical inactivity approximately doubles the relative risk of premature death, regardless of cause (called all-cause **mortality**). **Relative risk (RR)** is an epidemiological term that quantifies the incidence of some event (in this case, premature death) in one group compared with another (e.g., inactive compared with active populations). An inverse relationship between physical activity and mortality appears to be dose related; that is, the higher the level of activity, the lower the rate of mortality. Most studies have focused on all-cause mortality and the risk of cardiovascular disease (CVD), **coronary heart disease (CHD)** and cerebrovascular disease (stroke) in particular. The relationship between physical activity and mortality holds true even when different measures of physical activity are used.

Major Causes of Death and Disease in Australia and in Other Developed Countries

Table 2.2 lists the leading causes of death and disability in Australia. Combined, all forms of CVD

(CHD, cerebrovascular and blood vessel diseases) are clearly the most common cause of death, accounting for nearly 40% of deaths each year. The death rate due to CVD has declined steadily since the late 1960s in Australia and in other countries such as the United States and Canada, primarily because of advances in medical treatment and medication and changes in lifestyle factors such as diet. It still remains the major killer, however, and consumes hundreds of millions of dollars in health care costs each year. Moreover, the decline in incidence of CVD has not been evenly spread across the population but has been concentrated in the higher socio-economic levels. That is, the death rate due to CVD has declined to a lesser extent among socio-economically disadvantaged groups, leaving a widening gap in death and disease rates between income levels and between indigenous and non-indigenous populations.

After CVD, cancer is the next leading cause of death, accounting for about one-quarter of deaths each year. Other major diseases or conditions follow, such as chronic obstructive pulmonary disease (COPD) and diabetes. Of these diseases, physical activity has potential to aid in the treatment and management of CVD, CHD, COPD, stroke and diabetes (type 2 mainly).

A National Health Priority Areas (NHPA) initiative has been developed with collaboration between Commonwealth, State and Territory government and non-government organisations to develop an effective and coordinated approach to improving health outcomes in major areas of concern (Australian Institute of Health and Welfare 2000). NHPA lists six areas:

▶ Cardiovascular health

▶ Cancer control

▶ Injury prevention and control

▶ Mental health

▶ Diabetes mellitus

▶ Asthma (added in 1999)

While simple death rates (mortality) give some indication of the consequences and prevalence of serious disease, other epidemiological measures give a better overall description of the total burden of disease. For example, the relative risk (RR) gives an indication of the strength of the relationship between a particular risk factor and the risk of disease (e.g., the ratio between an inactive lifestyle and the risk of dying from CVD). However, it does not give any information about the prevalence of the risk in the population. Another epidemiological measure,

---

TABLE 2.2—Major Causes of Death, Disease and Disability in Australians

10 leading causes of death (% of deaths)	10 leading causes of DALYs	10 major risk factors contributing to DALYs
Malignant neoplasms (cancer)[a] (26.5%)	Ischaemic heart disease[ab]	Tobacco use
Ischaemic heart disease[ab] (22.5%)	Stroke[ab]	Physical inactivity[a]
Cerebrovascular disease (stroke)[ab] (9.4%)	COPD[b]	High blood pressure[ab]
COPD and allied conditions[b] (5.0%)	Depression[b]	Alcohol
Pneumonia and influenza (3.9%)	Lung cancer	Obesity[ab]
Accidents (3.5%)	Dementia	Diet lacking in fruit and vegetables
Diseases of blood vessels[b] (2.3%)	Diabetes[ab]	High blood cholesterol level[ab]
Type 2 diabetes[ab] (2.2%)	Colorectal cancer[a]	Illicit drugs
Suicide (2.1%)	Asthma[b]	Occupation
Hereditary and degenerative CNS diseases (1.6%)	Osteoarthritis[b]	Unsafe sex

[a]Physical activity is beneficial in preventing this disease/condition (primary prevention).

[b]Physical activity is beneficial in the management of this disease/condition (secondary prevention).

Abbreviations: DALYs = disability-adjusted life years, or the number of potential years of life lost because of premature death, poor health or disability. The DALY provides an estimate of the overall burden of disease; COPD = chronic obstructive pulmonary disease; CNS = central nervous system.

Compiled from M.B. Van Der Weyden, 1999, "The burden of disease and injury in Australia: Time for action," *Medical Journal of Australia* 171 (11-12): 581-582; Australian Bureau of Statistics, 2000, *Australia now—a statistical profile: health and mortality*. **www.abs.gov.au/Ausstats**.

---

the **population attributable risk (PAR),** reflects both the relative risk and the prevalence of that risk among the population. The PAR is the proportion of a given health outcome attributable to a risk factor in the population. Recent estimates indicate that 44% of Australian adults are insufficiently active to derive any health benefits. Thus, nearly half the adult population is at increased risk of CVD and other diseases because of physical inactivity. By knowing the RR of inactivity and the number of inactive adults, we can calculate the proportion of major diseases attributed to physical inactivity (PAR). For all deaths each year, regardless of cause, the PAR of physical inactivity is 18%, that is 18% of all deaths each year can be attributed to physical inactivity. Physical inactivity is the second most important modifiable risk factor for disease, second only to tobacco use (mainly cigarette smoking, which has a

PAR of 24%) (Stephenson et al. 2000). The PARs for various diseases attributed to physical inactivity among the adult Australian population are presented in the middle column of table 2.3.

The PAR also gives an indication of the potential to prevent disease by altering the prevalence of a particular risk factor among the population (e.g., by decreasing the number of people who are inactive). It has been estimated that 5,335 (18%) of the 29,637 deaths due to coronary heart disease (CHD)[1] in Australia in 1996 were attributable to physical inactivity (Stephenson et al. 2000). When CHD, diabetes and colon cancer are considered together, the 1996 estimates indicate that 6,395 deaths due to these diseases could be attributable to physical inactivity. These values give some perspective as to the magnitude of the health problems associated with physical inactivity and, in turn, the potential to have a

---

[1]Coronary heart disease (CHD) is the most prevalent form of cardiovascular disease. CHD includes coronary artery disease (CAD), and the terms are sometimes used interchangeably. CAD, and most cases of CHD, are caused by a reduction in blood flow to the myocardium (heart muscle) as a result of atherosclerosis, a pathological degenerative process causing obstructive lesions in the main coronary arteries. The risk factors for CHD and CAD are similar. In general, this text will use the broader term CHD, except when presenting information from a source that specifically uses the term CAD.

TABLE 2.3—Proportion of Diseases and Hospital Admissions Attributable* to Physical Inactivity Each Year in Australia

Disease or condition	Incidence (%)	Hospital admissions (%)
CHD	18	24
Stroke	16	35
Type 2 diabetes	13	6
Breast cancer	9	3
Colon cancer	19	10
Falls	18	6
Depression	10	15

*Data are expressed as population attributable risk (PAR) for each disease/condition (i.e., 18% of the incidence of disease and 24% of hospital admissions due to CHD are attributable to physical inactivity).

Compiled from J. Stephenson, A. Bauman, T. Armstrong, B. Smith, and B. Bellew, the Commonwealth Department of Health and Aged Care and the Australian Sports Commission, 2000, *The costs of illness attributable to physical inactivity in Australia: A preliminary study.* (Canberra: Commonwealth of Australia). Accessed via the Active Australia Web site **www.dhac.gov.au/pubhlth/publicat/document/phys_costofillness.pdf**.

large impact on death by increasing the proportion of the population that is physically active. These issues are discussed in further detail in the next chapter.

Because the many costs of disease are generally borne by the community, it is also important to account for the total burden of disease. For example, many diseases do not result in imminent death but may cause disability sufficient to limit or prevent employment and a normal lifestyle. The burden of disease then falls on the person's family (which loses income), the person's employer (which loses an experienced employee) and the community (which must fund disability payments and costs of medical and rehabilitative care). The **disability-adjusted life year (DALY)** estimates potential life years lost because of premature death, disability and poor health (van der Weyden 1999). The DALY can be further subdivided into years of life lost to poor health (YLL) and years of life lost to disability (YLD). According to recent Australian statistics, premature mortality (a person dying sooner than expected) is responsible for more than 50% of the total burden of disease (van der Weyden 1999). The leading causes of YLL are CVD (including heart disease and stroke), cancer and injury.

The 10 leading causes of DALYs in Australia in 1996 are presented in table 2.2. Of these 10 conditions or diseases, physical activity has potential to prevent 4 (ischaemic heart disease [CHD plus some other forms of heart disease], stroke, diabetes mellitus and colorectal cancer) and has potential benefit in the management of another 4 (COPD, asthma, depression and osteoarthritis). Table 2.2 also lists the 10 major risk factors contributing to the burden of disease in Australia in 1997; physical inactivity is second only to tobacco use. In addition, physical activity is an effective treatment for 2 other major risk factors, obesity and high blood pressure. These statistics reveal the tremendous potential benefits of increasing the number of physically active people across the population: decreased mortality and morbidity, lowered health care costs and reduced consequences of disease and premature death. Considering that a physically active lifestyle is a cost-effective strategy to positively influence the nation's health, it is not surprising that many countries have recently initiated public health campaigns to increase participation in regular physical activity (discussed further in the next chapter).

Key Studies on Physical Activity and Mortality

It is useful to consider a few of the key studies showing a relationship between physical activity and reduced incidence of premature death (mortality) and disease (morbidity). The data from these and many other studies have been instrumental in demonstrating the strong association between physical inactivity and adverse health outcomes and in convincing governments to fund initiatives to encourage physical activity in the wider population. In addition, these studies also provide useful information concerning the amount of activity needed to positively affect health, which is an important public health issue. Before a discussion of these studies, it is helpful to summarise some of the methods used to quantify physical activity status in large study populations.

Methods to Quantify Physical Activity

The most common means to assess the relationship between physical activity and health or mortality are physical fitness, **leisure-time physical activity (LTPA)** and direct monitoring of activity. Physical fitness includes components of **cardiorespiratory fitness (CRF),** muscular fitness and body composition. An often assessed measure of CRF is **maximum oxygen uptake,** or aerobic power **($\dot{V}O_2$max),** either measured directly in a maximal exercise test or estimated from submaximal testing. CRF may also be assessed by a test of exercise tolerance, or time to fatigue at a specified work rate. Muscular fitness includes measures of muscular strength, flexibility, endurance and neuromuscular factors such as balance, coordination and agility. These tests have special relevance to studies of functional capacity in aging and disabled individuals. Body composition measures include estimates of body fat and lean body mass, anthropometry (girths, skinfolds) and fat distribution (especially abdominal fat). Some of these methods to measure physical fitness are discussed further in chapter 6.

Measuring LTPA is a complex task because it involves assessing human behaviour (i.e., performance of physical activity), which can be highly variable. Assessment of LTPA often involves self-report by the study population using an activity diary, recall survey or retrospective quantitative exercise history. Diaries require the subjects to record daily physical activity for a specified time, usually only a few days. These require good subject compliance, are labour intensive for the research team and, although very accurate, are generally not used for large studies. Recall surveys ask subjects to recall the types and amount of activity undertaken during a specified period. These require little effort by the subject but may be influenced by the accuracy of the subject's memory. The retrospective quantitative physical activity history requires more comprehensive and detailed recall of previous participation, often in the year preceding the survey. The latter two methods (recall survey and retrospective quantitative history) are often used in large surveys of physical activity participation (e.g., national surveys).

Direct measurement of physical activity may involve observation (the experimenter records all activity observed), electronic monitoring (e.g., heart rate monitors or pedometers) and other physiological monitoring. The latter may involve the use of portable oxygen analysers or estimation of energy expenditure through ingestion of stable (harmless) isotopes; although highly accurate, both of these methods are expensive and labour intensive for the research team. Each of these methods has advantages and disadvantages in terms of ease of administration, cost, and reliability and validity of data. No single measure can give a comprehensive and accurate view of physical activity levels, especially at the population level. Misclassification of activity level (e.g., classifying someone as active who is not) tends to increase the variability of measurements and thus obscures or underestimates the relationship between physical activity and health. The more precise a measure of physical activity used, generally the stronger the association between physical activity and health. As expected, the strongest relationship has been observed between measures of CRF and health. This is most likely because methods used to measure CRF are more reliable and accurate and because considerable physical activity is required to improve CRF.

Influential Studies Showing a Relationship Between Physical Activity and Reduced Mortality

One of the first studies to demonstrate a dose-response relationship between physical activity and mortality followed more than 16,000 alumni of Harvard University (Paffenbarger et al. 1986). Alumni who entered university between 1916 and 1950 were followed for 12 to 16 years during the period from 1962 to 1978. Physical activity levels were estimated from self-reports of total activity including sports, walking, stair climbing and other activities. A significant dose-response relationship was observed between the amount of energy expended in physical activity each week and death due to cardiovascular disease, even after adjustment for possible confounding variables such as age, smoking and hypertension. Death rates declined consistently with increasing total weekly energy expenditure from physical activity of 500 to 3,500 kcal/wk. Compared with inactive men (<500 kcal/wk), death rates were 25 to 33% lower in men whose physical activity energy expenditure exceeded 2,000 kcal/wk. Physical activity energy expenditure had an independent effect on mortality even in those with other risk factors for disease, such as family history of CHD, hypertension, smoking and obesity. In addition, the largest reductions in relative risk of death occurred in the older age groups (>60 years), those who are at greater risk of disease and death.

In 1995 and 1996, Blair et al. published two important studies on thousands of American men and women whose fitness levels were classified based on an exercise tolerance test (time to fatigue during treadmill walking) (Blair et al. 1995, 1996). In the first study, the men's fitness levels were assessed and then reassessed after 5 years. The largest differences in death rate due to CVD were between those who remained in the lowest fitness category (lowest 20th percentile) during the 5 years compared with those in the middle fitness category (20th-60th percentile). Men who improved their fitness level from the lowest category over the study period demonstrated a 50% reduction in mortality. For each minute of improvement in the treadmill test, the mortality rate due to CVD decreased about 8%. This study provides strong evidence that significant health benefits accrue from even modest improvements in CRF that can be achieved through regular moderate physical activity.

In the 1996 follow-up study, more than 25,000 American men and more than 7,000 women were followed for 8 years after an initial exercise tolerance test (Blair et al. 1996). Low fitness at the start of the study was an independent predictor of mortality among men and women. The RR for low fitness (1.5 in men and 2.1 in women) was similar to that observed for other documented risk factors such as smoking (both men and women) and (for men only) abnormal ECG, elevated systolic blood pressure and increased blood cholesterol level. Even in the presence of other risk factors, there was an inverse relationship between mortality and physical fitness. More important, death rates were lower in fit people with one or more CVD risk factors compared with low-fit people with no risk factors (see table 2.4). The largest decline in death rate was noted for people in the moderate fitness category compared with the lowest fitness category (middle 40% compared with bottom 20% on exercise tolerance test). Only slight further decreases in mortality were observed between the middle and high fitness categories (middle 40% and upper 40%, respectively). This study shows that

TABLE 2.4—Relationship Between All-Cause Mortality and Cardiorespiratory Fitness

MEN'S AGE-ADJUSTED DEATH RATES[a]

Number of risk factors	Low fitness	Moderate fitness	High fitness
0	27	15	14
1	42	26	23
2 or 3	58	43	24

WOMEN'S AGE-ADJUSTED DEATH RATES[a]

Number of risk factors	Low fitness	Moderate-high fitness
0	26	7
1	20	18
2 or 3	42	17

Sample size = 25,341 men and 7,090 women. Fitness levels are assigned as low fitness = least fit 20% on exercise tolerance (time to fatigue) test; moderate fitness = next 40% (20th-60th percentile); high fitness = most fit 40%. For women, because of the smaller sample size, the moderate and high fitness categories are combined. Risk factors = number of risk factors for heart disease such as cigarette smoking, total cholesterol level ≥6.2 mmol · L^{-1} and systolic blood pressure ≥140 mmHg.

[a]Age-adjusted death rate = deaths per 10,000 person-years. Data are adjusted for possible confounding variables such as age, year of measurement, chronic illness, family history of cardiac disease, fasting blood glucose level and body mass index.

Data from S.N. Blair, J.B. Kampert, H.W. Kohl, C.E. Barlow, C.A. Macera, R.S. Paffenbarger, and L.W. Gibbons, 1996, "Influences of cardiorespiratory fitness and other precursors on cardiovascular disease and all-cause mortality in men and women," *JAMA* 276: 205-210.

low fitness is an important independent predictor of all-cause and CVD mortality in both men and women. Moreover, even moderate physical fitness seems to protect against premature death in individuals with other risk factors for CVD, including family history.

The relationship between low CRF and CVD and all-cause mortality risk was assessed in a recent prospective study of more than 25,000 adult American men classified by body mass (Wei et al. 1999). Low CRF was a strong predictor of CVD and all-cause mortality. RR observed for low fitness was of similar magnitude to RR for diabetes and other CVD risk factors such as hypertension, smoking and high blood cholesterol levels. The RR of CVD and all-cause mortality ranged from 1.6 to 2.3 in low-fit men; that is, low-fit men were 1.6 to 2.3 times more likely to die during the study period compared with fit men. The RR of CVD and all-cause mortality was related to body mass, increasing from 1.6 to 1.7 in men of normal weight (body mass index (BMI) <25 kg · m^{-2}) to 2.0 to 2.3 in obese men (BMI ≥30 kg · m^{-2}); BMI, a simple method to determine an optimal body weight range, is the ratio of body mass (in kg) to height (in metres squared), expressed as kg · m^{-2}. This study confirms the significance of physical inactivity as a health risk and points out the potential health benefits of physical activity in overweight and obese men.

The four studies discussed previously are representative of a large body of literature showing that physical inactivity is a strong independent predictor of premature death due to all causes and especially CVD. The magnitude of the risk associated with physical inactivity is equal to that associated with other major risk factors for CVD such as hypertension, high blood cholesterol levels, elevated BMI and smoking. Even in individuals with one or more of these risk factors, physical activity lessens the risk of dying. It is important to note that the largest benefits seem to accrue from moderate levels of activity and physical fitness, with only modest additional gains from higher intensity exercise. Given the low rate of participation in regular moderate physical activity in most developed countries (40-60% of the population), there is tremendous potential to influence the health of entire nations by encouraging a physically active lifestyle among the population. A larger proportion of Australian adults is at risk from physical inactivity than from most other major risk factors, with the exception of excess body mass. Moderate physical activity is a relatively inexpensive intervention to change CVD risk factors, cheaper than medication or surgery. Thus,

considerable effort has been directed at facilitating the adoption of a physically active lifestyle across the wider population. This is discussed further in chapter 3.

How Active Are We?

Before further discussing the relationship between physical activity and health or disease prevention, it is necessary to first look at the prevalence of physical activity in modern Australia and other developed countries.

Activity Levels of Australians

A number of surveys have been undertaken in the past 20 years to gauge participation in physical activity of the Australian population. Most surveys use self-reported activity, usually by querying a representative sample about recent physical activity, such as over a given time period immediately preceding the survey. Two recent comprehensive surveys are the 1997 and 1999 National Physical Activity Surveys. These were telephone-based surveys of a representative sample of approximately 4,000 adults in 1997 and 3,000 adults in 1999, aged 18 to 75 years, who were asked about their physical activity in both the preceding week and the preceding 6 months (Armstrong, Bauman and Davies 2000). Using established methods for estimation of energy expenditure, activity levels were categorised as high, moderate, low and sedentary. Table 2.5 presents a summary of some 1997 and 1999 data for adult Australians differentiated by age and sex.

Overall, the 1997 survey found that 62.2% of adults were "sufficiently active", defined as at least 150 min per week of walking or moderate to vigorous physical activity. This is considered the minimum amount of activity required to derive health benefits (discussed later in this chapter). The remaining 37.8% were classified as either sedentary or insufficiently active. These individuals would be considered at risk of premature mortality and the many diseases associated with physical inactivity. Table 2.5 also shows that participation in physical activity declines with age in both sexes. In addition, within each age category and overall, men are more likely than women to participate in physical activity, especially vigorous activity.

The 1999 survey used essentially the same methods as in 1997, and thus the data can be compared to provide a short-term view of participation trends

TABLE 2.5—Percentage of Australian Adults Who Are Physically Active

Age and sex	Sedentary[a]		Insufficient time[b]		Sufficient time[c]	
	1997	**1999**	**1997**	**1999**	**1997**	**1999**
18-29 yr	7.3	6.3	25.0	25.0	74.0	68.7
30-44 yr	11.7	16.9	29.6	29.6	63.6	53.5
45-59 yr	18.1	18.2	31.9	31.9	53.8	50.0
60-75 yr	19.2	17.9	28.1	28.1	53.4	54.1
Men overall	13.7	14.6	25.9	25.9	63.4	59.6
Women overall	13.1	14.7	31.5	31.5	61.1	53.8
Adults overall	13.4	14.6	28.7	28.7	62.2	56.6

[a]Sedentary is defined as those who reported no leisure-time physical activity in the previous week.

[b]Insufficient time is defined as undertaking some physical activity but not enough to be categorised as sufficient.

[c]Sufficient time is defined as >150 min per week of walking or moderate to vigorous physical activity.

Compiled from T. Armstrong, A. Bauman, and J. Davies, 2000, *Physical activity patterns of Australian adults. Results of the 1999 National Physical Activity Survey.* (Canberra: Australian Institute of Health and Welfare). **www.aihw.gov.au/publications/health/papaa/papaa.pdf**.

over the 2 years (see table 2.5). Alarmingly, participation rates declined between 1997 and 1999 in adults overall and in all age groups except the oldest surveyed (60-75 years). The age group 30 to 44 years showed the largest decline in participation in sufficient activity (nearly 10%); participation in sufficient activity also declined more in women than in men. There are several possible reasons for the decline in participation rates, although no one single factor has yet been identified. In contrast to the younger age groups, participation rates in the older age group were maintained between 1997 and 1999, which may be partially attributable to educational and media campaigns to promote physical activity targeted at older individuals during this time (1999 was the International Year of Older People). Both surveys also show an inverse association between educational level or occupational status and participation.

These recent data show that about 40% of the Australian adult population is insufficiently physically active to derive health benefits. The prevalence of physical inactivity is nearly twice that of smoking and three times that of hypertension among the population. That is, almost twice as many people are at increased health risk from physical inactivity than from smoking, and three times as many people are at risk from physical inactivity than from hypertension.

Activity Levels in Other Countries

Data from other developed countries, such as the United States, the United Kingdom, New Zealand and Canada, suggest that Australia is not alone in having a substantial proportion of the population at risk of disease because of physical inactivity. In the United States, up to 50 to 60% of the population is considered to be insufficiently active to achieve health benefits, and up to 30% may be considered sedentary (no leisure-time physical activity) (U.S. Department of Health and Human Services 1996). As in Australia, participation rates are lower across all age groups in women compared with men (and girls compared with boys); participation also declines with age. Physical activity participation rates also tend to be inversely related to educational level and income and to vary by race or ethnicity (e.g., lower in African Americans and Hispanic Americans than in white, non-Hispanic Americans).

A recent survey by the Hillary Commission for Sport, Fitness and Leisure in New Zealand shows similar trends (National Health Committee of New Zealand 1998). About 64% of adults were classified as active (150 min per week of leisure-time physical activity); 21% were considered to be physically inactive and 15% sedentary (no leisure-time physical activity). Inactivity was more prevalent in women than in men and in Maori (especially men) than in non-

Maori. These data were essentially unchanged between 1990 and 1996.

The data from Australia and overseas indicate that a significant portion of the population in developed countries is at risk of disease because of physical inactivity. Participation rates have either remained relatively constant (New Zealand) or declined (United States, Australia) over the past decade, suggesting that despite awareness of the health benefits of physical activity, many are not willing to, or are unable to, incorporate such advice into their lifestyles. Many countries, alarmed by the high number of inactive people and the accompanying risks (and costs) to health, have developed national campaigns to promote physical activity among the wider population. This topic is explored further in the next chapter.

Effects of Physical Activity on Risk Factors for Cardiovascular Disease

Cardiovascular disease (CVD) includes coronary heart disease (CHD, the major form of CVD), stroke and other diseases of the circulatory system such as peripheral vascular disease. When all aspects of the disease are considered together, CVD is the major cause of death and disability in most developed countries, accounting for 40 to 50% of all deaths each year. In Australia, CHD is the second leading cause and stroke the third most common cause of death. The economic and social burden of CVD is staggering: in 1998, direct health care costs were $894 million for coronary heart disease, $216 million for type 2 diabetes and $630 million for stroke (Stephenson et al. 2000).

Although age, sex and genetic predisposition are important factors in development of CVD and CHD, many of the **risk factors** for these diseases are related to lifestyle (see table 2.6 for risk factors). Thus, it is possible to significantly affect the rates of morbidity and mortality, and their associated costs, of the entire population by attending to lifestyle-associated risk factors. The PARs of physical inactivity to CHD and stroke are 18% and 16%, respectively, indicating the relative contribution of physical inactivity to development of these diseases.

Studies measuring CRF to assess risk of premature death from CVD report relative risk of physical inactivity in the range of 2 to 3; that is, physically inactive people are two to three times more likely to die of CVD compared with active people. These numbers are similar to RR values showing a relationship between CVD/CAD risk and other

TABLE 2.6—ACSM Risk Factors for Coronary Artery Disease (CAD)

Risk factor	Criteria
Family history	Diagnosed CAD or myocardial infarction before 55 years in male first-degree relative or before 65 years in female first-degree relative (parent, child or sibling)
Cigarette smoking	Current smoker or have quit within previous 6 mo
Hypertension	140/90 or greater, confirmed by measurement on two or more separate occasions, or on antihypertensive medication
Dyslipidaemia	TC >5.2 mmol · L^{-1} or HDL-C <0.9 mmol · L^{-1} or on lipid-lowering medication
	(HDL-C >1.6 mmol · L^{-1} is considered a negative risk factor; if present, subtract 1 from total of other risk factors)
Impaired fasting glucose	Fasting blood glucose concentration ≥6.1 mmol · L^{-1}, confirmed by measurement on two or more separate occasions
Obesity	BMI >30 kg · m^{-2} or waist girth >100 cm
Sedentary lifestyle	Not participating in regular exercise or meeting minimum physical activity recommendations by USSG

Abbreviations: TC = total cholesterol; HDL-C = high-density lipoprotein cholesterol; BMI = body mass index.

Compiled from American College of Sports Medicine, 2000, *ACSM's guidelines for exercise testing and prescription*, 6th ed. (Lippincott Williams & Wilkins), 24.

major risk factors such as hypertension, smoking and **dyslipidaemia** (abnormal blood lipid profile). Thus, physical inactivity is as much of a health risk, at least for development of CVD, as these other conditions. Among the adult population, the prevalence of physical inactivity is much higher than these other risk factors. That is, there are more people at risk of premature CVD and death because of physical inactivity than smoking, hypertension or other conditions; this is reflected in the high PAR associated with physical inactivity (refer to table 2.3, discussed earlier in the chapter). This suggests that there is considerable potential to reduce CVD incidence by increasing the number of active adults.

Mechanisms by Which Physical Activity Reduces the Risk of CVD

Physical activity is thought to reduce the risk of CVD by a number of mechanisms (summarised in figure 2.1). Regular endurance-type exercise reduces the work of the heart by lowering resting and submaximal exercise heart rate (HR) and systolic blood pressure (SBP); the product of these two factors (HR × SBP), called the rate pressure product, reflects the work of the heart. Resting and exercise stroke (ejection) volume also increase as a result of regular exercise. Increased vascularity in skeletal muscle helps to lower total peripheral resistance, contributing to the decrease in blood pressure. In addition, blood viscosity decreases because of expansion of plasma volume, which, combined with decreased platelet aggregation, reduces the risk of clot formation, one trigger of myocardial infarction and stroke.

There are many indirect effects of regular physical activity on risk factors for CVD. Physical activity may prevent obesity or assist in weight loss by increasing total daily energy expenditure, by metabolising fats and by increasing **basal**, or resting, **metabolic rate**. Exercise favourably alters the blood lipid profile by increasing the protective high-density lipoprotein (HDL) level and reducing triglyceride concentration. Combined dietary and exercise intervention leading to weight loss reduces total cholesterol and low-density lipoprotein (LDL) concentrations. Insulin sensitivity and glucose uptake increase acutely for up to 24 to 48 h after exercise, contributing to better **glucose tolerance** and prevention of type 2 diabetes. Resting and submaximal exercise blood pressure is reduced by regular moderate physical activity. By preventing obesity, physical activity also indirectly helps prevent type 2 diabetes and hypertension. Finally, physically active people may be more likely to adopt other healthy behaviours such as consuming a healthy diet or not smoking cigarettes.

EFFECT OF REGULAR EXERCISE ON CVD RISK FACTORS

Lowers blood pressure at rest and during exercise

Induces favourable blood lipid profile (increases HDL-C, lowers triglycerides)

Reduces body mass and abdominal fat levels

Enhances insulin sensitivity and glucose tolerance

EFFECT OF REGULAR EXERCISE ON CARDIOVASCULAR FUNCTION

Enhances stroke volume and ejection fraction

Increases myocardial function by decreasing "afterload"

Reduces myocardial oxygen demand by lowering blood pressure and heart rate at rest and during submaximal exercise

Reduces blood viscosity and platelet aggregation

Enhances capillary density in skeletal muscle

Decreases circulating catecholamine levels during submaximal exercise

Compiled from A.S. Leon (ed.), 1997, *Physical activity and cardiovascular health: A national consensus.* (Champaign, IL: Human Kinetics), 21; American College of Sports Medicine, 2000, *ACSM's guidelines for exercise testing and prescription,* 6th ed. (Lippincott Williams & Wilkins), 5-6.

FIGURE 2.1   Biological mechanisms by which exercise prevents cardiovascular disease (CVD).

Physical Activity and Obesity

In Australia, the incidence of overweight and obesity has been estimated at over 60% for adult men and nearly 50% for adult women; nearly 20% of children are also considered overweight or obese. Over the past 20 years, the incidence of overweight and obesity has risen in most developed countries, including the United States, Australia and the United Kingdom. Surprisingly, this has occurred despite a steady or declining consumption of fat in the diet; this trend has been attributed to an increasingly sedentary lifestyle. Of even more concern, the incidence of overweight and obesity is increasing at alarming rates in children and adolescents, which has serious implications for their health as adults. Approximately 80% of obese children remain obese as adults.

Obesity is a risk factor for a number of diseases or impairments including cardiovascular disease, hypertension, type 2 diabetes, certain forms of cancer (breast, bowel, prostate), osteoarthritis and low back pain. Significantly, these conditions are major causes of death, disease and disability in Australia (refer to tables 2.2 and 2.3). Thus, there is a potential for wide-ranging health benefits by preventing or lessening the incidence of obesity.

Regular physical activity is an important intervention for prevention and treatment of obesity. A combination of dietary intervention and physical activity is the preferred treatment because dieting alone is rarely successful for inducing permanent weight loss. The amount of activity recommended as part of a healthy lifestyle (discussed in detail later in the chapter) of 150 to 300 kcal (630 to 1260 kJ) per day or 1,000 to 2,000 kcal (420 to 8400 kJ) per week is thought to be sufficient to prevent the typical 0.5 kg per year weight gain associated with aging. This energy expenditure can be accomplished by 30 to 60 min brisk walking, 15 to 30 min jogging or 30 to 60 min aerobics or resistance training each day.

Body fat distribution may be more important for determining health risk of obesity than total body or fat mass. Abdominal obesity, an excess of fat deposited in the abdominal region, is associated with hypertension, abnormal blood lipid levels, insulin resistance and increased risk of type 2 diabetes, and increased risk of cardiovascular disease (called the metabolic syndrome; discussed in chapter 8). Exercise has been shown to effectively reduce abdominal fat levels in adult men and women and in adolescents. Even a small reduction in abdominal fat deposition (as measured by waist measurement or waist to hip ratio) is associated with improved insulin sensitivity, favourable changes in blood lipids and reduced risk of cardiovascular disease.

For most overweight or obese individuals, a combination of dietary and exercise intervention is required for permanent loss of excess body fat. Physical activity appears to be a key component to maintaining weight loss. Weight loss through dieting alone often leads to reduction in basal metabolic rate (BMR); regular exercise prevents this decline in BMR by helping to maintain or even increase lean body mass. More detailed guidelines for exercise prescription in obesity are discussed in chapter 8.

Physical Activity and Hypertension

In Australia, it is estimated that up to 20% of the population may have elevated blood pressure (defined as >140/90 mmHg). Since hypertension has no overt symptoms, many hypertensive individuals are unaware of their condition. Hypertension is a risk factor for cardiovascular disease, stroke, peripheral vascular disease, retinopathy and renal failure. Epidemiological and intervention studies show that physical activity reduces the risk of developing hypertension by 30 to 50%. Even moderate levels of physical activity effectively reduce mild to moderate hypertension (resting blood pressure of 140-180/90-105 mmHg). Exercise by itself is ineffective for reducing severe hypertension when blood pressure is above these values, and medication is required to reduce blood pressure toward the recommended levels. However, for severe hypertension, there is some evidence that moderate exercise may reduce the dose of medication required to control blood pressure.

There appears to be a dose-response relationship between blood pressure and the amount of physical activity; that is, blood pressure levels are related to the amount of physical activity performed or physical fitness level. In hypertensive individuals, moderate physical activity (i.e., <70% $\dot{V}O_2$max) reduces both systolic and diastolic blood pressure by about 6 to 7 mmHg; more intense exercise does not confer any further changes in blood pressure. It is not clear which mechanisms underlie the beneficial effects of exercise on blood pressure. Reduced activity of the sympathetic nervous system, leading to reduced peripheral vascular resistance, is likely to be at least partially involved. Physical activity also acts indirectly to reduce blood pressure by helping to control body weight and possibly stress levels. Further details for exercise prescription for hypertensive individuals are presented in chapter 8.

Physical Activity and Diabetes

Physical inactivity is a major independent risk factor for type 2 diabetes, the eighth most common cause of death and seventh leading contributor to DALYs (refer to table 2.2). Diabetes is also a risk factor for CHD, blood vessel diseases, kidney failure, retinopathy (degeneration of the retina, leading to blindness) and neuropathy (degeneration of peripheral nerves). Type 2 diabetes begins later in life, usually in middle to old age, although there is now a disturbing trend for younger people (teens and 20s) to present signs of this form of diabetes. Type 2 diabetes is characterised by high blood glucose levels resulting from a relative insulin insufficiency, caused by insulin insensitivity in peripheral tissues. Over the past 20 years, the incidence of type 2 diabetes has increased alarmingly, possibly doubling; it is now estimated that 5% and perhaps as many as 7% of the Australian population exhibits signs of type 2 diabetes such as impaired glucose tolerance or hyperinsulinaemia. Obesity (especially abdominal obesity), physical inactivity, impaired glucose tolerance, hyperinsulinaemia and family history are the strongest risk factors for type 2 diabetes. Those at increased risk of diabetes include the elderly, the indigenous population and some overseas-born populations.

The preferred first treatment options for most people with type 2 diabetes include weight loss, dietary modification and physical activity. Regular activity reduces body fat levels, increases insulin sensitivity and enhances insulin-independent glucose uptake from the blood. Insulin sensitivity may be improved by regular exercise even without weight loss, and even slight loss of body mass significantly improves glucose tolerance. Regular moderate endurance-type activities (e.g., 30-60 min of walking), especially when performed daily, are effective for enhancing glucose tolerance. Recent evidence suggests that a combination of moderate-intensity circuit-resistance training and aerobic exercise may be more effective than aerobic exercise alone. Further information on physical activity for those with type 2 diabetes is discussed in chapter 8.

Physical Activity and Blood Lipid Disorders

Dyslipidaemia (abnormal blood lipid levels) is a major risk factor for CVD and contributes to hypertension. It is estimated that 39% of adult women and 47% of adult men have elevated blood cholesterol concentration (>5.5 mmol $\cdot$ L^{-1})(Armstrong, Bauman and Davies 2000). Dyslipidaemia is associated with obesity, especially abdominal obesity, physical inactivity, type 2 diabetes and family history. Regular endurance physical activity is recognised as an important intervention to increase blood levels of the cardioprotective lipid fraction (high-density lipoprotein [HDL]) and to reduce triglyceride levels. Blood levels of total cholesterol and low-density lipoprotein (LDL) decrease if physical activity leads to weight loss (usually also involving dietary intervention). The total amount of energy expenditure seems to be important for determining the effect of physical activity on blood lipid levels; a minimum of 1,000 to 1,200 kcal per week is required to induce favourable changes in HDL levels.

Physical Activity and Cancer

Cancer is the single most common cause of death in Australia and many developed countries, accounting for about 25% of all deaths each year. The incidence of cancer is increasing; in Australia, one in three men and one in four women will be directly affected by some type of cancer in their lifetime. Cancer is a complex group of many diseases, all originating from the uncontrolled growth of a single cell. The most common forms in men are cancer of the airways (trachea, bronchus, lung), prostate and colon; in women, cancer of the breast, airways and colon are the most common. Australia also has the highest incidence of skin cancer in the world. Different cancers are associated with different risk factors and causes, some of which are preventable and others of which are related to genetic influence. Cigarette smoking is the most important preventable cause of cancer of the airways and may contribute to other forms of cancer.

Epidemiological evidence suggests an inverse relationship between physical activity or physical fitness and the incidence of cancer. This relationship is strongest for colon cancer. There is some evidence, although not conclusive, that physical activity reduces the risk of breast and reproductive system cancers in women and prostate cancer in men. Physical activity may reduce by half the risk of colon cancer in men, but fewer studies on females make it unclear whether this also holds true for women. Moderate physical activity, as generally recommended for good health, is associated with reduced risk of cancer, although more intense exercise appears to give additional benefits.

There are many possible mechanisms by which physical activity may reduce the risk of cancer, such as

> ▶ enhanced movement of, and reduced colon exposure to, potential carcinogens in fecal material (colon cancer);
> ▶ lower body fat levels (endometrial, breast, colon cancers);
> ▶ lower levels of sex steroids (breast, prostate cancers); and
> ▶ enhanced immune function and reduced stress levels (in theory, all cancers).

In addition, individuals who choose to exercise may be more likely to adopt healthier lifestyles overall, possibly reducing the risk of cancer associated with factors such as cigarette smoking or high-fat diets. Some common genetic factors may also predispose an individual to both a physically active lifestyle and a low risk of cancer. Physical activity recommendations for cancer patients are discussed in more detail in chapter 9.

Physical Activity and Mental Health

Mental health is one of the six National Health Priority Areas. Depression is a disease of major and growing importance worldwide; the World Health Organization estimates depression will be the second leading cause of DALYs by the year 2020. Depression is a major contributor to disease and disability in Australia, and physical inactivity contributes 10% to the incidence and 15% to the number of hospitalisations resulting from depression each year.

Compared with the number of studies on physical activity and physical health, there is a relative lack of high-quality controlled studies on the benefits of physical activity for mental health. Population and cross-sectional studies associate regular physical activity with better indices of mental health in both healthy individuals and those with certain types of mental illness, such as anxiety or depressive disorders (U.S. Department of Health and Human Services and CDC 1996). Beneficial effects include lower anxiety and stress levels and improved self-esteem, self-efficacy, mood-state and well-being. Moderate physical activity is now advocated as adjunct therapy for treatment of clinical anxiety and depression.

Psychological well-being may be defined as the extent to which people experience mainly positive, as opposed to negative, emotions in their daily lives and the extent to which individuals feel satisfied with their life circumstances (Gauvin, Spence and Anderson 1999). There are relatively few studies on the effects of physical activity on global psychological well-being, and most studies have focused on the responses of individual components of well-being such as anxiety or depression.

Cross-sectional and population studies suggest that physically active people experience less anxiety, although it is unclear whether there is a causal relationship. It is possible that individuals with low anxiety (or high psychological well-being) are also those who are attracted to regular exercise. Recent meta-analysis of intervention studies suggests that small decreases in anxiety result from regular exercise training (Gauvin, Spence and Anderson 1999). Acute exercise seems to induce positive effects on anxiety that last up to 2 to 3 h after exercise. Compared with studies on anxiety, the data are stronger for a relationship between physical activity and depression. Epidemiological data suggest that physically inactive people are at increased risk of depression compared with the physically active (RR of 1.3 to 1.8). Intervention studies also show decreases in measures of depression that seem to be greater than the decreases in anxiety associated with physical activity. In addition, greater beneficial effects on indices of depression occur in those experiencing symptoms of clinical depression as opposed to healthy individuals. The general consensus among those who treat individuals with depression is that physical activity is best used in concurrent treatment, that is, in addition to rather than instead of some form of psychotherapy.

Little is known about the dose-response relationship between the amount of physical activity (e.g., duration, frequency, intensity, mode) and psychological well-being. It is very difficult to perform well-controlled, long-term studies while also manipulating exercise variables such as frequency or intensity. In addition, there are many possible social and biological confounding variables that may interfere with interpretation of data from such studies. It is likely that positive effects of physical activity on psychological well-being relate more to the individual's perception of changes in physical fitness than to the actual amount of exercise. There seems to be agreement among mental health professionals that the levels of physical activity recommended by recent public health campaigns are sufficient to provide beneficial effects on psychological well-being (Gauvin, Spence and Anderson 1999). It is important to note, however, that this consensus is not necessarily based on solid empirical evidence and that further research is needed to clearly establish the links between regular moderate physical activity and psychological well-being. The mechanisms responsible for the psychological health benefits of physical activity are not clearly understood. Some propose that exercise induces favourable changes in brain neurotransmitters or neuroreceptor function. Others postulate that physical activity may be beneficial by providing social interaction and support, relief from daily stressors, or the chance to develop self-efficacy.

Physical Activity and Quality of Life (QOL)

Quality of life (QOL) is a psychological construct that can be defined as an individual's perception of his or her position in life. This is a subjective term since it relies on the individual's perception rather than on specific measures. QOL is difficult to quantify because it is multidimensional, containing facets of physical, psychological and social health. There is a difference of opinion as to what should be assessed in measuring QOL, and there are over 300 different scales in use to measure various aspects of QOL (Trine 1999). Health-related QOL (HQOL) includes concepts such as the individual's perception of his or her health-related quality of life, life satisfaction, happiness and well-being.

The issue of whether physical activity influences HQOL has been addressed among different populations. However, research on healthy adult populations is inconclusive. Larger studies tend to show a positive, but low, correlation between physical activity and HQOL. Intervention studies sometimes, but not always, show a positive relationship, but these tend to be short term (10-30 weeks), and it is possible that a longer period is needed to influence HQOL. Physical activity is likely to affect HQOL by improving psychological and physical well-being, physical function and perhaps cognitive function.

The evidence showing that physical activity may beneficially alter HQOL is probably stronger in populations with diseases or conditions affecting physical capacity than in healthy populations. For example, multifactorial cardiac rehabilitation, which includes physical activity among other interventions, enhances HQOL measures in the first few months after myocardial infarction, although this effect persists only as long as the patient is actively involved in the intervention (Oldridge 1997). The extent of improvement in HQOL seems to be related to initial health status—compared with healthy individuals, those with significant health impairment tend to show larger improvements in HQOL associated with physical activity. Since HQOL is influenced by the individual's perception of physical capacity and physical health, this perception is likely to be positively affected by actual improvements in physical capacity induced by regular exercise.

What Is Appropriate Physical Activity? Minimum and Optimum Recommendations

People often ask, "What is the optimum amount of physical activity needed for good health?" Implied is the other aspect of this question: "What is the minimum amount?" If we are to increase the number of people who are physically active, it is important to be able to answer these questions. It is essential that exercise managers and other health professionals are able to give clear advice to convince people that they can achieve health benefits by being physically active.

As expected, the answer to these seemingly simple questions is complex and depends entirely on the individual and the desired outcome(s). In recent years, guidelines about the recommended level of physical activity for good health have been advanced by several agencies, including the following:

▶ The American College of Sports Medicine (ACSM)

▶ The U.S. Department of Health and Human Services' Office of the Surgeon General (USSG)

▶ The National Heart Foundation of Australia (NHFA)

▶ The Australian Sports Commission in conjunction with various State and Federal agencies (**Active Australia**)

▶ The World Health Organization (WHO)

Current Recommendations for Physical Activity for Good Health

Summaries of guidelines by ACSM, the U.S. Surgeon General (USSG), Active Australia and National Heart Foundation of Australia (NHFA) are presented in figures 2.2 to 2.5 and are discussed in detail in the following sections. Since these guidelines have a public health focus, they are usually rather broad in terms of the amount and type of activity recommended. While seemingly broad, however, these are based on a large volume of scientific literature on the relationship between physical activity and various health outcomes.

Some terms used in these recommendations must be defined before discussing them in detail (see figure 2.6). There are slight variations in specific terms used in the different guidelines. The ACSM's definitions tend to be more precise and quantifiable, possibly because they have been written for professionals with exercise science training. The definitions used by the USSG, NHFA and Active Australia were written with a public health focus and tend to be more easily understood by the lay public.

Exercise mode: large muscle group activity that can be maintained continuously and is rhythmic and aerobic in nature, such as running/jogging, swimming, cycling, walking/hiking, aerobic dance/group exercise, cross-country skiing, rowing, rope skipping, stair climbing, skating and various endurance games

Frequency: three to five times per week

Duration: 20 to 60 min per session (minimum of 10-min bouts accumulated throughout the day)

Intensity: 40/50-85% $\dot{V}O_2$max or heart rate reserve, equivalent to approximately 55/65-90% age-predicted maximum heart rate (the lowest intensity is for unfit individuals)

Muscular strength and endurance training: two to three times per week, 8 to 10 exercises using large muscle groups, 1 to 2 sets of 8 to 12 repetitions of each exercise

Flexibility training: at least two to three times per week to stretch major muscle groups

Compiled from American College of Sports Medicine, 1998b, "The recommended quantity and quality of exercise for developing and maintaining cardiorespiratory and muscular fitness, and flexibility in health adults," *Medicine and Science in Sports and Exercise* 30: 975-991.

FIGURE 2.2   Summary of the American College of Sports Medicine's recommendations for exercise for healthy adults.

▶ All people over the age of 2 years should accumulate at least 30 min of endurance-type physical activity of at least moderate intensity on most, preferably all, days of the week.

▶ Additional health and functional benefits of physical activity can be achieved by adding more time in moderate-intensity activity or by substituting more vigorous activity.

▶ Persons with symptomatic CVD, diabetes or other chronic health problems who would like to increase their physical activity should be evaluated by a physician and given an exercise program appropriate for their clinical status.

▶ Previously inactive men over age 40, women over age 50, and people at high risk for CVD should first consult a physician before embarking on a program of vigorous physical activity to which they are unaccustomed.

▶ Strength-developing activities (resistance training) should be performed at least twice per week. At least 8 to 10 strength-developing exercises that use the major muscle groups of the legs, trunk, arms and shoulders should be performed at each session, with 1 to 2 sets of 8 to 12 repetitions of each exercise.

Reprinted from U.S. Department of Health and Human Services and Centers for Disease Control and Prevention, 1996, *Physical activity and health: A Report of the Surgeon General*. (Atlanta, GA: USDHHS/CDC/National Center for Chronic Disease Prevention and Health Promotion), 28-29.

FIGURE 2.3   Summary of the U.S. Surgeon General's physical activity recommendations.

► Think of movement as an opportunity, not an inconvenience.

► Be active every day in as many ways as you can.

► Put together at least 30 min of moderate-intensity physical activity on most, preferably all, days.

► If you can, also enjoy some regular, vigorous exercise for extra health and fitness.

Reprinted from Active Australia, The Commonwealth Department of Health and Aged Care and Australian Sports Commission, 1999, *National physical activity guidelines for Australians*. Accessed via Web site **www.health.gov.au/pubhlth/publicat/document/physguide.pdf.**

FIGURE 2.4   National physical activity guidelines for Australians.

1. Physical inactivity is a major risk factor for CVD, second only to smoking as a health risk.

2. Physical activity improves other CVD risk factors and decreases all-cause mortality. Benefits include reducing risk of diabetes, preventing falls and maintaining bone mass.

3. The benefits occur soon after beginning a physically active lifestyle and apply to men and women of all ages.

4. Physical activity should be a lifelong habit begun in childhood.*

5. Physical activity is an important component of cardiac rehabilitation after myocardial infarction, cardiac procedures or surgery.

6. The total amount of physical activity seems to be most important. The current recommendation is at least 30 min of moderate activity, such as walking, on most if not all days.*

7. It may be possible that accumulated bouts of 10 min activity may provide benefits, although more research is needed on this point.*

8. The moderate physical activity message suggests a lifestyle approach, including increasing incidental activity, brisk walking and other types of active recreation.

9. Moderately intense and vigorous exercise may give additional health benefits.*

10. Physical activity may assist in weight control, although dietary intervention may also be needed.

11. Health professionals are able to effectively advise patients on physical activity.

12. Policy and practice to provide supportive environments for physical activity should be developed.

13. The overall goal is to increase participation by the entire population, although special efforts may be directed to particular groups such as sedentary individuals.

14. Further research is needed to determine the effectiveness of strategies to increase participation in physical activity among the population.

*Similar to other published recommendations for physical activity (refer to figures 2.2-2.4).

Compiled from NHFA Physical Activity Policy 2000 (**www.heartfoundation.com.au/prof/index_fr.html**).

FIGURE 2.5   Summary of the National Heart Foundation of Australia (NHFA) Physical Activity Policy.

These definitions put forward by different groups, like their recommendations, are more similar than dissimilar. Where they differ tends to be in the interpretation and examples given. For example, both the NHFA and ACSM describe moderate activity in terms of the individual's comfort level during activity but use different ways to convey this—in the NHFA definition conversation can be maintained, whereas the ACSM states a time frame (45 min) of comfortable activity. The important thing is that these recommendations give the public and health professionals a starting point for individuals and groups to develop appropriate physical activity programs to meet specific needs. The extension of these guidelines to develop exercise prescriptions for healthy individuals is discussed in detail in section

PHYSICAL ACTIVITY

▶ NHFA: Any movement involving large skeletal muscles (e.g., walking, stair climbing, gardening, playing sports, work-related activity).

▶ USSG, ACSM: Bodily movement that is produced by the contraction of skeletal muscle and that substantially increases energy expenditure.

EXERCISE

▶ NHFA: Planned physical activity for recreation, leisure or fitness with a specific objective such as improving fitness, performance, health or social interaction.

▶ USSG: Planned, structured and repetitive bodily movement done to improve or maintain one or more components of physical fitness.

MODERATE ACTIVITY

▶ NHFA: Activity that is energetic but at a level at which a conversation can be maintained.

▶ ACSM: Absolute moderate exercise is in the range of 3-6 METs for most healthy individuals. Since this may vary by individual, it can also be defined as an exercise intensity well within the individual's capacity, one which can be comfortably sustained for a prolonged period of time (~45 min), which has a gradual initiation and progression, and is generally noncompetitive. If exercise capacity is known, it may be defined as 40-60% $\dot{V}O_2$max.

VIGOROUS ACTIVITY

▶ NHFA: Activity at a higher intensity, which may, depending on fitness level, cause sweating and "puffing".

▶ ACSM: Activity >6 METs (metabolic equivalents) for most healthy individuals or >60% $\dot{V}O_2$max if exercise capacity is known or exercise intense enough to represent a substantial cardiorespiratory challenge.

PHYSICAL FITNESS

▶ USSG, ACSM: A set of attributes that people have or achieve that relates to the ability to perform physical activity.

Abbreviations: ACSM = American College of Sports Medicine; NHFA = National Heart Foundation of Australia; USSG = U.S. Surgeon General.

Sources: National Heart Foundation of Australia Physical Activity Policy, 2000. **www.heartfoundation.com.au/prof/index_fr.html**; U.S. Department of Health and Human Services and Centers for Disease Control and Prevention, 1996, *Physical activity and health: A Report of the Surgeon General.* (Atlanta, GA: U.S. Department of Health and Human Services); American College of Sports Medicine, 2000, *ACSM's guidelines for exercise testing and prescription*, 6th ed. (Lippincott Williams & Williams).

FIGURE 2.6   Some definitions used in recommendations for physical activity.

2 and for individuals with diseases or impairments in section 3.

Comparisons of the Various Physical Activity Recommendations

Table 2.7 makes some simple comparisons between recent physical activity recommendations by the USSG, ACSM, Active Australia and NHFA.

Several variables must be considered when developing an appropriate activity program for individuals or groups, depending on skill, fitness level, access, goals, preferences and health status. Program variables that may be manipulated include mode (type of activity), intensity (how physiologically taxing the activity is), duration (each session or total per day), and frequency (how often per week). In the following section, each of these will be discussed in the context of

TABLE 2.7—Comparison of Recommendations for Physical Activity for Healthy Adults

Activity component	Recommendation	Major reasons for recommendation
Mode	**USSG:** not specified; variety implied **ACSM:** large muscle groups; various activities appropriate **Active A, NHFA:** not specified; variety implied; lifestyle approach	Facilitate enjoyment Less likely to cause injury Increase fitness and energy expenditure
Intensity	**USSG:** moderate intensity in general; further benefits from vigorous exercise **ACSM:** 40/50-85% $\dot{V}O_2$max or HRR **Active A:** moderate intensity in general; further benefits from vigorous exercise **NHFA:** both moderate and vigorous contribute to health benefits	Moderate: to enhance enjoyment, adherence, fat loss and control of blood pressure; also less likely to cause injury Vigorous: additional health benefits from increasing fitness
Duration	**USSG:** accumulate ≥30 min/day; further benefits from longer duration **ACSM:** 20-60 min per session **Active A, NHFA:** accumulate ≥30 min/day; does not need to be continuous	≥30 min/day associated with decreased mortality/morbidity; minimum to lose body fat Benefits related to exercise volume
Frequency	**USSG:** most, preferably all, days **ACSM:** 3-5 d/wk **Active A, NHFA:** most, preferably all, days	Benefits related to exercise volume Acute effects beneficial (e.g., blood glucose control) Encourage people to incorporate into daily life
Resistance training	**USSG:** 2 d/wk, 8-10 exercises using major muscle groups, 1-2 sets of 8-12 reps **ACSM:** 2 d/wk, 8-10 exercises using major muscle groups, 1-2 sets of 8-12 reps **Active A, NHFA:** not specified	Minimise loss of muscle mass and bone density with age Help maintain strength, coordination, balance and functional capacity during aging

Abbreviations: USSG = United States Surgeon General; ACSM = American College of Sports Medicine; Active A = Active Australia; NHFA = National Heart Foundation of Australia; HRR = heart rate reserve.

Sources of recommendations: USSG = Physical Activity and Health: A Report of the (US) Surgeon General, 1996; ACSM = American College of Sports Medicine, 1998, "The recommended quantity and quality of exercise for developing and maintaining cardiorespiratory and muscular fitness, and flexibility in health adults," *Medicine and Science in Sports and Exercise* 30: 975-991; Active A = Active Australia, Commonwealth Department of Health and Aged Care and the Australian Commission, 1999, **www.health.gov.au/pubhlth/publicat/document/physguide.pdf**; NHFA = National Heart Foundation of Australia, 2000, NHFA Physical Activity Policy. **www.heartfoundation.com.au/prof/index_fr.html**.

the four sets of current recommendations regarding physical activity (ACSM, USSG, Active Australia, NHFA). Chapter 7 covers the general principles of exercise prescription for healthy people, and chapters 8 to 10 discuss the general principles of exercise prescription for people with diseases or impairments.

Recommended Modes of Physical Activity

There is no single ideal mode to achieve physical fitness or health benefits, and all guidelines tend to be flexible when suggesting modes of activity. Health benefits of activity are more related to the combination of frequency, intensity and duration (or total energy expenditure), and positive adaptations tend to be independent of mode. The choice of activity for any given individual depends on many factors, including access and convenience, personal preference, skill and experience, climate, personal safety, age, and illness or disability. Population surveys generally indicate walking and aerobics (i.e., group exercise to music) as the most popular activity modes, but many others also attract significant interest.

The ACSM guidelines (refer to figure 2.2) are the most detailed in terms of suggested activities, indicating that any rhythmic activity using large muscle groups, or primarily aerobic in nature, that can be sustained continuously is suitable. Suggested activities include "walking/hiking, running/jogging, cycling/bicycling, cross-country skiing, aerobic dance/ group exercise, rope skipping, stair climbing, swimming, skating and various endurance game activities". When selecting activity mode, factors such as the risk of injury (e.g., from high-impact activities) should also be considered.

Similarly, the USSG suggests a wide range of activities that may meet the minimum recommendation of 30 min of moderate activity on most days (refer to figure 2.3). It suggests that the minimum may be accomplished through various tasks both occupational or nonoccupational and tasks of daily living if performed at moderate intensity. Examples of suitable activities include "brisk walking, cycling, swimming, home repair, and yardwork". This report notes the importance of personal preference and the ability to sustain the chosen activity.

Active Australia's guidelines focus on encouraging people to incorporate physical activity into work, family, social and community life and are thus also broad in recommended activity modes (refer to figure 2.4). Suggested activities include brisk walking, cycling, gardening and lawn mowing, dancing and swimming. The NHFA Physical Activity Policy does not recommend any specific modes but notes the importance of a lifestyle approach that includes "incidental physical activity, brisk walking and other forms of active recreation" (refer to figure 2.5).

Recommended Intensity of Physical Activity

All current guidelines recommend a minimum of moderate-intensity activity on a regular basis. Only a relatively small proportion of people regularly participate in vigorous activity—approximately 20% of adult Australians according to 1999 Active Australia data. The recommendation of moderate activity is based on the consideration that most people prefer and are more likely to adhere to a program of

moderate activity and that significant health benefits accrue from this level of activity. The definition of *moderate intensity* and its perception by the public are important. There is a common misconception that only intense exercise confers health benefits, yet this level of activity is not attractive to most adults. Thus, it is vital that the general public is aware of the health benefits of moderate activity and that such benefits are easily achievable. All of the guidelines note, however, that further health benefits may be achieved through more vigorous activity. The four sets of guidelines discussed here use slightly different wording to convey basically the same message as to appropriate intensity of activity.

The 1998 and 2000 ACSM recommendations suggest exercise intensity in the range of 55/65 to 90% **maximum heart rate (HRmax),** equivalent to 40/50 to 85% of **heart rate reserve (HRR)** or maximum oxygen uptake reserve ($\dot{V}O_2R$)(ACSM 1998b, 2000). ($\dot{V}O_2R$ is defined as the difference between $\dot{V}O_2$max and $\dot{V}O_2$ at rest; this method improves the accuracy of the relationship between oxygen uptake and heart rate reserve [ACSM 1998b]). The lowest value (55% HRmax or 40% HRR) is an appropriate starting intensity for individuals with low fitness and reflects recent research showing training effects at this intensity. In contrast, individuals of average fitness level require a higher training stimulus (e.g., minimum of 65% HRmax or 50% HRR). The wide range of exercise intensities (i.e., up to 90% HRmax or 85% HRR) allows flexibility for inclusion of virtually any type of activity. The higher intensities are appropriate for those already active and fit who wish to achieve fitness- and performance-related goals (e.g., training for sport or a specific event).

The 2000 ACSM recommendations define moderate exercise as activities in the range of 40 to 60% $\dot{V}O_2$max, equivalent to 3 to 6 METs (**metabolic equivalent,** or multiple of resting metabolic rate)(ACSM 2000). An alternative definition is that a moderate-intensity activity is "well within the individual's capacity, one which can be comfortably sustained for a prolonged period of time (45 min), which has a gradual initiation and progression and is generally noncompetitive" (ACSM 2000).

The USSG, although less specific in defining intensity, recommends moderate-intensity activity that can either be sustained or accumulated for 30 min per day. Noting the health benefits and attractiveness to most people of moderate-intensity exercise and the potential injury risk of higher-intensity exercise, it suggests that moderate intensity is more achievable by the wider population. This report does suggest, however, that greater health benefits may accrue from more vigorous activity.

Like the USSG, Active Australia also recommends moderate-intensity physical activity for the general public, but it also encourages those interested and able to "enjoy some regular, vigorous exercise for extra health and fitness". Regular vigorous exercise is advocated for children and teenagers under 18 years and for those wishing to improve physical fitness and sports performance in demanding high-energy activities. Vigorous exercise is defined as activity that makes one "huff and puff" or makes conversation difficult. It is further defined as 70 to 85% of **age-predicted maximum heart rate (APMHR)** (220 – age).

NHFA defines moderate activity as "activity that is energetic, but at a level which a conversation can be maintained" (the so-called "talk test"). Vigorous activity is defined as "activity at a higher intensity, which may, depending on fitness level, cause sweating and puffing"; these are similar to the Active Australia definitions. Moderate-intensity activity is recommended for the wider population because of the established health benefits, but it is noted that more vigorous activity may confer further health benefits.

TABLE 2.8—Metabolic Equivalent (MET) of Some Physical Activities

Activity	Pace or intensity	MET
Aerobics	Light intensity	5
	High intensity	7
Circuit training	General	8
Cycling	Leisure, <16 km · h⁻¹	4
	Moderate, 16-22 km · h⁻¹	8
	Vigorous, >30 km · h⁻¹	10-12
General home duties	E.g., cleaning, laundry	2.5-4
General lawn and garden	E.g., mowing lawn, raking leaves, trimming	4-6
Golf	General	8
Jogging/running	8 km · h⁻¹	8
	10 km · h⁻¹	10
	13 km · h⁻¹	13.5
Sitting, light office work		1.5
Social dancing		4.5
Swimming laps	Moderate	8
	Vigorous	10
Walking	Moderate, 5 km · h⁻¹	3.3
	Brisk, 7 km · h⁻¹	3.8
	Walking hills or backpacking	6-7
Tennis	General	6-8

Compiled from B.E. Ainsworth, W.L. Haskell, A.S. Leon, D.R. Jacobs, H.J. Montoye, J.F. Sallis, and R.S. Paffenbarger, 1993, "Compendium of physical activities: classification of energy costs of human physical activities," *Medicine and Science in Sports and Exercise* 1: 71-80; B.E. Ainsworth, W.L. Haskell, M.C. Whitt, M.L. Irwin, A.M. Swartz, S.J. Strath, W.L. O'Brien, D.R. Bassett, K.H. Schmitz, P.O. Emplaincourt, D.R. Jacobs, and A.S. Leon, 2000, "Compendium of physical activities: an update of activity codes and MET intensities," *Medicine and Science in Sports and Exercise* 32: S498-S516.

Recommended Duration or Volume of Physical Activity

Exercise duration is a function of intensity; that is, lower-intensity exercise requires a longer duration to achieve similar results. A moderate amount of physical activity associated with health benefits is 150 to 300 kcal (630-1,260 kJ) per day or ≥1,000 kcal per week (in addition to energy expenditure in activities of daily living). This could be accomplished by various combinations of intensity and duration (e.g., 37.5 min at 4 kcal $\cdot$ min^{-1}, or walking on a flat surface at 6 km $\cdot$ h^{-1}) or 21 min at higher intensity (jogging at 9 km $\cdot$ h^{-1}.

The ACSM recommends a wide range of activity duration, from 20 to 60 min; the choice of duration depends on exercise intensity and mode. Thirty min of moderate-intensity activity appears to be the minimum to elicit significant health benefits, especially in terms of weight control. The risk of musculoskeletal injury increases when duration exceeds 60 min of high-impact activities such as jogging or aerobics. The other sets of recommendations (USSG, NHFA, Active Australia) are consistent in suggesting a minimum accumulation of 30 min of moderate-intensity activity each day, although more vigorous or longer duration activity is encouraged for those who are interested and able.

Continuous Versus Intermittent Activity

The question of whether activity needs to be continuous to be beneficial is still a matter of debate. All four sets of recommendations imply (or state overtly) that activity may be accumulated through shorter sessions (e.g., 10-15 min at a time) repeated throughout the day. There is some evidence that multiple bouts of shorter activity may yield health benefits, but this issue is still controversial, and interpretation depends on the desired and measured outcomes. For example, in one recent study, 56 middle-aged, previously sedentary men and women were randomly allocated into groups that performed the same total amount of activity over an 18-week period but had differences in the duration and frequency of each bout (Woolf-May et al. 1999). Long walkers walked 20 to 40 min, intermediate walkers 10 to 15 min, and short walkers 5 to 10 min per bout. Total exercise time (about 150-160 min $\cdot$ wk^{-1}) and heart rates (about 74% of age-predicted maximum) were similar between groups over the 18-week study. Compared with a non-exercise control group, all three groups improved physical fitness to a similar extent. However, only the long and intermediate

walkers showed improvements in the blood lipid profile. It was concluded that accumulated bouts of shorter duration, moderate activity (e.g., 15 min walking) may provide benefits in terms of improved physical fitness and some CHD risk factors but that not all risk factors may be improved to a similar extent by shorter compared with longer bouts.

A recent review (Hardman 1999) noted inconsistent evidence that repeated shorter bouts of activity are as effective in conferring health benefits as the more traditionally recommended single longer bout. On the other hand, given that repeated shorter bouts provide at least some health benefits and are not harmful, this form of activity should not be discouraged in those who find it a more attractive means to be physically active. In other words, it is more important for people to become physically active in ways that suit their lifestyles and to which they are more likely to adhere. The more traditional prescription of 20 to 40 min of continuous activity per day is likely to yield more benefits in terms of physical fitness and favourable changes in disease risk factors. There are, however, fewer but significant benefits to be gained from shorter bouts of activity totalling at least 30 min per day.

Recommended Frequency of Physical Activity

The recommended frequency of activity depends on a variety of factors including desired outcomes, personal preference, access, time commitments and mode. In general, health benefits and training adaptations are a function of the volume of activity (i.e., a combination of duration, intensity and frequency). Low-intensity or shorter duration activities require more frequent sessions to achieve the same benefits as high-intensity or longer duration activities.

The ACSM recommends three to five sessions of aerobic or cardiovascular conditioning each week. Three sessions per week is the minimum frequency to induce a training effect, such as an increase in physical fitness (although unfit people may benefit from twice-weekly exercise at the onset). On the other hand, only minimal additional benefits are associated with more than five sessions per week, and the risk of musculoskeletal injury increases exponentially with more than five sessions per week of high-impact activity. For individuals with very low functional capacity (e.g., <3 METs), more than one bout of activity spaced throughout the day may be needed. For those of normal functional capacity, exercising all days of the week is not discouraged, provided it does not increase the risk of injury. For example, in addition to up to five sessions per week of aerobic activity, the ACSM also recommends two sessions of resistance training. For those wishing to exercise daily, choosing a variety of low-impact or complementary activities (cross-training) reduces the risk of injury.

The other three sets of recommendations (USSG, Active Australia, NHFA) are consistent in suggesting moderate activity, such as brisk walking, on most, if not all, days of the week. These recommendations encourage the incorporation of physical activity into the daily lifestyle. From the adherence viewpoint, activity is more likely to be maintained if it is a regular part of each day.

Resistance Training

The ACSM and USSG recommend similar forms of regular **resistance training** to enhance muscular fitness (refer to figures 2.2 and 2.3). The ACSM recommendations state that resistance training is an "integral part of the adult fitness program" and should aim to increase muscle strength and maintain fat-free mass and bone mineral density (ACSM 1998b). Resistance training should be progressive, individualised, and performed once to twice per week. Training more than twice per week is unlikely to lead to significant further increases in strength but may increase the risk of injury and may also limit time for aerobic activities. Since strength gains are specific to the body part exercised, training should include 8 to 10 exercises using all major muscle groups of the legs, trunk, arms and shoulders.

One to two sets per session of 8 to 12 repetitions to near fatigue are recommended for healthy adults, although more repetitions at a lower resistance (e.g., 10-15 repetitions) may be suitable for older individuals. Although greater gains in strength occur with higher resistance and fewer repetitions, high-intensity resistance training also increases the risk of orthopaedic injury. Emphasis is placed on developing total body strength and muscular endurance, since these are important for maintaining muscle mass, bone density and functional capacity, and on preventing muscular injury (e.g., low back pain). Because gains in strength are also specific to joint angle, exercises should involve movement through the entire range of motion. Dynamic rather than isometric exercises are recommended because they more closely simulate activities of daily living. Resistance training using weights (free or machine)

generally leads to greater increases in strength, although appropriate calisthenics using the body weight as resistance can be effective for those unable to access weightlifting equipment. Safety issues, such as proper technique and breathing, are also noted by the ACSM recommendations (ACSM 2000).

Evolution of Physical Activity Recommendations

In the previous section, we discussed the current recommendations on the appropriate type and amount of physical activity to achieve health benefits. It is important to recognise the historical basis for these recommendations, because they have evolved over the years with advances in research on the relationship between physical activity and health. In 1978, the American College of Sports Medicine published its first statement on the recommended type and amount of exercise for cardiovascular health and control of body weight (ACSM 1978). A summary of these recommendations is provided in table 2.9. This position was revised in 1990 and again in 1998 (ACSM 1990, 1998b). In the meantime, other health organisations with an interest in physical activity (American Health Association, World Health Organization, National Heart Foundation of Australia, Active Australia, among others) have also published recommendations. A close look at these recommendations shows changes in several key areas over time, especially with regard to the recommended intensity and duration of exercise.

In the earlier ACSM recommendations, the main focus was on exercise as a means to develop physical fitness (in particular, cardiorespiratory fitness). This emphasis was based on research in the 1960s and 1970s that showed a relationship between measures of physical fitness and health-related outcomes (e.g., lower mortality). In the past 20-plus years, however, it has become clear that lower intensity physical activity helps decrease the risk of all-cause mortality and of developing many diseases, without necessarily inducing large improvements in physical fitness. At the same time, research on exercise adherence (i.e., how likely people are to continue to exercise) has shown that low- to moderate-intensity exercise is preferred by most adults; only a small proportion of the population is attracted to the higher intensity exercise needed to improve physical fitness.

TABLE 2.9—Earlier and Current ACSM Recommendations for Exercise

Year	Type/mode	Frequency	Intensity	Duration	Resistance training
1978	Endurance, large muscle group	3-5 d/wk	50-85% $\dot{V}O_2$max or HRR 60-90% APMHR	15-60 min	Not included
1990	Endurance, large muscle group, strength	3-5 d/wk	50-85% $\dot{V}O_2$max or HRR 60-90% APMHR	20-60 min	1 set 8-12 reps 8-10 exercises 2 d/wk
1998	Endurance, large muscle group, strength	3-5 d/wk	40/50-85% $\dot{V}O_2$max or HRR 55/65-90% APMHR	20-60 min >10-min bouts accumulated throughout day	1-2 sets 8-12 reps 8-10 exercises 1-2 d/wk plus flexibility training

Compiled from American College of Sports Medicine, 1978, "The recommended quantity and quality of exercise for developing and maintaining fitness in healthy adults," *Medicine and Science in Sports and Exercise* 10:vii-x; American College of Sports Medicine, 1990, "American College of Sports Medicine position stand: the recommended quantity and quality of exercise for developing and maintaining cardiorespiratory and muscular fitness in healthy adults," *Medicine and Science in Sports and Exercise* 22: 265-274; American College of Sports Medicine, 1998b, "The recommended quantity and quality of exercise for developing and maintaining cardiorespiratory and muscular fitness, and flexibility in healthy adults," *Medicine and Science in Sports and Exercise* 30: 975-991.

To give some examples, low- to moderate-intensity activity (e.g., 3-6 METs or 40-60% $\dot{V}O_2$max) performed with sufficient duration and regularity is associated with benefits such as loss of body mass, lower resting blood glucose and blood pressure, and favourable changes in blood lipids and bone density. The ACSM (and other groups) now considers health-related exercise/physical activity in the context of an exercise "dose". That is, the health benefits depend on the amount of physical activity undertaken. As discussed previously, epidemiological evidence shows that the greatest health benefits occur in moving from a sedentary to low/moderately active lifestyle, with slight additional benefits accruing from a larger dose (i.e., longer duration or higher intensity) of activity (refer to table 2.4). The recent emphasis, therefore, is on a physically active lifestyle rather than on improving physical fitness. The focus is on physical activity (a broader term that includes all bodily movement that increases energy expenditure) as opposed to exercise (planned activity to enhance physical fitness). This is a subtle yet important distinction, especially for acceptance by the wider population, most of whom are not regularly active.

Another change in the general recommendations was the inclusion of resistance exercise training from 1990 onward (ACSM 1990, 1998b; U.S. Department of Health and Human Services and CDC 1996) as an integral feature of the activity program. As previously noted, the specific recommendations as to frequency, mode and training volume are based on scientific literature showing beneficial effects on body composition and weight control, bone density, muscle mass and strength, and functional capacity. Maintenance of muscle mass is especially important for maintaining functional capacity and the ability to lead an independent life during aging.

Recent public education campaigns (e.g., Active Australia) should be viewed as consistent with, and not in contradiction to, current ACSM recommendations. These campaigns suggest a *minimum* amount of physical activity recommended for good health (30 min of moderate-intensity exercise on most days); this is in the lower range of activity recommended by the ACSM. The public health campaigns also encourage those who are interested to perform exercise at higher intensity or for longer duration for additional health benefits. The most important point is that all of these recommendations provide adaptable goals that are attractive to and achievable by most people and thus aim to increase the number of people who are physically active *in some way*. Ultimately, this should greatly reduce the percentage of the population that is sedentary and the social and economic burdens of disease associated with physical inactivity.

Risks of Physical Activity

Although there are myriad health benefits of regular physical activity, the possible adverse outcomes must also be considered. There are two major areas of concern in terms of risk of physical activity—musculoskeletal injuries and cardiac events. While neither can be completely prevented, their occurrence can be minimised through proper health-risk screening, informed consent, appropriate and individualised activity prescription, and client education. These topics are discussed in detail in sections 2 and 3.

Physical fitness testing carries a risk of cardiac event, although the risk is considered to be extremely low. The risk of death as a result of maximal exercise testing performed according to established guidelines has been estimated at no more than 0.01%, and the risk of a complication requiring hospitalisation at no more than 0.2% (ACSM 2000). The risks associated with submaximal testing are considered to be even lower. Vigorous exercise also has associated risks of cardiac events, but again these are considered to be low and to vary with exercise intensity and frequency, fitness and health status of the exerciser. The relative risk of myocardial infarction is two to six times higher in vigorous (≥6 METs) compared with moderate activity; however, the risk is about 60% lower in individuals who regularly perform vigorous activity compared with those who do so infrequently (ACSM 2000). Overall, the risk of a cardiac event occurring during physical activity is far smaller than the risk associated with an inactive lifestyle; the benefits of appropriate regular physical activity far outweigh the risks of an untoward event during performance of that activity.

An increased risk of musculoskeletal injury is also associated with fitness testing and regular physical activity, although it is much harder to quantify because of its variable nature (e.g., it is unlikely to be reported because it is usually transitory and not often serious). Risk of musculoskeletal injury is greater in high-impact or weight-bearing activities such as jogging/running, high-intensity aerobics and free weight training. The risk also increases with duration, intensity and frequency of activity. Novice exercisers who undertake too strenuous a program and those who avoid proper warm-up and cool-down procedures are especially at risk of injury. Appropriate, individualised exercise prescription and client education are fundamental to preventing or lessening the risk of musculoskeletal injury (discussed further in sections 2 and 3).

Summary

It is now well accepted that there are many health benefits of regular moderate to vigorous physical activity, in particular, lowered risk of cardiovascular disease, obesity, hypertension, type 2 diabetes and some forms of cancer. Physical inactivity is as strong a predictor of cardiovascular disease as other major risk factors such as cigarette smoking, hypertension and dyslipidaemia. However, a significantly higher proportion of the population is at risk because of physical inactivity than these other risk factors. The population attributable risk (PAR) implicates physical inactivity in 10 to 18% of deaths or disability due to cardiovascular disease, cancer, diabetes, stroke and depression each year in Australia. Physical activity is a relatively low-cost strategy to enhance the health of entire populations and thus reduce costs associated with disease, disability and premature death. About only 60% of the adult Australian population is sufficiently active to achieve these health benefits, and this number seems to be decreasing in all but the older age groups. The majority of Australians recognise the importance of regular physical activity to good health yet are unable to incorporate this into their daily lives. How best to increase the proportion of physically active Australians (and citizens of other countries) remains a major challenge for the community.

Selected Glossary Terms

Active Australia—An Australian public health initiative to promote and improve participation in sport and physical activity across the population; founded in 1996.

age-predicted maximum heart rate (APMHR)—Estimated maximum heart rate, calculated as 220 minus age; used to determine recommended exercise intensity (e.g., exercising at a pace that elicits a heart rate equivalent to 60% of APMHR).

basal metabolic rate (BMR)—The lowest rate of energy expenditure to maintain the body in its basal state, measured in the morning in a fasting state under controlled laboratory conditions.

cardiorespiratory fitness (CRF)—The ability to perform prolonged exercise, quantified in a test of maximum oxygen consumption ($\dot{V}O_2max$) or time to fatigue at a certain work rate.

coronary artery or heart disease (CAD or CHD) risk factor—A health, behaviour or lifestyle factor that, based on epidemiological evidence, is known to be associated with the development of coronary artery disease (or narrowing of the coronary arteries).

disability-adjusted life year (DALY)—An estimate of potential life years lost because of premature death, disability and poor health.

dyslipidaemia—Blood lipid levels outside the recommended levels; in particular, concentrations of total cholesterol, high-density lipoprotein cholesterol, low-density lipoprotein cholesterol and triglycerides.

functional capacity—A general term referring to cardiorespiratory fitness and the ability to perform tasks of daily living.

glucose tolerance—The ability of the body to maintain the blood glucose level within the recommended range of <6.1 mmol $\cdot$ L^{-1} (fasting).

heart rate reserve (HRR)—A method to calculate recommended exercise heart rate based on the difference between maximum heart rate and resting heart rate.

leisure-time physical activity (LTPA)—A common measure of participation in physical activity in large studies, usually by self-report using physical activity diaries or other types of surveys.

maximum heart rate (HRmax)—The highest heart rate achieved during fatiguing exercise; can be estimated by 220 minus age, although there is considerable individual variation.

maximum oxygen uptake ($\dot{V}O_2max$)—Maximum capacity of the body to utilise oxygen during exercise; a good predictor, although not the best, of endurance exercise capacity; also known as aerobic power.

metabolic equivalent (MET)—A unit used to express the energy cost of physical activity, expressed as a multiple of resting metabolic rate; by definition, 1 MET = resting metabolic rate, or ~3.5 ml O$_2 \cdot$ kg$^{-1} \cdot$ min^{-1} (e.g., 10 METs = energy cost of 10 times resting metabolic rate).

mortality—An epidemiological term to quantify death rate.

population attributable risk (PAR)—An epidemiological measure of the proportion of a given health outcome attributable to a risk factor in the population; includes both relative risk and the prevalence of that risk among the population.

quality of life (QOL)—A psychological construct to assess an individual's perception of his or her position in life; it is multidimensional, including facets of physical, psychological and social health.

relative risk (RR)—An epidemiological measure of the strength of relationship between a risk factor (e.g., physical inactivity) and the risk of disease (e.g., cardiovascular disease).

resistance training—Exercise training designed to enhance at least one component of muscular fitness (e.g., muscular strength, power or endurance), often but not always involving weightlifting.

Student Activities and Study Questions

1. Access the most recent data on the relationship between physical activity, disease prevention and health. Compare these to the data provided in this chapter. Have there been any changes? If so, what reasons can you give for these changes? Make some predictions as to what future data may show.

2. Obtain printed material (e.g., brochures) on physical activity from health organisations (e.g., Heart Foundation, Cancer Fund, Diabetes Association). What type and level of exercise or physical activity do they recommend? How do they present information about physical activity? What are the reasons behind their recommendations regarding exercise or physical activity?

3. Read the previous ACSM guidelines for exercise (i.e., before 1998) for healthy adults. What changes in these recommendations have occurred over the years? What are the reasons for these changes?

4. Is it necessary to improve physical fitness to improve health and prevent disease? Or can physical activity prevent disease without changes in physical fitness? You will need to review the relevant literature to answer this question.

CHAPTER 3

Activating the Community

The previous chapter discussed the benefits of physical activity, its role in disease prevention and the recommended amounts of physical activity to achieve good health. Recent surveys indicate that the vast majority of Australians (as well as citizens in other countries) recognise the many health benefits of regular physical activity; in stark contrast, actual participation rates are remarkably low. This raises the obvious questions as to why, despite most recognising the need to be active, few put this knowledge into regular practice and, perhaps more important, what can be done to increase the proportion of the population that is sufficiently active to gain the many health benefits.

There is no doubt that modern industrialised society and its associated social and physical environments contribute to and possibly encourage an increasingly sedentary lifestyle. Work has become more sedentary, with fewer employed in occupations requiring physical labour. Entertainment and leisure pursuits, especially among the young, have also become more sedentary (e.g., computer games, television). The growth of large cities, with many people living in suburbs, has increased dependence on the automobile. At the same time, concerns about personal safety in the busy urban and suburban environment limit the attractiveness of outdoor recreation (especially for children) and reduce the use of walking or cycling as routine means of transportation to work, school and shops.

In recent years, especially since the 1996 release of the landmark U.S. Surgeon General's Report on Physical Activity and Health (discussed in the previous chapter), governments in Australia and throughout the world have developed policies and programs to try to increase participation in physical activity across the wider population. Because so much of the population is sedentary or insufficiently active, interventions at the population and community level are needed to have an impact on the nation's health. This chapter will first review the economic costs of physical inactivity in the context of disease prevention and then discuss some of the current concepts and programs aimed at increasing the number of active citizens.

Why Be Concerned With the Rate of Participation in Physical Activity?

Physical inactivity is a major health risk that contributes to the overall burden of death, disease and disability in most developed countries. Physical inactivity also takes an economic toll, costing billions of dollars each year. In most developed countries, health care costs are shared among the population, through government-supported medical care (as in Australia and many European countries) or through private and employer-sponsored health insurance (as in the United States and to a limited extent in Australia). Thus, the burden of the costs of disease and death attributed to physical inactivity is met by society as a whole.

Table 3.1 presents recent Australian data on the estimated costs of physical inactivity in Australia, as described in a report titled "The costs of illness attributable to physical inactivity in Australia: A preliminary study" (Stephenson et al. 2000). In estimating costs of physical inactivity (or any health risk or illness), three classifications are used:

▶ Direct costs—Costs of prevention, treatment and diagnosis of disease.

▶ Indirect costs—Costs associated with the value of human life or potential productivity (e.g., salary) lost through disease or premature death.

▶ Intangible costs—Social and personal costs to the individual and family who experience reduced quality of life as a result of illness, disability or premature death.

Direct costs are the easiest to measure since they are based on health and epidemiological data collected by government. Indirect and intangible costs are more difficult to estimate in dollar terms but are important to include in order to assess the full impact of disease and disability on society. All of these costs are important for identifying the relationship between lifestyle factors and disease, identifying the potential for disease prevention and health improvement through interventions such as physical activity, and directing policy development. For example, data show that physical inactivity is second only to tobacco use as a modifiable risk factor contributing to the total burden of disease (discussed in chapter 2). Successfully reducing physical inactivity could thus provide major benefits to the health and economy of the nation, justifying government efforts to increase participation in physical activity.

At What Levels Can We Promote Physical Activity?

As discussed in chapter 2, about only 60% of the Australian adult population is physically active on a regular basis. Approximately 40% of the population is therefore at risk of premature death and disease from insufficient physical activity; about 20% of the total population can be considered sedentary. The rates of inactivity are equivalent or even somewhat higher in other countries such as the United States and the United Kingdom. In Australia, participation rates either increased slightly or remained relatively constant from the 1980s to mid-1990s (depending on the particular survey). In contrast, recent Australian Institute of Health and Welfare (AIHW) data show that rates of participation de-

TABLE 3.1—Costs of Illness Attributable to Physical Inactivity

Disease/ condition	Position as cause of DALYs	Total direct costs[a], 1993-1994	Costs[a] attributable to physical inactivity (PAR of physical inactivity)
All-cause mortality	—	$31,397.0	$5,651.0 (18%)
CHD	1st	$894.0	$161.0 (18%)
Breast cancer	—	$183.9	$16.0 (9%)
Colon cancer	8th	$81.6	$15.7 (19%)
Stroke	2nd	$630.0	$101.0 (16%)
Type 2 diabetes	7th	$216.7	$27.5 (13%)
Depressive disorders	4th	$562.0	$56.2 (10%)

[a]In millions of dollars.

Abbreviations: DALYs = disability-adjusted life years, or the number of potential years of life lost because of premature death, poor health or disability; CHD is the most prevalent cause of DALYs (1st), colon cancer the 8th, and so on; PAR = population attributable risk (refer to chapter 2); CHD = coronary heart disease.

Data compiled from J. Stephenson, A. Bauman, T. Armstrong, B. Smith and B. Bellew 2000, "The costs of illness attributable to physical inactivity in Australia: A preliminary study," Commonwealth Department of Health and Aged Care and the Australian Sports Commission, Canberra. **www.dhac.gov.au/pubhlth/ publicat/document/phys_costofillness.pdf**.

clined from 1997 to 1999 across nearly all age groups (except for those over 65 years), especially among women. These decreases occurred despite high recognition by adults (>85%; Armstrong, Bauman and Davies 2000) of the importance of physical activity to good health. It appears that increasing the number of active adults is a complex problem requiring more than a single solution. Simply educating the public about the importance of physical activity is not enough to reverse the trend toward a sedentary lifestyle. Providing opportunities for people to maintain a physically active lifestyle requires a coordinated approach involving government, the health care system, non-government agencies, schools, businesses and the wider community. Although this concept is well accepted, there is presently not enough known to clearly identify the best ways to activate entire populations.

The following sections discuss recent thinking and research into effective interventions and programs to increase participation in physical activity, beginning with recent examples of national initiatives—the Healthy People 2000 and 2010 initiatives in the United States, Active Australia, and the Hillary Commission for Sport, Fitness and Leisure programs in New Zealand. It is important to note that they are representative examples only; it is not implied that these are the only initiatives. In addition, since each is an ongoing program, it is likely that changes may have occurred since the writing of this text (early 2002). Web sites are listed at the end of this chapter so that readers may access current information about these programs.

Healthy People 2000 and 2010 (United States)

Healthy People 2000 outlined a national strategy to improve the health of all Americans (U.S. Department of Health and Human Services [USDHHS] and Department of Education 2000). It listed various health objectives, including physical activity, to be achieved by the year 2000. Specific targets were set for various health issues such as mortality from cardiovascular disease, prevalence of obesity, and participation in physical activity.

Launched early in 2000, Healthy People 2010 builds on the previous initiative to provide future health objectives that "challenge individuals, communities and professionals to take specific steps to ensure that good health, as well as long life, are enjoyed by all" (USDHHS and Department of Education 2000). It emphasises the health benefits and disease prevention that can be achieved through

lifestyle improvements and proper preventive care; physical activity is identified as one of 10 leading health indicators. Healthy People 2010 encourages cooperation between the public, health care providers, government (national, state and local), schools, businesses and non-government organisations to develop and coordinate programs that support healthy and physically active lifestyles. Resources are provided to assist these groups, and prominent people are involved in community promotion.

Some of the physical activity objectives of Healthy People 2010 are to

- increase to at least 30% the proportion of people aged 6 and older who regularly participate in at least 30 min of light to moderate physical activity,
- decrease to no more than 15% the proportion of people who perform no leisure-time physical activity,
- increase to 40% the proportion of people performing regular muscular strength exercise,
- increase to 50% the proportion of overweight people adopting sound dietary practice in combination with physical activity,
- increase to 50% the proportion of school physical education class time spent in physical activity,
- increase the number of worksites offering physical activity programs, and
- increase to 50% the proportion of primary care physicians who counsel their patients to become physically active (Healthy People 2010 Web site).

Within each objective are special targets for specific segments of the population (by age, gender, ethnic/racial group, income level, and so on). For example, targets for adults include an objective to reduce to 20% the proportion of adults who engage in no leisure-time physical activity and to increase to 30% the proportion of adults who engage in vigorous activity (Healthy People 2010 Web site). Also included are targets for children and adolescents, such as the objectives to increase to 25% the proportion of middle schools providing daily physical education for all students and to increase to 85% the proportion of "adolescents who engage in vigorous physical activity that promotes cardiorespiratory fitness 3 or more days per week".

To achieve its physical activity objectives, Healthy People 2010 has developed specific programs aimed at such target groups as youth, the elderly and the general community. "Ready, Set, It's Everywhere You

Go" is aimed at promoting physical activity among adults. Resources are provided to assist in marketing, reaching target audiences, attracting media promotion, planning local events and lobbying local government. On-line resources also suggest ways for adults to incorporate physical activity into a busy life. "Promoting Lifelong Physical Activity" provides guidelines and recommendations to encourage young people to adopt and maintain a physically active lifestyle. Ten recommendations suggest ways that schools and community sports can encourage physical activity, for example, by involving the family, developing accessible facilities, providing adequate training for teachers and coaches, and changing physical education curriculum to emphasise enjoyable lifetime physical activity. For all of its programs, Healthy People 2010 advocates a partnership approach, discussed later in the chapter.

Active Australia

Active Australia was launched in December 1996 as a public health initiative ("national participation framework") to promote participation in regular moderate physical activity and sport across the population. The program involves both direct promotion of physical activity to the public and action through public policy to facilitate change. At the government level, it represents a partnership involving the Australian Sports Commission, the Commonwealth Department of Health and Family Services, the National Association of Local Government, and sport and recreation departments in all States and Territories. Since its launch, both national and state campaigns have been implemented.

Active Australia's vision is to have "all Australians actively involved in sport, community recreation, fitness, outdoor recreation, and other physical activities" (Sport and Recreation Ministers' Council 1997). There are three main goals:

▶ To increase and enhance lifelong participation
▶ To realise the social, health and economic benefits of participation
▶ To develop quality infrastructure, opportunities and services to support participation

Active Australia works through three networks—schools to provide the link with youth, clubs and organisations to provide the link with the community, and local government to enhance opportunities for and access to physical activity programs.

Monitoring participation rates is an important part of Active Australia, hence the 1997 and 1999 surveys of physical activity patterns mentioned earlier in this chapter and in the preceding chapter.

Active Australia provides key stakeholders with a national framework for actively supporting and influencing opportunities to participate in physical activity and sport. Key stakeholders are identified as government and non-government groups and commercial and non-profit agencies at the national, state and local levels. Active Australia does not offer activity programs as such; rather, it is a network that links direct providers, allowing local councils, schools, clubs and organisations to work closely with each other to meet the community's needs. It also offers resources, advice and assistance to its network of Active Australia providers. National initiatives include educational resources to assist physical activity providers, Active Australia Awards to support and recognise innovative program delivery, and Active Australia Day.

The Active Australia Local Government Network is a network of councils committed to supporting and promoting opportunities for physical activity and sport at the community level. Its aims are to encourage more people to become physically active and to "create better places for sport and physical activity in the local community".

The Active Australia Indigenous Sport Program (ISP) aims to improve Aboriginal and Torres Strait Islander participation in physical activity and sport. It is a national framework to provide opportunities for sport and recreation for indigenous groups in the context of community development. The ISP offers a variety of programs to foster youth sport development, a mentor scheme, cross-cultural awareness in sport, sports training and scholarships for indigenous athletes, and a national conference.

The Active Australia Schools Network is a national network of schools committed to supporting and promoting sport and physical activity that is "fun, safe, challenging, rewarding, well-managed, focused on learning, and linked to the community". The Schools Network program provides participating schools with a planning framework and assistance for enhancing delivery of physical activity programs, access to support and assistance for staff training, resources and materials designed to promote physical activity in the community, and links to other programs such as the local government network. Focus is placed on the "whole school" approach to physical activity, in which a broad range of activities are incorporated into a school's life.

Hillary Commission for Sport, Fitness and Leisure of New Zealand

After the 1996 U.S. Surgeon General's report on physical activity and health, the **Hillary Commission for Sport, Fitness and Leisure** was asked to form an intersectoral task force to develop strategies to increase physical activity participation in New Zealand. The task force first collected data describing participation rates in New Zealand (low, as in most developed countries) and possible health benefits to be realised from increased participation. Based on these findings, the National Health Commission recommended that physical activity is an important health concern for New Zealand and that government should play an active role in promoting moderate physical activity in conjunction with healthy eating and body weight maintenance.

In response, the Hillary Commission for Sport, Fitness and Leisure has initiated a variety of programs to promote physical activity throughout the community (Hillary Commission Web site 2002). "Push Play" promotes active lifestyles among adults. It provides on-line and print information to link individuals with local councils or groups providing physical activity services and events. Individuals can phone or e-mail an Active Living Coordinator to discuss physical activity. "Kiwi Walks" is a community-based walking program in conjunction with local authorities and regional sports trusts. It sponsors a series of free walks throughout New Zealand that are easily accessible, less than 60 min duration and suitable for most ages and fitness levels. Walking maps for specific areas can be accessed on-line.

"Green Prescription" encourages general practitioners to give patients written advice to be physically active as part of their health management. Resources and case studies are provided to GPs to help them prescribe physical activity for their patients. "Healthy Maori Lifestyles (He Oranga Poutama)" focuses on developing healthy lifestyles for Maori people through sport and physical leisure. Continuing a series of recreation and sport programs begun in the late 1980s, this program promotes physical activity through a holistic approach involving local Maori communities. Local community coordinators act as catalysts within their communities to create awareness and opportunities for active recreation. Programs include grants and funding for specific programs and scholarships for tertiary training in sport, physical education and recreation.

"Young People First" aims to ensure that an active lifestyle is developed early in life, and "KiwiSport" offers young children opportunities to develop skills in a wide variety of sports. "SportsMark" endorses school programs that have adopted best practice models for physical activity and sport. Many active leisure opportunities in sport and non-traditional activities (e.g., extreme sports) are offered through "Sportfit". Each program also offers a Maori dimension in an effort to ensure equity to access. The interactive *Hyperzine* on-line magazine offers creative information about sport and physical activity participation for young people. Many other programs encourage development of coaching and sport administration skills and women's participation in sport and physical activity.

Key Factors for Promoting Physical Activity at the Population Level

Changing the health behaviour of an entire population is a complex task requiring more than simply educating the public about the benefits of changing specific health behaviours such as physical activity. Unfortunately, there is general consensus among those working in the health field that it is too early to clearly identify the best approaches for promoting physical activity among the wider population. Although many programs have been attempted throughout the world, it takes years to fully evaluate the effectiveness of large-scale community programs and to identify what makes programs succeed or fail. There is agreement, however, that effective population-based promotion of physical activity requires cost-effective, multifaceted programs involving a variety of methods to educate the community and support behaviour change. Effective programs appear to emphasise low- to moderate-intensity activity, promote unsupervised activity (as opposed to structured programs), adopt a partnership approach involving various stakeholders in the community and provide local, easily accessible interventions within the community.

The U.S. Department of Health and Human Services (USDHHS et al. 1999) identifies five levels of social structure at which physical activity interventions may be targeted:

▶ Individual level: increase awareness, motivation and commitment; build skills and self-efficacy to change physical activity behaviour

▶ Interpersonal or group level: create or enhance social networks and support for physical activity in the community or workplace

▶ Institutional or organisational level: change organisational structures and develop policies to encourage physical activity

▶ Community level: address social norms and enhance community resources and inter-organisational communication and coordination; use mass media and regional planning to promote physical activity

▶ Societal or public policy level: enact policies, regulations, incentives and social reinforcement to encourage participation

It is generally agreed that, to be effective, future efforts must involve coordination at all of these levels if we are to significantly increase the proportion of people who are regularly physically active. The following sections discuss various methods to promote physical activity and particular needs that must be addressed.

Environmental and Policy Interventions

Our physical and social environments are important factors influencing the ability to maintain a physically active lifestyle. For example, perception of personal safety can be a major barrier to exercising within the community, such as walking within one's neighbourhood. Government policy and provision of recreational facilities may either hinder (e.g., lack of accessible and safe facilities) or enhance (e.g., providing cycle paths or recreation reserves; funding for community sport) participation in physical activity. The 1986 Ottawa Charter for Health Promotion defined five types of possible interventions to promote health across the population—public policy, supportive environments, community action, personal skills and involvement of health services. Of these, four (all but personal skills) can be directly influenced by environmental and policy approaches, usually involving some level of government (Sallis, Bauman and Pratt 1998).

According to the ecological model of human behaviour, environment may influence health behaviours such as physical activity (Sallis, Bauman and Pratt 1998; Sallis and Owen 1999). For example, the urban environment with busy roads may inhibit cycling as a means to incorporate physical activity into the daily routine; provision of bike paths may encourage more people to use cycling as a mode of physical activity. Poor weather or the perceived lack of safety on footpaths or in parks may discourage

the elderly from regular physical activity such as walking; recent initiatives to open indoor shopping malls for community walking programs address such concerns. Although any health behaviour reflects a complex interaction of many factors, environment and government policies can positively or negatively influence participation in physical activity. Based on the ecological model of human behaviour, Sallis, Bauman and Pratt (1998) propose four general guidelines for interventions to promote physical activity among the wider community:

▶ Health behaviour is determined by a complex interaction of many factors, so a combination of methods to promote physical activity is needed.

▶ Interventions must be specific to the setting. Some may involve removing impediments, such as lack of safety, whereas others may involve providing facilities where none existed previously.

▶ Environmental interventions may be needed before introducing other types of interventions, such as educational programs. For example, a program promoting walking would be unsuccessful if citizens do not have access to safe areas in which to walk.

▶ Educational and environmental interventions need to be specific to the setting and should be coordinated when possible. Some settings are suitable only for educational interventions, for example, information brochures in a doctor's office. On the other hand, some settings provide opportunity for both physical activity and educational interventions, as in a recreation centre, school or community centre.

In developed countries, the government exerts control over much of the environment and public policy through direction of resources for infrastructure (e.g., roads, cycle paths, parks), programs (e.g., community sports), education (e.g., funding for physical education and school sports), aged care, zoning regulations and town or regional planning. Because most governments in developed countries are elected, community support for environmental and policy interventions is important. Figure 3.1 lists some of the ways that environment and government policy may positively influence the ability to maintain a physically active lifestyle.

There are many possible ways to change environment and government policy to promote physical activity; some are expensive (e.g., infrastructure),

- ▶ Accessible and safe footpaths and cycle paths
- ▶ Coordinated and affordable public transport
- ▶ Funding for accessible infrastructure and programs, especially in underserved and low socio-economic areas
- ▶ Facilities appropriate to all ages (e.g., skateparks for the young) and climate (e.g., indoor facilities in extreme climates)
- ▶ Addressed issues of safety in public recreation space (e.g., adequate lighting)
- ▶ Zoning laws to require pedestrian access to shops and businesses and between neighbourhoods
- ▶ Building designs that provide access to open and safe stairs and signs encouraging their use
- ▶ Change rooms and showers at worksites
- ▶ Health insurance rebates for physical activity participation
- ▶ Reduction of taxes on physical-activity-related items (e.g., sports shoes, employer subsidy)
- ▶ Employer-sponsored programs or subsidised memberships to non-employer programs
- ▶ Use of media to promote participation
- ▶ Coordination between different levels of government (local, regional, state, national)

FIGURE 3.1 Environmental and policy factors that may positively influence physical activity.

whereas others can be effective yet cost relatively little. Signs to encourage the use of stairs rather than lifts or escalators at work is a simple, low-cost intervention that may increase stair usage (but only as long as the signs remain posted). Most current research in this area is limited by experimental design and lack of appropriate control groups (reviewed by Sallis, Bauman and Pratt 1998), but studies throughout the world suggest that providing accessible infrastructure appropriate to the community has a positive influence on participation in physical activity. For example, provision of accessible walking tracks in a low-income rural region of the United States (southeastern Missouri) was associated with increases in weekly walking time (Brownson et al. 2000). More important, access to the trails increased walking times in groups that generally show low participation rates, such as women, the elderly and those with low income. For the trail users, the most attractive aspects of the trails were scenic beauty, no cost, convenience, safety and lighting, indicating the importance of design and free access.

It should not be inferred, however, that the individual must remain passive and wait for government or large organisations to act; individual behaviour modifications and interventions to change the environment should complement each other (USDHHS et al. 1999). Community action initiated by citizens acting locally, regionally and nationally can be an important impetus for change. For ex-

ample, citizens can work with local government to alter traffic patterns to facilitate pedestrian access, use public facilities (e.g., schools, sports reserves) for community activity programs and develop community activity programs administered by volunteer workers (e.g., see National Heart Foundation's "Just Walk It" program described later in the chapter).

Partnership and Coordinated Action

Coordination between major stakeholders in the community is also essential to promote physical activity in the wider population and to lobby for changes in public policy and resources. One of the first programs to take this approach was the Canadian PARTICIPation program in the 1970s, which coordinated efforts by the public service, health professionals and private sector to raise awareness about the benefits of physical activity. Healthy People 2000 and 2010 in the United States and the recent Active Australia program involve coordination between national, state and local agencies (e.g., national and state departments of health, sport, recreation and education; local councils; and non-government groups such as sports clubs and the National Heart Foundation). Throughout the world, coalitions are forming between organisations with core interests in physical activity, environmental groups and urban and transport planners. In the United States, for example, these groups played an active role in enabling recent legislation to expand national and local transport policy beyond simple provision of roads to also include funding for integrated mass transport, pedestrian access and bicycle facilities. Decreasing reliance on the automobile not only increases physical activity but also contributes to a cleaner environment.

Role of the Family Physician

In Australia and many developed countries, the family medical practitioner plays a central role in health care delivery to the community and provides a vital source of health information. Advice from a family physician is one of the most influential factors in convincing an individual to change health behaviour. Several potential benefits of promoting physical activity through family medical practitioners include

- ▶ a high degree of public confidence in doctors,
- ▶ the strong influence of a doctor's advice on health behaviour,
- ▶ the placement of physical activity within the context of other health risks (e.g., control of blood pressure or diabetes), and
- ▶ the opportunity for long-term follow-up.

Recent research has focused on the effectiveness of promoting physical activity through the family physician. In the United States, the Physician-centered Assessment and Counseling for Exercise and Nutrition (PACE) program, based on the stages of change theory of behaviour change (refer to chapter 4), involved patients receiving from their physicians 3 to 5 min of exercise counselling, written materials and phone calls. Follow-up assessment showed a significant increase in physical activity (participation rates and minutes walked per week) in the intervention group compared with the control group (Long et al. 1996). In a recent Australian study, 763 formerly sedentary adults were given advice about physical activity by their family physicians (Bull and Jamrozik 1998). Counselling consisted of 2 to 3 min of verbal advice on exercise together with a pamphlet on exercise sent to the patient within 2 days. Physicians advised patients on the importance of regular activity and the recommended inclusion of moderate exercise and discussed any concerns, such as injuries. As determined by postal surveys and telephone interviews during the subsequent 12 months, the proportion of adults who were

"now active" and the amount of time spent exercising were significantly higher in the intervention group (given advice) compared with the control group (not given advice). In New South Wales, recent evaluation of a project titled "Active Practice", in which GPs gave written physical activity prescriptions to their patients, showed short-term improvements in physical activity when the prescription was supplemented with mailed booklets matched to the stage of change of individual patients (New South Wales Department of Health 1999).

As mentioned previously, the "Green Prescription" program in New Zealand encourages general practitioners to provide written advice on ways to become physically active as part of a patient's health management (Hillary Commission for Sport, Fitness and Leisure Web site). Over one-third of doctors are now providing physical activity advice to their patients, encouraged by a partnership between general practice groups and funding from the national health ministry.

While promoting physical activity in the primary health care setting may be effective, there are several barriers to its use. Time constraints in a standard consultation and lack of financial remuneration are two barriers identified by medical practitioners. In addition, few doctors receive formal training in exercise prescription, which may limit their ability to give more than general advice about appropriate exercise (i.e., to write an individualised exercise program that progresses over time). Supplementing doctor advice with additional resources, such as information booklets, enhances patient participation. Referral to an exercise scientist, or group health care practice that includes an exercise scientist, is becoming a viable alternative that involves the family physician but also meets the needs of patients requesting or needing more detailed advice and information.

Increasing Participation of Immigrants, Minority Groups, and Those of Non-English-Speaking Backgrounds

Participation in physical activity is not evenly distributed across the population but rather is strongly influenced by demographic variables such as age, sex, socio-economic status, education level, race, ethnicity and country of origin (Armstrong, Bauman and Davies 2000). In Australia, participation is higher in Australian-born individuals of European descent and lower in indigenous Australians, immigrants and those from non-English-speaking backgrounds. For example, participation in sufficient activity to benefit health is 22 to 27% lower in people whose main language spoken at home is not English (Armstrong, Bauman and Davies 2000). Participation is also directly correlated with education level and socio-economic status. Differences between races or ethnic groups in physical activity participation have also been noted in other developed countries, in particular the United States. In addition, conditions such as type 2 diabetes, cardiovascular disease and hypertension are more prevalent in some minority groups, for example, the higher incidence of hypertension among African Americans or the higher incidence of type 2 diabetes in Native Americans and Indigenous Australians. Decreasing the number of sedentary individuals among these populations may thus have a beneficial effect on disease rates.

The disparity in physical activity patterns between different racial or ethnic groups has prompted recent studies of efforts to enhance participation targeted at specific groups (for the United States, reviewed by Taylor, Baranowski and Young 1998). In Australia, one study focused on women of the Polish-Australian community in the Hunter Valley, one of the largest ethnic communities in this area (Brown and Lee 1994). A program of regular moderate exercise, mainly walking, and group discussion of relevant topics was developed and delivered through an existing social network within the community; some aspects were given in Polish to enhance comprehension. Follow-up assessment showed improvements in physical fitness and reductions in blood pressure and dietary fat consumption. As already mentioned, national strategies in Australia (Active Australia's Indigenous Sport Program) and New Zealand (the Hillary Commission's Healthy Maori Lifestyles) incorporate specific programs to enhance participation in physical activity among the indigenous communities.

Increasing Participation Among Women

Participation in physical activity is lower overall in women compared with men and in every age group except in the range 45 to 59 years where values are roughly equal; participation by women also declines with age (Armstrong, Bauman and Davies 2000). Overall, women are 20% less likely to participate in sufficient physical activity to benefit health compared with men. The proportion of individuals who are classified as sedentary or who perform insufficient activity is also higher in women (about 57%

for women and 53% for men). Although women are more likely to participate in walking as a form of activity, women have a much lower rate of participation in more vigorous activity, which is most likely to yield health benefits. Participation rates also declined to a greater extent between 1997 and 1999 in women than in men (7-10% and 4-6% declines, respectively, depending on the type of vigorous activity measured) (Armstrong, Bauman and Davies 2000).

There are many possible reasons for the lower participation rates of women than of men, and it is impossible to isolate any one factor. The largest drop in participation occurs in the age groups 18 to 29 and 30 to 44 years. These data likely reflect trends of women with children increasingly being employed outside of the home while still maintaining the role of primary care-giver for the family, the consequence of which is limited discretionary time for many things including physical activity. In addition, it is likely that current surveys fail to adequately measure the amount of physical activity involved in household duties undertaken by most women; thus, these surveys may be consistently underestimating the amount of physical activity performed by women.

Most recent national initiatives such as Active Australia incorporate strategies specifically designed to address the disparity in participation between men and women. In Australia, the National Policy on Women and Girls in Sport, Recreation and Physical Activity provides guidelines, case studies and strategies to "foster a culture that encourages and supports the full involvement of all women and girls in every aspect of sport, recreation and physical activity" (Australian Sports Commission 1999a, 1999b). Factors identified as influencing participation in physical activity by women include equity of access, programs and facilities; availability and accessibility of childcare services; culturally-appropriate programming; privacy; and safety.

Marketing and Promoting Physical Activity: Use of Mass Media and Information Technology

While individualised, face-to-face interventions may be ideal to promote physical activity behaviour change, it is simply impossible to have a major impact at the population level with this approach given the large number of inactive people and the cost of individualised programs. A more effective method is the use of mass media.

Various forms of mass media have been used for at least 20 years to promote physical activity, such as

- ▶ posters and brochures in relevant locations (e.g., educational materials in doctors' offices and shopping centres),
- ▶ direct mailing of physical activity information to a specified community,
- ▶ television and radio advertising (e.g., the "Life—Be In It" campaign in Australia in the 1980s),
- ▶ promotional community events (e.g., Heart Week, Active Australia Day), and
- ▶ promotion via telephone calls or via telephone information "hot lines" in association with promotion through other media such as television.

Follow-up research indicates high recall by the public associated with various campaigns; that is, a large proportion of the public (generally about 70%) remember the campaign and its message. For example, the National Heart Foundation of Australia initiated two mass media campaigns in 1990 and 1991 with the slogans "Exercise: Make It Part of Your Day" in the first campaign and "Exercise: Take Another Step" in the second campaign. Based on the social cognitive, social marketing and transtheoretical models (described later in this section and in further detail in chapter 4), these campaigns were designed to reach mainly inactive people. National promotion occurred through paid television advertising, public service announcements on radio, posters and other educational materials, publicity tours by experts, magazine articles and inclusion of physical activity themes in two national television drama shows. Local initiatives included promotional activity days and competitions. Follow-up interviews with a representative sample indicated high recall after each campaign and a significant increase in self-reported walking, especially among the elderly and least active, in the first campaign only (reviewed by Sallis and Owen 1999).

The ability of these campaigns to influence physical activity behaviour is not always consistent. Many studies show little impact of simple mass media campaigns, in the absence of supporting programs, on behaviour change. Clearly, then, more specific targeting and tailoring of mass media campaigns to specific groups, in conjunction with support from other directions, are needed to effectively promote physical activity at the population level.

To be effective, mass media promotion must be based on a sound theoretical framework. Psychological theories such as the social marketing model, the transtheoretical model and the social cognitive theory have been used recently to develop mass media campaigns to promote physical activity (Marcus et al. 1998). Health and physical activity promotion campaigns have used modified models originally developed to market and promote commercial products and services. Promotion of health or physical activity is marketed as any new or existing commercial product. These models can be briefly described in the context of physical activity promotion as follows (Marcus et al. 1998, 2000):

- ▶ **Social marketing model**—Social marketing is the application of marketing techniques to social and health issues in an attempt to change health behaviour of a particular group or groups of people. Programs should be tailored to reach particular target groups, taking into consideration that socio-demographic characteristics of these groups influence physical activity behaviour (e.g., physical activity is lower in groups with lower income and education level). Models of consumer behaviour are also used to develop promotional strategies.

- ▶ **Social cognitive theory**—Behaviour, such as physical activity, is strongly influenced by individual and environmental factors, and the ability to change depends on the individual's perception of his or her ability to control these factors and behaviour. Programs thus focus on facilitating individual behaviour change through techniques such as goal setting, social support and enhancing self-efficacy.

- ▶ **Transtheoretical (or stages of change) model**—Behaviour change is a process of five stages of motivational readiness to change. These stages range from precontemplation (inactive people not yet thinking about becoming active) to preparation (those preparing to become active) to maintenance (those who are able to remain physically active over the long term). Different interventions are targeted for people in different phases of change.

"Targeted" intervention strategies involve directing a program to promote physical activity at one or more particular groups, usually those with low participation rates (Marcus et al. 2000). Physical activity behaviour has been shown to increase with targeted strategies aimed at people in particular stages of motivational readiness. For example, Active Australia targeted older individuals through the "Rusty the Tin Man" media campaign in 1999, the Year of the Older Person. Because physical activity participation declines with age (discussed in the previous chapter), the campaign encouraged older Australians to improve health and well-being by maintaining a physically active lifestyle. At first, the tin man was rusty and squeaky, but through moderate physical activity he improved his "energy and get-up-and-go". It is thought that this campaign may explain why rates of physical activity participation were maintained between 1997 and 1999 in older people, while they declined in all younger age groups.

Targeted strategies assume that all individuals in a particular group may be influenced in a similar manner by a similar message. In contrast, "tailored" intervention strategies can be more specific by customising the message to become physically active to individuals within a targeted group. For example, interventions aimed at promoting physical activity among adults could be made more specific (tailored) by providing different information and support based on current physical fitness levels and activity patterns (active compared with inactive people) or health status (healthy people compared with those with disease or impairment). It is proposed that tailored interventions increase the likelihood that the receiver will pay attention to the message and initiate behaviour change.

Promotion of Physical Activity in the Workplace

Most adults and many adolescents are employed, often spending considerable time at some type of workplace. Thus, the workplace seems a logical location to reach a major part of the population with the health message about physical activity. Worksites can be considered communities with established communication networks and other organised structures and resources that can be effectively used to educate and support behaviour change.

Worksite health promotion and physical activity programs have been available for the past 20 to 30 years, especially in North America and, in fact, predate many national efforts to promote physical activity among the population. One of the goals of the U.S. Healthy People 2000 and 2010 objectives is to increase the number of worksites offering company-sponsored physical activity programs (USDHHS 2000).

Some of the benefits associated with worksite physical activity programs include

▶ enhanced corporate image and community relations;

▶ enhanced employee recruitment, satisfaction and retention;

▶ increased employee productivity and reduced absenteeism and disability;

▶ enhanced ability of employees to cope with stress and conflict at work; and

▶ reduced health care costs (USDHHS et al. 1999).

Ideally, promotion of health and physical activity in the worksite should result in healthier, more satisfied and more productive employees, which in turn enhances the company's viability and profits.

Support for worksite programs varies in different countries and is influenced by a variety of factors such as taxation laws, the local work culture, costs to the company, and the health care system. For example, in the United States, companies pay a substantial portion of private health insurance for their employees, and thus there is an incentive for employers to reduce health care costs through worksite health and physical activity programs. Differences in taxation laws among countries also influence the feasibility of offering such programs to employees, for example, whether the company receives any tax reduction or incurs a tax liability for providing such services to its employees. The perceived costs of initiating worksite programs may be unattractive to management. However, there are many options for providing these programs to employees, some of which may be very inexpensive to initiate and maintain. Data from the United States suggest that most programs are cost-effective; that is, the rate of return exceeds the initial investment. The fact that U.S. Healthy People 2000's target of increasing the number of worksites offering such programs was met well before the year 2000 indicates that worksite programs are not necessarily too expensive to maintain, at least in the United States.

Management support is essential to the success of a worksite program. Top management must not only fund the program, but managers at all levels must also be seen to be actively involved. Successful programs require management support to transform the corporate culture into one that values health and physical activity as a long-term investment. Sometimes environmental and policy changes are needed (e.g., selling healthy foods at the company cafeteria, allowing employees to use flexible schedules to fit physical activity into lunch breaks). Figure 3.2 lists some simple ways that companies can encourage their employees to become physically active.

Worksite physical activity programs have been criticised for attracting too few in the workforce (often less than 20%) and for serving those who are already active and fit (Dishman et al. 1998). In the past, many programs offered structured activities that do

---

POLICY SUPPORT OF PHYSICAL ACTIVITY

Use flexible work schedules to permit physical activity before or after work or during lunch breaks

Use flexible work schedules to permit employees to use public transport

Encourage management to actively support and participate in programs

Coordinate efforts to promote physical activity with other nearby businesses (e.g., sharing costs or facilities)

Send company teams to organised events such as Corporate Cup, fun runs

ENVIRONMENTAL SUPPORT OF PHYSICAL ACTIVITY

Provide showers and change rooms

Provide secure bicycle storage for employees who cycle to work

Provide suitable space for physical activity when feasible

Encourage use of stairs instead of lifts

COMMUNICATION SUPPORT OF PHYSICAL ACTIVITY

Encourage group activity during breaks (e.g., walking during lunch break)

Allow the use of company communication channels (e.g., e-mail, newsletters, meetings) to promote programs and educate employees

Encourage formation of committees to organise programs and special events

---

FIGURE 3.2   Strategies for employers to encourage physical activity among employees.

---

not attract the majority of workers (e.g., gym-based programs or high-intensity aerobics classes). More recent thinking about worksite programs centres on offering low-cost, moderate activity programs that incorporate lifestyle changes such as using the stairs, walking during breaks at work or bicycling to work. More structured programs may be helpful by allowing already active employees to gain additional benefits from vigorous exercise (e.g., gym-based programs) and by providing ongoing support in a social setting (e.g., aerobics classes or walking groups).

Home-Based and Lifestyle Interventions to Promote Physical Activity

Many people prefer to be active on their own or with a small group of friends in their local neighbourhood. Many find attending a structured program, for example, at a fitness centre, inconvenient and unattractive. Home-based activity is consistent with the recent recommendations for incorporating moderate-intensity activity, especially walking, into daily living. Many interventions have been tested to determine whether home-based promotion of physical activity is effective for increasing and supporting participation (reviewed by Sallis and Owen 1999). Such programs might start with a face-to-face meeting to introduce participants to the program, followed by mailed material or phone calls to provide additional educational information and ongoing support. Frequent (i.e., once per week or fortnight) phone call reminders from activity counsellors seem to be effective because they provide ongoing support while remaining convenient yet unobtrusive. Lifestyle physical activity, that is, incorporating regular moderate-intensity activity into one's lifestyle, has also been shown to be as effective as structured exercise sessions in terms of participation rates (reviewed by Dunn, Anderson and Makicic 1998; Sallis and Owen 1999). Promotion of home-based lifestyle physical activity through combined use of face-to-face meetings, ongoing support through frequent phone call reminders and mailed educational material thus appears to be an effective, low-cost strategy to enhance participation in physical activity across the wider population.

Promoting Physical Activity for Children and Youth

Children need to develop skills and attitudes that encourage a physically active lifestyle. Unfortunately, modern lifestyles often work against physical activity in children. Many factors contribute to this, including

- concerns for safety (e.g., children no longer walk to school),
- declines in physical activity programs within schools in some areas (e.g., less time for physical education; reduction in number of specialist physical education teachers),
- increased popularity of sedentary leisure-time pursuits (e.g., video games, television), and
- increased number of dual-income families with limited parent availability to transport children to programs.

Moreover, participation rates decline from primary to secondary school; once in high school, girls are less likely than boys to participate in general, especially in vigorous activity. School is central to a child's early development and, together with other groups in the local community, can be an important force in promoting physical activity in children and families.

In the past decade, a number of guidelines have been put forward in several countries focusing specifically on physical activity for children and youth. In the United States, the Healthy People 2010 objectives include specific goals for physical activity for children. Goals include increasing the number of children and youth participating in regular moderate and vigorous physical activity through school physical education and other programs and reducing the number of children and youth who are not regularly active (USDHHS 2000). There is also an effort to combine programs to promote physical activity with other lifestyle factors such as good nutrition. As described previously, both Active Australia and the New Zealand Hillary Commission initiatives incorporate specific programs to encourage participation in physical activity by children in schools and in community sports.

The U.S. Centers for Disease Control and Prevention published strategies to promote physical activity among children and youth (Sallis and Owen 1999; USDHHS and Department of Education 2000). These recommendations suggest that

- policies and environments should focus on promoting and encouraging safe, physically active lifestyles;
- physical and health education policies and programs should be consistent with the desire to promote physical activity; and
- the combined efforts of parents, educators, other trained personnel, health care providers and community groups is needed.

School-based physical activity through physical education classes and other programs can provide many of the skills young people will need to maintain a physically active lifestyle through adulthood. Physical education has many objectives in addition to health-related goals, including developing social, cognitive, motor and sports skills. It may be difficult to incorporate all of these aspects into a single physical education curriculum given the financial and time constraints. However, intervention studies in primary schools show that changes in curriculum and teacher training may positively influence children's physical activity patterns (reviewed by Sallis and Owen 1999). Employment of specialist physical education teachers and ongoing education and support of classroom teachers with regard to physical activity have been shown to increase physical activity in children. Health-related physical education programs that focus on lifetime skills, that can also be performed outside of school, that are noncompetitive and that children find enjoyable also seem to be effective for promoting physical activity among children and youth.

Promoting physical activity among children does not have to be limited to formal physical education classes. There is much that schools can do to incorporate physical activity into other aspects of the curriculum and to involve family members and community groups as well (see figure 3.3). For example, walking tours of local historic sites can be incorporated into history/cultural studies lessons; biology classes can include active collection of specimens for study. Most excursions can be designed to require walking, and all of these activities may also include parental participation.

Although most children are exposed to physical education at school, the majority of physical activity occurs outside of school. Studies of physical activity patterns in children show a strong correlation between time spent outdoors and physical activity (reviewed by Sallis, Bauman and Pratt 1998), suggesting that simply getting children outdoors may increase participation rates. There are, however,

▶ Include daily physical activity in the curriculum

▶ Train older children to act as activity leaders for younger children

▶ Develop links with local sports clubs (e.g., invite coaches to offer sports skill clinics during lunch)

▶ Offer single-sex classes, especially for high school girls

▶ Focus on active recreation rather than just on sport

▶ Offer non-traditional activities such as in-line skating, aerobics, dance and beach volleyball

▶ Offer motor skill and physical activity training for classroom teachers

▶ Encourage teachers to guide children in active use of playground equipment and other facilities

▶ Involve parents in physical activity programs

Not all initiatives need to be adopted in a single school.

Compiled from Australian Council for Health, Physical Education and Recreation, 2000, *Active Australia Children and Youth Schools Network*. Hindmarsh, SA: ACHPER.

FIGURE 3.3   Examples of successful school initiatives to increase participation in physical activity.

many obstacles to a physically active lifestyle in the built environment of many urban, suburban and rural communities, and some of these are especially discouraging to children and youth. Lack of safe pedestrian access or bike paths means that children are dependent on parents to drive them to many leisure activities, even their own sporting events. In rural Australia, children may spend hours each day travelling to and from school seated in a bus. One recent encouraging trend in Australia is the provision of local neighbourhood parks that incorporate facilities for active play by children and youth, such as playground equipment for younger children and skateboard parks or BMX bike tracks for teenagers.

Compared with adults, children and youth are attracted to and motivated by different forms of physical activity. Children are motivated more by fun and social interactions and less by the perceived need to improve fitness or health through physical activity. In children, predictors of physical activity include self-efficacy, social norms about activity, beliefs about physical activity outcomes and involvement in community programs (Trost et al. 1999). Effective programs for children and youth need to focus on enjoyment and social interactions, facilitate skill development and social support, and remove real and perceived barriers such as lack of transport and funds. In addition, research suggests the most effective programs are those that aim to reduce time spent in sedentary leisure pursuits while increasing the opportunity for lifestyle physical activity, such as cycling or walking (Sallis, Bauman and Pratt 1998).

Case Study 3.1

It is the summer holidays. Ben is 13. His parents both work and are concerned about how he will spend his holidays. He usually spends them with a few friends, indoors watching videos, playing video or computer games and eating junk food. While not a top athlete, he does not mind being active but feels he needs a break from organised sport in which he participates during the school year.

What would you recommend to Ben and his parents?

(*Note*: You should solve this case study in the context of this chapter, that is, using a community rather than an individual approach to promoting physical activity.)

Key Issues

1. What do you think might be Ben's parents' concerns and goals?

2. Where will you seek the information Ben needs to do something different this holiday? What organisations might be helpful? What programs are currently available for young people in your city/town?

3. What local infrastructure exists in your city/town to accommodate the interests of Ben and his friends?

4. What barriers to participation might Ben encounter? What solutions can you offer?

5. What factors do you think will be positive influences on Ben's participation in local programs?

What Makes Effective Promotion of Physical Activity in the Community?

Many national and international efforts to promote physical activity at the population level have begun since the 1996 U.S. Surgeon General's report on physical activity and health. Because long-term studies of participation rates and evaluation of particular programs require considerable time, it is still too early to clearly identify what works and what does not. However, it is generally believed that several common features are required to successfully change physical activity patterns across the wider community:

▶ Political and government endorsement at the national level

▶ Shared responsibility across governmental and non-governmental organisations

▶ Leadership of national government and organisations in providing a framework for collaboration between different groups

▶ Adequate resources, environment and strategies consistent with the message of encouraging moderate physical activity as part of daily life

▶ Focus on the entire population with targeting of specific groups with low participation rates

▶ Ongoing evaluation of the effectiveness of various strategies and programs (USDHHS et al. 1999; National Health Committee of New Zealand 1998)

Many groups should be involved in the planning, development, delivery and evaluation of promotional strategies, including (but not limited to) national, state and local government; regional planners; scientists and professionals with particular expertise (e.g., exercise, behavioural and social scientists and health care practitioners); providers of sport and recreation services (e.g., fitness centres, sports clubs); local business and community groups; and other social services such as libraries, social services organisations, aged care centres and places of worship. The key is for all of these groups to work together in a coordinated manner to remove barriers and give all citizens the ability to maintain a physically active lifestyle.

Evaluation is an ongoing process of asking meaningful questions and collecting relevant data to be used at all stages of program planning, delivery and modification. Because there can be diverse needs and interests and many stakeholders, evaluation is an essential function of community-based programs to promote physical activity. In fact, evaluation is critical for determining the effectiveness of a program—including the success of marketing and dissemination strategies, program delivery, program satisfaction, outcomes such as participation or changes in health, and cost-effectiveness. An ongoing process, evaluation uses feedback and data to monitor progress and continually refine the program. It is essential to plan the evaluation process from the onset along with other aspects of the program so that the most appropriate indicators to measure during the program can be chosen. For example, a community walking program that does not collect ongoing data on client satisfaction and concerns would not be able to determine the causes of a lower-than-expected participation rate.

On a simple level, the process of evaluating community-based programs can be categorised into five steps (USDHHS et al. 1999):

▶ Defining expectations

▶ Deciding what to evaluate

▶ Selecting evaluation measures

▶ Collecting and analysing data

▶ Collating and reporting results

Defining expectations includes deciding on the goals and objectives, vision, time line and desired outcomes (i.e., what the program hopes to achieve). The specifics of program delivery (e.g., education campaign, activity classes, special events) and partner involvement must be identified at this point. Planners must also decide on measurable objectives (for determining if the goals and objectives have been achieved). The evaluation process, which involves collecting quantitative and qualitative data on which to base decisions about program effectiveness and any needed modifications, can be broken down into three steps—process, impact and outcome evaluation (see table 3.2).

Process evaluation involves keeping track of what is happening in the program on a regular basis, allowing the planners to determine and control whether the program is being implemented as originally planned. Impact evaluation gathers information about the short- to medium-term effects of the program, such as changes in client attitudes about physical activity, fitness levels or participation rates. Outcome evaluation collects information about the long-term effects of the program, such as changes in health status, disease risk, morbidity or mortality, and long-term trends in participation rates. This

---

TABLE 3.2—Evaluating and Monitoring Community Physical Activity Programs

Steps	Purpose	Examples of questions to ask
Process evaluation	Ongoing review of program Identify effective aspects Identify changes needed Make changes while program is running	Is program running as planned? Who is participating? Are targets being met? Should any changes be made now? Are partnerships effective? Have barriers been encountered?
Impact evaluation	Compare data with objectives Determine short-term effects Measure extent of change(s) in target group	What has been accomplished? Were objectives achieved? Did target group's attitudes or behaviour change? What differences did the program make to target group? Are participants healthier? What aspects of program worked well? What aspects didn't work? What should be changed?
Outcome evaluation	Identify long-term and permanent changes Compare outcomes with objectives Determine if there is a long-term impact on health behaviour	Has the program influenced policy? Have effective partnerships been established? Are people healthier? More active? Have disease risk factors changed? How expensive and cost-effective was the program?

Compiled from USDHHS et al., 1999, *Promoting physical activity: A guide for community action.* (Champaign, IL: Human Kinetics), 152-155.

---

information can be compared with the outcome objectives (e.g., to increase participation, to decrease the prevalence of risk factors) to help determine the program's effectiveness. Many of these measures are complex and costly to assess, and outcome evaluation may not always be undertaken.

Evaluation measures are indicators that assess over time the program's specific goals and objectives. For example, if an objective is to increase the proportion of a community's children that is active in sport or physical activity, specific data must be collected on how many children live in the community, their participation rates before and at different times during the program, the types of activities in which they participate and the children's perceptions of the program. Reporting the results of evaluation is important because it shares the data and outcomes with stakeholders, especially those who funded the program (e.g., government, local business). This may take the form of written or oral reports, press releases or news conferences, presentations to various stakeholders, or educational materials.

Like evaluation, data analysis and report writing should also be ongoing processes. Efficient community programs can quickly incorporate client satisfaction and effectiveness to change programs as needed. For example, a program with declining attendance should be able to quickly identify responsible factors (e.g., conflicts with other events, program not addressing the clients' needs) and make adjustments to reverse the trend or else face a likely outcome of not achieving the program's objectives and expectations. It is far better to make corrections while the program is running than to wait until the end of what has become an unsuccessful program. Ultimately, a program's success and effectiveness rely on timely feedback at each step of the decision-making process to ensure consistency between program planning, goals, delivery and outcomes.

Examples of Programs to Promote Physical Activity to the Wider Community in Australia

In recent years, there has been a tremendous effort to promote physical activity on the local, regional, state and national levels in Australia and overseas; the Active Australia campaign was described briefly in a previous section of this chapter. It is beyond the scope of this book to provide a comprehensive description of all these efforts, but it is instructive to present a representative sampling of these programs to illustrate the creative approaches taken to promote physical activity. It is important to note that many of these programs have not been thoroughly evaluated because of time or budgetary constraints, so it is difficult at this point to draw firm conclusions as to the effectiveness of one particular approach over another. This section is provided simply to illustrate to students (and other interested readers) the variety of approaches that have been taken throughout Australia. Although this section focuses on recent programs up to the time of writing (early 2002), by the time you, the reader, read this section, some of these programs may have changed dramatically, may have ceased or may have been replaced by other types of programs.

Promoting Walking As a Form of Physical Activity Throughout a State

Queensland has a lower rate of participation in physical activity than other States, in particular, walking as a leisure-time activity. The National Heart Foundation (Queensland Division) developed "Just Walk It" (JWI) to increase the community's participation in physical activity by encouraging individuals to walk together in small groups within their neighbourhoods. The program works with local community organisations, such as local government and community health centres, to tailor an appropriate walking program for its residents. Within a neighbourhood, volunteer organisers develop local walking paths and lead small groups on regular group walks (usually three times per week). These organisers are recruited and supported by local co-ordinators and a local committee of stakeholders, which in turn liaise directly with the Heart Foundation's State JWI coordinator and staff. The program is free of charge.

Promoting Physical Activity Among the Elderly

In recognition of the International Year of the Older Person (1999), the city of Melville, West Australia, established the "Older People, Active Living" project to promote heart health through physical activity and education. "Active at 50" incorporates circuit weight training, aquatic exercise and walking components with education about health, fitness, exercise and heart health. Highly commended as an outstanding physical activity project by the National Heart Foundation's Local Government Awards in 1999, this program served as a model for other local governments to establish similar programs.

The "Be Active, Stay Strong" project operated by the Warringah Council, NSW, offered a series of special events to encourage physical activity and healthy lifestyles among the elderly. Physical activity components introduced participants to gentle resistance training, circuit training, aquatic exercise, walking and tai chi. Eighty percent of participants committed to continue their participation in physical activity.

Case Study 3.2

Margaret is a 65-year-old pensioner in good health who has recently moved to your city/town. She moved after the sale of her family's large rural property to be near her married daughter and her family. She wants to meet people her age and to remain physically active. She is not familiar with the new area in which she lives (your city/town). She does not drive but lives near access to public transport.

continued

continued

As a regional health promotion officer in your city/town, you are asked to provide some ideas to help meet Margaret's goals.

Key Issues

1. What are Margaret's main goals?
2. Where will you seek the information Margaret needs to get started? What organisations might be helpful? What programs are currently available for people like Margaret?
3. What local infrastructure exists in your city/town to accommodate her interests?
4. What barriers to participation might Margaret encounter? What solutions can you offer?
5. What factors do you think will be positive influences on Margaret's participation in local programs?

Promoting Physical Activity Among Ethnic Girls and Women

In Victoria, the Dandenong Oasis Leisure Centre modified its programs and facilities to encourage African and Asian Muslim women to participate in physical activity. It first established what barriers limited access to physical activity among these women and then developed programs to address these barriers. For example, in some Muslim societies, women must not be seen unveiled by adult men, so a curtain was installed over parts of the pool so the girls and women could swim in privacy (Australian Sports Commission 1999a). The centre has also developed programs to encourage participation by other ethnic groups in the area. The Dandenong Leisure Centre won the 1998 Active Australia Innovation Award for these programs.

Promoting Sports Participation Among Girls

The city council of Whittlesea, Victoria, determined that two major barriers limited girls' participation in sport—the girls felt their sports skills were inadequate, and they were unfamiliar with role models in the community. As a partner in the Active Australia Local Government Network, the city council used its links with other Active Australia partners to develop a working party. A two-part approach was initiated to address these barriers. First, girls-only school clinics were developed in non-traditional sports such as cricket, golf, futsal, Australian Rules football, table tennis and bocce; these games were chosen because the girls were unlikely to have encountered these sports before and because there were strong local clubs. Girls who developed interest in one or more of these sports were then linked with

the relevant sports club(s), which offered these girls weekend clinics to further advance their skills.

Wilderness Programs for At-Risk Young People

Recent evidence suggests that physically active recreation and sport have potential for crime prevention, especially in at-risk youth (Cameron and MacDougall 2000). Appropriate sport and activity programs can reduce crime by providing accessible, alternative activities in a supportive social context. "Operation Flinders" in South Australia provides "wilderness therapy" for young men and women who have either breached the law or are at risk of doing so. The objective of the program is to develop character and a sense of accomplishment, trust and cooperation through experience in a wilderness setting. Throughout Australia, wilderness and cultural trail camps for Aboriginal youth show that appropriate sport programs can decrease crime and delinquency in rural and remote communities. An Adelaide-based service for homeless youth provides team sports and physical activity programs with the aim of offering support networks and providing these youth with a sense of belonging (Cameron and MacDougall 2000).

Local Government Initiatives to Develop Infrastructure to Support Physical Activity

The Maroochy Shire Council, Queensland, developed an innovative strategy called "Get on your bike!" to encourage cycling as a form of physical activity. After community consultation, the council integrated its pedestrian and cycle paths, producing an on- and off-road bikeway network within the shire. A pamphlet identifies the cycle paths, provides information on local cycle clubs and gives safety tips; this strategy is now integrated into the shire planning scheme. This project won a 1999 National Heart Foundation Local Government Award for outstanding policy for structural change.

The Frank McEllister Community Park in Alice Springs encourages active recreation by providing playground equipment, open grassed areas, tables and seating, a fitness trail and a concrete path. The park is used by a variety of people, including people with disabilities, for diverse activities such as cycling, in-line skating and walking/jogging. Developed by the town council after community consultation, the project included a 5-year plan, and there are plans for future development. This project won a 1998 Local Government Award from the National Heart Foundation.

"TravelSmart" is an innovative initiative by the WA Department of Transport aimed at preserving the environment and enhancing quality of life by reducing reliance on automobile travel (Western Australia Department of Transport 2000). The approach educates and motivates people to use alternatives such as walking, cycling, public transport and car pooling. In partnership with local business, government and community groups, "TravelSmart" offers advice and information to raise awareness of how simple behavioural changes can positively influence health and the environment. Evaluation of a pilot program showed 14% less car travel, 16% more walking, 91% more cycling and 21% increased use of public transport; these changes in travel behaviour were sustained for at least 2 years.

Case Study 3.3

As a regional health promotion officer, you have been asked by the State Department of Health to help a rural town establish a community physical activity program. The town has a population of 10,000, is located >250 km from a large city and is the regional centre serving the adjoining rural areas. Compared with state or national averages, income is below average, and the incidence of heart disease and health risks such as obesity, hypertension and type 2 diabetes are above average. Infrastructure includes three primary schools and one high school, a public pool, tennis courts and soccer/football fields. The regional public hospital is located in the town.

Outline the different approaches you would take to establish a community physical activity program under three different sets of conditions, as follows:

a. Minimal funding for the program (a part-time project officer for 12 h per week plus the costs of photocopying and phone calls)
b. Moderate funding for the program (a full-time project officer plus the cost of modest equipment [up to $3,000 per year])
c. High level of funding for the program (a full-time project officer plus funds for infrastructure and equipment, subject to approval by the state government)

Key Issues

1. How will you identify and involve the major stakeholders in such a program? Who do you think will be the major stakeholders?
2. What steps will you take to obtain additional funding in conditions (a) and (b)?
3. How will you determine the program's goals, objectives and mission?
4. How will you staff a program in conditions (a) and (b)?
5. What type of infrastructure and equipment might be appropriate in condition (c)? How will you determine this?
6. How will you evaluate the program?

Summary

Most people in developed countries recognise the benefits of regular physical activity, yet as many as half of the population is insufficiently active to derive these health benefits. Since the landmark 1996 U.S. Surgeon General's Report on Physical Activity and Health, many developed countries have initiated national, regional and community programs to widely promote physical activity in the hope of having a positive impact on preventable disease. Many approaches have been used, although it is still too early to conclusively define the best ways to activate entire communities. Among the current, most relevant programs to students of exercise management are Active Australia, programs initiated by the Hillary Commission for Sport, Fitness and Leisure in New Zealand, and the U.S. Healthy People 2010 physical activity initiatives. Each of these programs aims to develop coordinated approaches involving partnerships with major stakeholders in the community. There is much that governments can do, both locally and nationally, to promote physical activity, including providing policy, strategies and infrastructure consistent with the message to maintain a physically active lifestyle. Other approaches include promoting physical activity in daily living and transport; using advances in communications technology and mass media, such as the Internet; tailoring programs for particular segments of society; urging general practitioners to include advice on physical activity in health care settings; and linking schools and community sports to promote physical activity among children and families. The challenge is to provide a coordinated approach that removes access barriers and enhances opportunities for all citizens to enjoy a physically active lifestyle.

Selected Glossary Terms

evaluation—A process to collect and analyse important information to guide decision making; in the exercise context can be applied to development of programs for individuals, groups, communities or organisations.

Healthy People 2000, 2010—A national strategy by the U.S. Department of Health and Human Services to improve the health of all Americans by encouraging cooperation between all government and non-government stakeholders to develop programs that support healthy lifestyles.

Hillary Commission for Sport, Fitness and Leisure—The government body that supports sport and active living in New Zealand by creating opportunities for its residents to be physically active through sport and other means.

social cognitive theory—A theory that a behaviour, such as physical activity, is strongly influenced by individual and environmental factors, and the ability to change depends on the individual's perception of his or her ability to control these factors and behaviour.

social marketing model—The application of business marketing techniques to social and health issues in an attempt to change health behaviour of a particular group or groups of people.

transtheoretical (or stages of change) model—A model theorising that behaviour change is a process of five stages based on the individual's motivational readiness to change. These stages range from precontemplation (not yet thinking about changing health behaviour) through to maintenance (maintaining long-term changes in health behaviour).

Student Activities and Study Questions

1. Find out details on recent mass media campaigns to promote physical activity in your community (if possible, at various levels—local, regional, state or national). These details should include which media were used for the campaign (e.g., television, print, brochures); the time frame and purpose of the campaign; which group(s) initiated and promoted the campaign; and success rates, if known. If you can, obtain materials (e.g., videotape of advertisements, brochures, posters) from these campaigns and evaluate them in terms of the theoretical models on which they are based, the target groups and other aspects.

2. Try to attend a community event that might be associated with promotional campaigns. Observe who organises these events (e.g., non-profit organisations, government, health care providers) and what roles they take. Who participates in these events (e.g., patients, the general public, doctors, entertainers) and what roles do these people take? What are the primary messages being conveyed? How successful do you think the event is? Why?

3. Find and attend at least two community-based physical activity programs. (Programs run through commercial or corporate fitness centres are generally not considered community based). Who organises and administers these programs? How much input is through volunteer participation? Identify yourself and talk with participants to find out what they think about the programs.

4. Find out which local, state or national non-governmental organisations promote physical activity (there are foundations specific to heart disease, such as the Heart Foundation, and other conditions such as asthma, arthritis and diabetes). Obtain some of their information brochures. Who are their target groups? What are their recommendations regarding physical activity? Is there a consistent message about physical activity across these diverse groups?

5. Observe whether physical activity is promoted in your local area and, if so, how? (Start with shopping centres, doctors' surgeries, schools, sports clubs and entertainment centres.) How could current promotional materials be improved?

Web Sites of National Organisations Promoting Community-Level Physical Activity Interventions

Organisation	Web site address
Active Australia	www.activeaustralia.org
Healthy People 2010 (United States)	http://web.health.gov/healthypeople
Hillary Commission for Sport, Fitness and Leisure (New Zealand)	www.sparc.org.nz

PRINCIPLES OF PHYSICAL ACTIVITY SCREENING, ASSESSMENT AND PRESCRIPTION

The previous section discussed the profession of exercise management, health benefits and recommended amounts of physical activity, and efforts to promote physical activity across the population. We now turn our attention to methods of translating these recommendations into practical means by which most people can achieve a physically active lifestyle. The general term for this is *exercise prescription and programming* or, in keeping with the recent recommendations, *physical activity prescription and programming*.

As noted in the previous section, the current recommendations are very broad and are intended as a public health message aimed at the general population. For many, these broad recommendations will suffice—that is, some people are content to enjoy regular brisk walking and activities of daily living that incorporate physical activity. On the other hand, others will want more specific guidance, sometimes individualised to their particular interests, needs and abilities. It is possible that, of the many people who are not regularly physically active, the lack of knowledge about particulars of *how* to be physically active is a deterrent to some.

Physical activity prescription encompasses a process beginning with health risk screening (to ensure safety), physical fitness assessment (when appropriate), and development and delivery of the activity program (the prescription and programming part). Underpinning each of these steps is the need to include strategies to promote adoption and ensure long-term compliance (adherence). These are interrelated processes; for any given individual, health risks identified in screening will influence the choice of fitness assessment, type of exercise prescription and strategies to enhance compliance. The process is also ongoing in that people's needs, interests and health status change over time. Thus, program evaluation and modification are essential parts of the process of physical activity prescription. Physical activity prescription is an integral part—indeed, the basis—of the profession of exercise management. The skills needed to effectively develop and deliver physical activity programs, whether for individuals, groups or entire communities, form a unique part of professional development in the exercise sciences.

This section discusses the basic process of physical activity prescription and programming, including the different aspects mentioned above, for healthy adults—those without disease or impairment that may influence their ability to be physically active. The next section (section 3) then extends these principles to exercise prescription across the lifespan and for individuals with disease or impairment. Regardless of the client for whom physical activity prescription is developed or the form it may take, the hallmark of an effective prescription is that it is based on sound scientific evidence and rationale.

CHAPTER 4

Encouraging Physical Activity and Facilitating Behaviour Change

The benefits of regular physical activity are known and accepted by many within society, but only a small percentage of adults participate in regular physical activity, and the percentage of children participating in regular physical activity is decreasing. The 1999 Physical Activity Survey (Armstrong, Bauman and Davies 2000) reported that almost 90% of Australian adults believed increasing physical activity would improve health; however, 15% were classified as inactive and less than 50% were sufficiently active to gain the health benefits of regular activity (accumulating at least 30 min on at least 5 days each week). There is a large discrepancy between the number of adults who know there are many health benefits of physical activity and the number who put this knowledge into action (i.e., are regularly active). For many, to become active requires a complete change in lifestyle, that is, a change in behaviour. Changing behaviour is a complex process, and many factors influence whether or not an individual is likely to change behaviour and then sustain that change. So, why do some people change behaviour and begin a regular activity program while others do not? Moreover, why do some who adopt a new behaviour continue while others stop? Research has attempted to answer these questions with the intention of developing methods of understanding **behaviour change.** An understanding of behaviour change, factors that support behaviour change and factors that inhibit behaviour change provides a framework to guide the development of **interventions** to help people adopt and maintain a new behaviour.

Health psychologists have provided insight into theories that address behaviour change and the interventions that may accelerate change. Some of these theories have been specifically examined in the context of physical activity. Because behaviour change is so complex, no single theory fully explains activity **adoption,** drop-out and maintenance. Theories and models used to understand why people are or are not active are aimed at the individual, interpersonal or environmental level. The social cognitive theory and theories of **reasoned action** and **planned behaviour** have been used to explain adoption and maintenance of physical activity.

The theories of reasoned action and planned behaviour explain intention to participate as the immediate determinant of action; the theory of planned behaviour also cites that perceived control influences action. Social cognitive theory explains that participation in physical activity will be supported or hindered by a combination of environmental factors (e.g., access, safety, time) and personal attitudes and beliefs (e.g., experience, knowledge, skills). The transtheoretical model of stages of change applies multiple theories of behaviour change and provides identification of actual behaviour in addition to intention to change behaviour. The transtheoretical model is a stage-based approach that identifies different phases of readiness and participation. These theories and model can be used as frameworks to explain behaviour change and guide the development of intervention strategies to increase participation in physical activity. Environmental models explain participation in physical activity through socio-cultural and environmental influences.

Given that less than one-half of adults are regularly active, one of the greatest challenges is to help accelerate behaviour change at the individual, group and environmental level. A key role of the exercise scientist is to assist with the adoption of physical activity and then to promote **adherence** to the new or revised program. Most textbooks examine the technical aspects of physical activity screening, assessment and prescription before addressing the importance of behaviour change concepts. Because of the continued high rates of physical inactivity and the positive benefits associated with implementation of behaviour change strategies, we think it is important to focus first on concepts relating to behaviour change and then use these concepts to underpin the more technical aspects of physical activity programming. This chapter provides an overview of factors associated with participation and adherence, barriers to participation, various psychological theories on understanding behaviour change, and interventions that may maximise participation in physical activity. Reflection on, and incorporation of, these concepts is integral for enhancing the effectiveness of screening, assessment and prescription.

Physical Activity Participation and Adherence

Identifying factors associated with both inactivity and participation in physical activity allows inactive groups to be identified and targeted. Many demographic and psychosocial factors differ between active and inactive individuals. Generally, inactive individuals tend to be less educated, older, blue-collar workers and smokers; they also have lower **self-efficacy,** lower socio-economic status and a negative decisional-balance (negative consequences of participating outweigh the positive). Some of these factors are modifiable (e.g., smoking, self-efficacy) and others cannot be changed (e.g., age). Intervention strategies can be designed to help change modifiable factors or to alter the environment to make physical activity more attractive to inactive groups.

Individual perceptions of enjoyment and satisfaction, health status, ability to perform the selected activity, access and time availability all contribute to whether or not an individual participates in physical activity. Participation can also be influenced by environmental factors such as weather, program flexibility, convenience, and support cues and prompts (e.g., active role models, accessible parks and walking paths). Past experience may provide a positive or negative influence on participation. If past experience was painless and enjoyable, the client is much more likely to readily adopt physical activity; if past experience was painful and boring, it may be more challenging to help the client adopt a recommended program.

After adoption of a physical activity program, approximately 50% of participants drop out within the first 3 to 6 months. Helping clients sustain physical activity is obviously a challenge. Once again, it is useful to identify reasons why some people adhere to physical activity and remain active while others begin activity and then drop out. Although some of the personal attributes for non-adherers are similar to non-participants (blue-collar worker, lower level of education, age), it appears that some environmental and program-based factors for maintaining activity are different from factors associated with adoption. Individuals are more likely to stick with a program if they have social support for participation, the program is fun, varied and of low-intensity, and it includes strategies to help with behaviour change (goal setting, relapse prevention, stimulus control).

Barriers to Participation

Both participants and non-participants have reasons for not exercising. However, participants have developed strategies to overcome or minimise these reasons, or barriers. Barriers can be real (e.g., injury) or perceived (e.g., exercise is too strenuous). Once barriers are identified, strategies can be developed to target the problem; these strategies, or interventions, create an easier path to exercise.

One real barrier to participation for most in Western cultures is the increasing interest in sedentary hobbies. Work hours are becoming longer, and people are welcoming hobbies that require less energy. Continued technological advances have resulted in the design of more efficient devices and services; this success in technology has made it easier to be sedentary. For example, the attractiveness of computer-based children's games creates competition for keeping children active. It has become increasingly challenging to help people overcome barriers to participation. Web-based services have enhanced the efficiency of some tasks, thereby reducing the need to be active. Until recently, for example, most people carried out supermarket shopping at the supermarket. This required transportation to the shop (walking, cycling or driving and then parking the car and walking) and then walking through the supermarket. This service is now offered via the World Wide Web, which certainly enhances efficiency but reduces regular physical activity. On the other hand, the enhanced efficiency of these services should result in more time for active leisure pursuits. Services developed and promoted on the World Wide Web to help increase physical activity may reach individuals with sedentary hobbies who have historically been difficult to reach with messages about physical activity. Research is needed to determine if Web-based promotions of physical activity increase activity in the population.

Real or perceived lack of time is the most frequently cited barrier to participation in regular physical activity. Work, family and social commitments all influence time availability and may be perceived as time constraints. Individualised, flexible prescriptions that address time availability and constraints will help clients incorporate physical activity into the weekly schedule. For some clients, a structured prescription with set days and times may be most effective, whereas others may require a prescription that is flexible in duration and frequency. Innovative prescriptions that encourage families, partners and friends to be active together may also increase participation. Finally, promoting the accumulation of several short bouts of activity may make physical activity goals more achievable.

Clients also cite numerous other barriers to participation, both real and perceived. Within distinct groups, such as older adults, barriers appear to be similar. For example, older people may not participate because of ill health, perceived risk of injury, perceptions of safety or problems associated with social isolation. Barriers for participation in the 18 to 39 age group include childcare responsibilities and lack of time and motivation. Specific interventions aimed at barriers for specific groups have been successful in increasing physical activity within the targeted group.

Consideration of the theories that explain behaviour change, and not just the factors associated with activity and inactivity, helps researchers understand reasons for, and barriers to, participation and evaluate changes in behaviour resulting from an intervention. Dishman and Buckworth (1996) performed a meta-analysis of interventions used to increase physical activity in sedentary adults. The results showed that interventions based solely on targeting a specific factor associated with inactivity were less successful than interventions that utilised behaviour modification techniques. For example, worksite fitness centres that target the barriers of lack of time and inconvenient facilities have had limited success in reaching inactive employees. Programs incorporating models of behaviour change such as targeting inactive employees with simple educational messages and helping them identify reasons for, and barriers to, participation have been more successful. Hence, current research recommendations suggest the inclusion of interventions derived from a theoretical framework and designed to accelerate behaviour change.

Theoretical Models of Behaviour Change

Psychological theories and models that explain behaviour change help provide a framework for understanding the processes involved in the adoption and maintenance of physical activity. Intervention strategies can then be designed to target these processes and accelerate activity adoption and maintenance. Put simply, theories are used to understand and guide the development of interventions. There are several theories that explain behaviour change, and the exercise scientist must evaluate each situation and choose one or more that appropriately assist the given population. It is not essential that only one theoretical framework be used to understand behaviour change. Brawley (1993) suggests that for a theory to be practical and applicable, it must posses the following six characteristics:

1. A focus on processes that are changeable
2. A description of the links between key factors so that these can be the targets of change
3. Associated and accurate assessment measures of these factors, links and change

4. Shown validity

5. Concepts translatable to interventions believed to affect cognitive or behaviour change

6. A framework for conceptualising why an intervention failed to produce change

The theories of reasoned action and planned behaviour, social cognitive theory, and the transtheoretical model of stages of change meet these six suggested characteristics and have all been used as frameworks to address adoption and maintenance of physical activity.

Theories of Reasoned Action and Planned Behaviour

The theory of reasoned action maintains that an individual's intention to change behaviour is the immediate determinant of behaviour. This intention is driven both by the individual's attitude toward the behaviour and by **social norms.** Attitude toward a certain behaviour results from self-evaluation of positive or negative performance of that behaviour; that is, an individual is more likely to have a positive attitude about a behaviour, such as physical activity, if he or she performs that activity well. Social norms are the individual's perception of social pressures to perform or not perform the behaviour. The importance of both of these traits is dependent on the individual and the behaviour in question and is therefore different for each situation

To explain physical inactivity, the theory of reasoned action assumes that individuals do not believe that participation in physical activity will produce the needed benefits or that individuals perceive that significant others do not wish them to participate. For example, a client is referred to a personal trainer by her general practitioner because she is overweight. She repeatedly fails to keep appointments. It is subsequently discovered that she played sports and was very active as a child and adolescent but remained overweight, so she believes that exercise will not help her lose weight. Thus, this client's attitude toward participation is negative, which explains her drop-out. Several studies have shown that intention to exercise does not account for all exercise behaviour; and it may not be a linear, one-way link from initiation to actual behaviour. Therefore, to fully explain exercise behaviour, reconfiguration of the model may be necessary.

The theory of planned behaviour is an extension of the theory of reasoned action. An additional factor, control, is believed to influence intention as well as attitude toward behaviour and subjective norm. Perceived control accounts for non-volitional internal and external factors that may influence behaviour; an individual is less likely to perform a behaviour if he perceives a lack of control over specific internal and external factors. Internal factors, such as skill, ability and knowledge, and external factors, such as time, availability and dependence on others, may influence exercise intention. Hence, if an individual perceives he has access to resources and opportunities to be active and encounters few obstacles, he is more likely to intend to become physically active. Although there is little research to support this model in explaining exercise behaviour, it does takes into account perceived barriers to exercise.

Social Cognitive Theory and Self-Efficacy

To explain behaviour change, social cognitive theory emphasises the interaction of environmental factors with personal attitudes and beliefs. Participation in physical activity can be helped or hindered by the environment and by beliefs that participation will result in selected goals. These beliefs are based on knowledge, skills and past experience. Individual belief in ability to participate, or self-efficacy, is one dimension of the social-cognitive theory.

Self-efficacy is an individual's confidence in his or her ability to perform a specific behaviour. It is proposed that individuals with high levels of self-efficacy attempt and persevere at more difficult tasks and apply more effort to each task. For example, a client would be considered to have high self-efficacy if she believed that she would continue to walk (physical activity program) during holidays and during rainy weather. Individual self-efficacy is influenced by four types of experiences:

1. Enactive experience (e.g., established experience): successful previous accomplishments

2. Vicarious experience: observation of others performing successfully

3. Verbal persuasion: the influence of others through verbal communication

4. Physiological states: the influence of periods of stress

Consequently, self-efficacy is dynamic and increases or decreases as a result of these experiences.

It has been suggested that for behaviour change to occur, an individual must strongly believe that he or she can engage in, and persevere with, the new behaviour. Specific to the physical activity setting, it is presumed that an individual will be unlikely to adopt physical activity if he does not believe in his ability to perform the activity prescribed. That is, the client may know what to do and how to do it, yet, if self-efficacy is low, he may not put this knowledge into action. **Outcome expectancy**, or the belief that goals will be attained through participation, is also an important construct shaping attitudes and beliefs. For example, a client states a desire to participate in physical activity, and a regular solo walking program is prescribed. The client walks one night and feels tired and lonely; as a result, the next night he does not walk (outcome expectancy). The client does not believe he can perform the activity and hence has a low level of self-efficacy toward walking; he is unlikely to continue his walking program. On the other hand, if self-efficacy toward an activity is high, continued participation in that activity is more likely. Self-efficacy and outcome expectancy influence the decision to attempt and sustain a behaviour change.

Numerous tools have been developed and validated to measure individual self-efficacy related to physical activity. Some of these tools measure exercise-specific self-efficacy, and other tools measure a more general confidence in physical skills. Exercise-specific tools assess confidence in performing a spe-

cific activity (e.g., walking) in increasingly difficult situations (e.g., increased length of time). The more general physical tools address confidence in overall physical ability (e.g., strength, agility, speed).

Exercise-specific self-efficacy has been measured and validated using an eight-item questionnaire (see figure 4.1) (McAuley, Talbot and Martinez 1999). The eight items measure confidence in performing increasingly difficult tasks (walk for 5 min to walk for 40 min). A 100-point scale in 10-point increments is used to rate confidence in performing the tasks, with 0% representing no confidence at all and 100% representing complete confidence. The sum of the confidence ratings is divided by the total number of items on the scale to calculate the total strength of self-efficacy. Scores range from 0 to 100, with 100 representing the highest level of self-efficacy.

Ryckman and colleagues (1982) developed and validated a more general physical self-efficacy scale. Responses to 22 items are given on a 6-point Likert scale, with 1 representing strongly agree and 6, strongly disagree (see figure 4.2). Eleven items are scored in reverse and all responses are added to yield a score from 22 to 132, with higher scores reflective of higher self-efficacy.

For each of the following amounts of time, please choose a number from the following scale to indicate your level of self-confidence. Your choices are:

0%	10	20	30	40	50	60	70	80	90	100%

No confidence   Complete confidence

I can walk for:

1. 5 minutes _____%
2. 10 minutes _____%
3. 15 minutes _____%
4. 20 minutes _____%
5. 25 minutes _____%
6. 30 minutes _____%
7. 35 minutes _____%
8. 40 minutes _____%

Responses are given using a 100-point scale in 10-point increments. The sum of all responses is calculated and divided by 8 to yield the self-efficacy score.

Adapted, by permission, from E. McAuley, H. Talbot and S. Martinez, 1999, "Manipulating self-efficacy in the exercise environment in women: Influences on affective responses," *Health Psychology* 18 (3): 288-294.

FIGURE 4.1   Sample eight-item questionnaire to assess exercise-specific self-efficacy.

Please circle the most appropriate response for each of the following questions. Your choices are:

1	2	3	4	5	6
Strongly agree	Agree	Somewhat agree	Somewhat disagree	Disagree	Strongly disagree

®1.   I have excellent reflexes.   1 2 3 4 5 6

2.   I am not agile and graceful.   1 2 3 4 5 6

®3.   I am rarely embarrassed by my voice.   1 2 3 4 5 6

®4.   My physique is rather strong.   1 2 3 4 5 6

5.   Sometimes I don't hold up well under stress.   1 2 3 4 5 6

6.   I can't run fast.   1 2 3 4 5 6

7.   I have physical defects that sometimes bother me.   1 2 3 4 5 6

8.   I don't feel in control when I take tests involving physical dexterity.   1 2 3 4 5 6

®9.   I am never intimidated by the thought of a sexual encounter.   1 2 3 4 5 6

10.   People think negative things about me because of my posture.   1 2 3 4 5 6

®11.   I am not hesitant about disagreeing with people bigger than me.   1 2 3 4 5 6

12.   I have poor muscle tone.   1 2 3 4 5 6

13.   I take little pride in my ability in sports.   1 2 3 4 5 6

®14.   Athletic people usually do not receive more attention than me.   1 2 3 4 5 6

15.   I am sometimes envious of those better looking than myself.   1 2 3 4 5 6

16.   Sometimes my laugh embarrasses me.   1 2 3 4 5 6

®17.   I am not concerned with the impression my physique makes on others.   1 2 3 4 5 6

18.   Sometimes I feel uncomfortable shaking hands because my hands are   1 2 3 4 5 6
      clammy.

®19.   My speed has helped me out of tight spots.   1 2 3 4 5 6

®20.   I find I am not accident prone.   1 2 3 4 5 6

®21.   I have a strong grip.   1 2 3 4 5 6

®22.   Because of my agility, I have been able to do things that many others   1 2 3 4 5 6
      could not do.

Responses are given using a six-point Likert scale, with items marked ® scored in reverse. The sum of all responses yields the self-efficacy score.

Adapted, by permission, from R. Ryckman, M. Robbins, B. Thornton and P. Cantrell, 1982, "Development and validation of a physical self-efficacy scale," *Journal of Personality and Social Psychology* 42 (5): 891-900.

FIGURE 4.2   Sample 22-item questionnaire to assess general physical self-efficacy.

Individuals who respond that they do not feel confident exercising in certain situations have a low self-efficacy and are less likely to adopt a new physical activity regime. These individuals can be targeted with specific interventions designed to increase their self-efficacy. Alternatively, individuals with a high level of self-efficacy are likely to attempt a behaviour change, and strategies to help them maintain high self-efficacy may help them maintain the adopted change. Both exercise-specific self-efficacy and gen-eral physical self-efficacy have been shown to increase with participation in physical activity and to be susceptible to manipulation. It may therefore be possible to structure the environment and implement strategies to enhance individual self-efficacy. An example is the attempt to attract a larger percentage of the population to physical activity by recommending the accumulation of 30 min of physical activity daily. Special skills are not needed, and the goal can be achieved simply by increasing nor-

Case Study 4.1

Claire, a 72-year-old healthy woman, decided to join a walking program at the local shopping mall with a friend. Part of the pre-participation questionnaire included a self-efficacy questionnaire. Claire scored 51 (out of a possible 100) on the exercise-specific self-efficacy scale. Given her level of self-efficacy, recommend an initial walking program for Claire.

Key Issues

1. What does Claire's self-efficacy score imply about her likelihood to adopt physical activity?
2. What strategies (e.g., programming) may help maximise adoption?
3. Is it expected that Claire's self-efficacy score would change? How?

mal everyday activities. The result may be an increase in individual self-efficacy for some people.

Adoption may also be enhanced by encouraging clients to choose their own physical activity. Client selection provides individuals with a sense of self-prescription, which may increase self-efficacy. Giving the client options such as climbing the stairs at work, walking the shopping centre at lunch, exercising in the morning before work and organising active vacations may reduce the barriers to participation. If a client feels able to achieve these recommendations, self-efficacy may be increased. Finally, providing clear instructions and opportunities for skill development, in addition to modelling the desired behaviour, may also help increase self-efficacy. For example, a previously inactive female who received a gift membership to a commercial fitness centre may be hesitant to join. Inviting her to have one-on-one instruction with a female exercise scientist before joining a low-intensity females-only class may help raise self-efficacy and increase the likelihood of attendance.

Transtheoretical Model of Stages of Change

The transtheoretical model of stages of change, which explains change as a process that involves a series of stages, is an extension of the social cognitive theory. This model identifies actual behaviour as well as intention to change behaviour (i.e., readiness). Identification of readiness to change behaviour and initiation of that change allow targeted prescriptions to be made. Prochaska and DiClemente (1983) were the first to propose a stages of change model to describe behaviour change. They suggested that an individual progresses through five distinct stages during the behaviour change process, culminating in maintenance of the new behaviour:

1. **Precontemplation:** no intention to change behaviour
2. **Contemplation:** thinking about changing
3. **Preparation:** beginning to change
4. **Action:** actively changing behaviour
5. **Maintenance:** sustaining change

Originally, this model was developed to explain changes in addictive behaviours such as tobacco smoking, but recently it has also been used to explain adoption and maintenance of physical activity. This model suggests that people use different **processes of change** to move from one stage to another, hence an individual may need a number of processes to attain the final stage of behaviour maintenance. Specific processes of change have been associated with specific stages within this model. Identification of these processes has initiated the development of specific intervention strategies that target each specific stage. For progression to occur, it is essential to match an intervention with an individual's stage of change.

An individual or community must be both physically and psychologically ready to begin a physical activity regime, or attempts to implement a physical activity program may be futile. The concept of determining an individual's readiness for activity emerged after the identification of demographic and psychosocial factors that differed between active and inactive individuals. The stages of change model evaluates readiness before challenging a client to change a behaviour. Addressing an individual's readiness to adopt a physical activity regime and implementing appropriate intervention strategies may assist the adoption process.

Stages of Change

The five-stage continuum, specific to the physical activity setting, appears as follows:

1. **Precontemplation:** no intention of beginning a physical activity regime
2. **Contemplation:** thinking about beginning a physical activity regime but still inactive
3. **Preparation:** beginning a physical activity regime although participation is irregular
4. **Action:** actively participating in regular physical activity although involvement has been for less than 6 months
5. **Maintenance:** regular participation for greater than 6 months

Progression through the stages is not always linear, and individuals progress at varying rates. Relapses may occur, and several attempts may be needed before an individual progresses to the next stage. This model is best viewed in cyclical format (see figure 4.3).

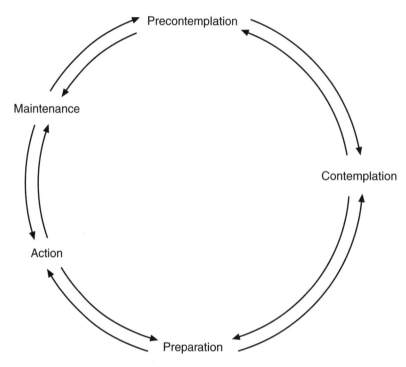

FIGURE 4.3   Stages of change model.

Case Study 4.2

In April, David, 45 years, was prescribed a walking program four times per week by an exercise scientist referred to by his GP. David maintained the walking program in the mornings for 10 weeks. However, due to darkness in the early morning and rain during June, he found early morning walking difficult and stopped, although he continues to think about walking weekly. Recommend a program to help him return to regular walking.

Key Issues

1. What stages of change has David cycled through?
2. How have environmental changes altered David's participation in physical activity? How can these "unchangeable" issues be addressed?
3. What strategies would you recommend to help David reach a maintenance stage?

Individual stage of change can be identified from a response to a single question (see figure 4.4). Clients select the statement that most accurately describes their current physical activity status; a number of studies have shown this response to be both a valid and reliable measure of exercise-related stage of change. Regular exercise has been defined as participating in at least three sessions per week, each for at least 20 min. Of concern is whether or not this question retains reliability and validity when assessed as an accumulation of at least 30 min of daily physical activity. It must be determined whether this model can also be applied to the more recent recommendations for physical activity.

Progression through the stages, stability within a specific stage and regression to a previous stage result from activities an individual uses in an attempt to change behaviour. These activities are considered processes of change.

Processes of Change

Processes of change are cognitive, affective and behavioural activities that may help an individual change behaviour. Table 4.1 defines 10 processes

---

How do you feel about your current level of physical activity? Regular physical activity is defined as at least 3 sessions per week, each for at least 20 minutes.

1	I do not intend to start.
2	I am thinking of starting.
3	I have started some activity but not regularly.
4	I have been regularly active for less than 6 months.
5	I have been regularly active for at least 6 months.

Adapted, by permission, from B. Marcus, C. Eaton, J. Rossi and L. Harlow, 1994, "Self-efficacy, decision-making, and stages of change: An integrative model of physical activity," *Journal of Applied Social Psychology* 24 (6): 493.

FIGURE 4.4   Sample question to identify stage of change.

TABLE 4.1—Processes of Change

Process	Definition
Consciousness raising	Trying to increase information and understanding about oneself and the problem
Self-reevaluation	Assessing feelings about oneself with respect to the problem
Dramatic relief	Experiencing and expressing feelings about the behaviour problem and its solutions
Environmental reevaluation	Assessing how the behaviour problem affects physical and social environments
Social liberation	Increasing awareness and access to alternatives for non-problem behaviours available in society
Self-liberation	Choosing and committing to act and believing in ability to change
Counterconditioning	Substituting alternatives for problem behaviours
Stimulus control	Controlling stimuli that elicit problem behaviours
Reinforcement management	Rewarding changes or being rewarded by others for making changes
Helping relationships	Accepting and trusting the support of important others during behaviour change

Adapted, by permission, from B. Marcus, S. Banspach, R. Lefebvre, J. Rossi, R. Carleton and D. Abrams, 1992, "Using the stages of change model to increase the adoption of physical activity among community participants," *American Journal of Health Promotion* 6 (6): 425.

that were selected from a variety of different theories to explain actions used to change behaviour, hence the term *transtheoretical*. There are two categories of processes of change, the experiential and the behavioural. Experiential processes appear to be more important for individuals in the early stages of change and include consciousness raising (I should get some information about exercise), self-reevaluation (maybe I can exercise after all), dramatic relief (physical inactivity may be endangering my health), environmental reevaluation (others may also be healthier if I exercise) and social liberation (more and more people are encouraging me to exercise). Behavioural processes are more important for individuals in later stages and include self-liberation (I will make time for exercise), counterconditioning (I exercise to help relieve stress when I feel anxious), stimulus control (I intentionally place reminders to exercise around my house), reinforcement management (I'll reward myself when I exercise more) and helping relationships (my friends support me when I exercise).

Individuals in the action and maintenance stages tend to use these processes the most, while precontemplators tend to use these processes significantly less. Adopters, or those moving positively through the stages of change, increase their use of these processes, whereas those relapsing to previous stages reduce their use of processes.

The identification of specific processes has led to the development of specific interventions that match each stage of change (see table 4.2). These interventions help accelerate progression through the stages. For example, in a community-wide study designed to target individuals in contemplation, preparation or action, specific resource manuals were designed for each of these three stages (Marcus, Banspach Lefebvre et al. 1992). Contemplators were mailed a document titled *What's in it for you?* that focused on increasing lifestyle physical activity (environmental reevaluation), learning to reward oneself for increasing activity (reinforcement management) and considering the personal and social costs and benefits of

---

TABLE 4.2—Examples of Interventions Based on Processes of Change and Matched to a Specific Stage of Change

Stage	Intervention	Process
Precontemplation	Simple education	Consciousness raising
	Medical practitioner support	Dramatic relief
Contemplation	Description of benefits	Self-reevaluation
	Choice	Environmental reevaluation
	Decision-balance sheet	Self-liberation
Preparation	Goal setting	Self-liberation
	Contract/reward	Reinforcement management
	Verbal praise	Helping relationships
Action	Goal setting	
	Environmental cues (shoes, time, buddy system)	Stimulus control
	Relapse prevention	Counterconditioning
Maintenance	Relapse prevention	
	Generalised training	Self-liberation

participation (consciousness raising). A document titled *Ready for action* was mailed to participants in the preparation stage; this document focused on costs and benefits (consciousness raising), setting short- and long-term goals (self-liberation), time management (stimulus control), rewards (reinforcement management) and program self-development (self-liberation). Participants in the action stage were mailed the *Keeping it going* document, which focused on troubleshooting situations (consciousness raising), goal setting, rewards, cross-training (self-liberation) and finding exercise partners (helping relationships). Over 60% of participants in each stage showed progression to the next stage (e.g., contemplation to preparation, preparation to action) or higher stages (e.g., contemplation to action) after the 6-week intervention. Thus, targeting specific stages with process-oriented interventions may expedite the progression to behaviour change.

Of particular concern is reaching individuals in precontemplation. Precontemplators are unlikely to read educational material pertaining to physical activity or to contact individuals or groups who may facilitate adoption of physical activity. Progression to contemplation and action stages often occurs after a health scare, for example, a myocardial event. In these cases, individuals rely on the medical profession for advice and direction. Clearly, innovative strategies are needed to attract precontemplators to physical activity and to assist with their progression to contemplation and action. One useful strategy may be to elicit support from the medical profession to target apparently healthy individuals. Liaison with a general practitioner plus follow-up from both an exercise scientist and the general practitioner may be one strategy to encourage adoption of activity by inactive groups.

Projects in the United States and Australia have studied physician-directed physical activity counselling. Bull and Jamrozik (1998) reported increased physical activity in sedentary patients after verbal advice from a family physician; patients were also given a written pamphlet on physical activity. Physicians in this study participated in a 30- to 60-min training program on physical activity counselling, behaviour change and barriers to regular exercise. Approximately 33% of patients in the intervention group (verbal advice + pamphlet) were active at 1 and 6 months compared to only 20% of controls (usual care, no specific ad-

vice). At 12 months, a similar percentage of patients from each group were active. These results confirm that physician-directed counselling may help initiate participation by sedentary individuals. In contrast to most studies, which report a 50% drop-out within the first 6 months, participation rates were still high at 6 months. This increased maintenance may be due to the recommendations for physical activity. The physicians in this study followed current recommendations and counselled clients to participate in moderate-intensity leisure activities in unsupervised settings.

The PACE (Patient-centered Assessment and Counseling for Exercise and Nutrition) program was a similar project based in the United States using the stages of change model. Sedentary patients were again the target, and participation in physical activity was increased after a brief counselling session (3-5 min), a stage-matched written pamphlet and a 10-min booster call (Long et al. 1996). Continued research is refining these strategies to encourage participation in physical activity and enhance activity adherence. Projects such as "Active Script" in Australia have attempted to refine the process by providing a prescription pad for physicians to recommend physical activity. Research is needed to determine if these types of strategies help individuals identified as irregularly active increase their daily activity to meet current recommendations (refer to chapter 2) and if these strategies help individuals maintain regular activity. Additional interventions have been designed to target individuals classified in other stages.

Interventions

Interventions are tools designed to facilitate adoption and maintenance of regular physical activity. The development and refinement of some of these tools have resulted from an understanding of the theories of behaviour change. These interventions can be tailored to the individual, group or environmental level; community-based interventions (targeting groups and the environment) such as Active Australia were discussed in chapter 3. The present section will concentrate on interventions aimed at the individual.

Recent research suggests that, to accelerate behaviour change, interventions must be based on theory but applied practically. It would be expected that multiple interventions targeted at specific stages of behaviour change would be most successful. The intervention strategies presented in table 4.2 are shown in relationship to a specific stage and process of change. These interventions and others have shown increases in short-term physical activity but limited increases over the long term. Interventions may help accelerate the behaviour change process and progression through the stages.

For those in precontemplation, the processes of dramatic relief and consciousness raising may help accelerate change. Strategies that may be implemented include enlisting medical practitioner support and providing simple education that debunks myths and clarifies reasons for, and barriers to, participation.

Individuals in contemplation may benefit from self-reevaluation and environmental reevaluation. Helping the individual choose the type of activity in which to participate, providing role models, intro-

ducing a decision-balance sheet (see figure 4.5) and emphasising benefits may help progression to preparation. The decision-balance sheet helps clients consider the negative and positive effects of regular participation in physical activity. This process helps the individual evaluate reasons for participating and begin to assess strategies to overcome potential barriers to participation.

Preparation is a stage in the behaviour change process where many interventions may help the client adopt regular physical activity. Recommendations for a slow and gradual increase in participation, verbal reinforcement, contracts and rewards may help the client become a regular participant. A sample contract is presented in figure 4.6. Specific goals should be targeted within a specified time frame; a self-selected reward is attained on achievement of the goal. This type of **extrinsic** reinforcement may be beneficial before the recognition of **intrinsic** rewards. Initially, most participants enjoy

---

Consider the positive and negative aspects of beginning or changing your physical activity program by completing all parts of the following table. An example is given for each part.

Gains to self	Losses to self
1. *lose weight*	1. *less time for other hobbies*
2.	2.
3.	3.
Gains to important others	Losses to important others
1. *more energy to play with kids*	1. *less time for lunch with friends*
2.	2.
3.	3.
Approval of others	Disapproval of others
1. *my family would like to see me more active*	1. *less time for overtime*
2.	2.
3.	3.
Self-approval	Self-disapproval
1. *feel better about myself*	1. *feel self-conscious*
2.	2.
3.	3.

Responses are given for advantages and disadvantages in each of the four categories: self, important others, approval of others and self-approval.

FIGURE 4.5   Sample decision-balance sheet with an example for each category.

James, a 28-year-old carpenter, visited a personal trainer for a swimming and cycling program. The personal trainer identified stage of change with all clients and encouraged clients to complete a decision-balance sheet. James circled "3", or preparation, on the stages of change questionnaire (figure 4.4). He was given a decision-balance sheet and stated that positive aspects of participating would include increased fitness, improved strength, and greater energy, while the negative aspects of participating would include less time for paid overtime, less time with family, missing lunch break with work mates, being tired or sore for work, and the pool entrance fee. Suggest a weekly exercise program for James.

Key Issues

1. What processes of change may be important for James?
2. How can these processes be targeted with specific interventions?
3. How can the information gained from the decision-balance sheet help in the development of a weekly exercise program?

CENTRE FOR PHYSICAL ACTIVITY & SPORT EDUCATION

School of Human Movement Studies–The University of Queensland

HEALTH CHALLENGE

Participant Contract for Physical Activity

I, *Joe Smith*, agree to comply with the following three goals from *12 June* to *12 August*.

GOALS

Goal #1: walk the dog for 30 minutes 5 days each week (Monday to Friday)

Goal #2: cut down my evening glasses of wine to one glass of wine and to not drink any alcohol on at least 2 days each week

Goal #3: swim for 25 minutes each Saturday

REWARDS

With successful adherence to these goals, I will purchase a 'fitball'.

Signed: Date:

Witness:

FIGURE 4.6   Sample contract for participation in physical activity.

exercise for extrinsic reasons (e.g., social interaction, rewards). To maximise program maintenance, it is important to help the client begin to recognise intrinsic factors (e.g., feel better, more energy).

Goal setting may also be beneficial for individuals in the action stage. Recognition of intrinsic rewards may begin at this point, so extrinsic rewards may no longer be necessary. Individuals have many varied reasons for participating in physical activity; common goals often include increasing fitness, improving health, losing/maintaining weight, increasing strength, changing appearance, reducing stress and increasing energy levels. An individual client may have many other goals, such as socialising or spending time alone. To be effective, goals must be

▶ clearly defined,
▶ specific,
▶ within a specified time frame,
▶ set with manageable strategies, and
▶ realistic.

Goals need to be clear and achievable rather than vague ("I would like to lift 20-kg boxes at work"

rather than "I would like to be stronger"). Goals with specific numerical targets are more likely to enhance motivation ("I would like to lose 5 kg" rather than "I would like to lose weight"). In addition, time frames for goals should be date specific ("from 23 March to 20 June") rather than vague ("for the next 2 months"). Each specific goal must have a targeted strategy to achieve the goal ("I will walk 45 min 6 days per week at an RPE of 12-13 for 4 weeks from 10 June to 8 July"). It is the role of the exercise scientist to help guide the client in setting realistic, achievable goals given the client's starting point, health concerns, if any, and time constraints.

Goals can be set over the short term (daily, weekly, monthly) and long term (>2 months). An exercise regime tailored to meet the clearly defined, specific and realistic short-term goals of the individual client will assist in maximising adoption and maintenance. Feedback on long-term goals and the strategies employed to achieve these goals is critical for assisting with exercise adherence. A sample goal-setting sheet is shown in figure 4.7.

For individuals in the maintenance stage of change, **relapse prevention** strategies, which are tools to help an individual return to regular activity

Start date:_____

Short-term goals: Date: _____ (4-6 weeks from start date)
(Targets I want to accomplish in 4 weeks.)
    1.
    2.
    3.
Strategies to achieve these goals:
(What I need to do *now* to reach my goals.)
    1.
    2.
    3.
Long-term goals: Date: _____ (3-6 months from start date)
    1.
    2.
    3.
Strategies to achieve these goals:
    1.
    2.
    3.

FIGURE 4.7   Sample goal-setting sheet.

after an interruption (e.g., holiday, inclement weather), can also be useful to introduce. Developing and enforcing environmental cues (e.g., stimulus control) may also encourage activity adherence. Environmental cues such as leaving walking shoes in the same visible location, monitoring activity on a calendar attached to the refrigerator and setting a specific time to exercise with a friend (e.g., buddy system) are easily implemented. In addition, the client should be encouraged to generalise participation so that he or she begins to be more active in other daily activities, such as using the stairs more, walking to a friend's house and taking active holidays. Encouraging more daily activity may help individuals develop a lifelong physical activity habit.

Environmental Approaches

Environmental approaches to behaviour change concentrate on the socio-cultural and environmental influences that affect participation in physical activity. Schools, worksites, health care institutions and communities may be targeted to create supportive environments for physical activity. These groups provide access to large numbers of people, and interventions targeted to specific physical settings have begun to show positive changes (see table 4.3). School support of initiatives such as the National Heart Foundation's "Jump Rope for Heart" encourages activity in a series of fun competitions. Many worksites provide a wide range of health and activity programs for employees. Several professional organisations (e.g., the National Heart Foundation [NHF], the American Heart Association, the American Academy of Pediatrics, the American Medical Association and others) in Australia and the United States advocate physician-directed counselling of physical activity. As such, health care settings may be an environment in which to accelerate the adoption and maintenance of physical activity. Finally, community support of safe bike paths and accessible parks helps increase activity across all age groups.

The NHF initiated an environmental approach to increasing physical activity through the Supportive Environments for Physical Activity (SEPA) project. The rationale of this project was that exercise needs to be accessible in four main areas: work, shopping, childcare, and leisure and recreation. After interviews with residents of one community, suggestions were made to improve road use, footpaths, public transport and seating in parks. Both government and non-government groups will be targeted with these suggestions. Future research is needed to evaluate whether such an approach is successful.

Summary

Despite general awareness of the benefits of regular physical activity, less than one-half of the adult population is regularly active. Personal and environmental barriers make it difficult for individuals to become active and remain active. Adoption and maintenance of regular physical activity requires a complex behaviour change process; several psychological theories attempt to explain this process. The theory of reasoned action states that intention to change is the determinant of behaviour. An extension of this is the theory of planned behaviour, which explains behaviour change by intention and

TABLE 4.3—Physical Settings Targeted to Accelerate Behaviour Change and the Benefits and Barriers of Each

Setting	Benefits	Barriers
School	Large groups of people, range of ages (students, parents, siblings, extended family), social support, role models	Teacher training, funding, addressing individual differences
Worksite	Easy access to employees, social support, easy changes to environment	Employment expectations, discrimination
Health care settings	Individual attention, follow-up	Feeling ill rather than well, transportation
Communities	Large groups of people, social support	Funding, addressing individual differences

perceived control of change. The social cognitive theory explains behaviour change as an interaction of environmental factors, individual attitudes and beliefs. The transtheoretical stages of change model incorporates the social-cognitive theory and describes behaviour change as a series of steps that an individual progresses through to attain behaviour maintenance. This model recognises that regression to previous stages may occur and different processes may be associated with each stage. By recognising the processes associated with each specific stage of change, interventions can be developed to accelerate the behaviour change process. Interventions targeted at specific stages such as simple education (precontemplation), decision-balance sheets (contemplation), contracts and rewards (preparation), goal setting (preparation and action) and relapse prevention (action and maintenance) may help accelerate this process. Although these interventions have been shown to accelerate change at the individual level, a large percentage of the population remains inactive or underactive. Environmental approaches to behaviour change address this problem through interventions aimed at settings with large target populations such as schools, worksites, health care institutions and communities. As Western societies become more sedentary, the challenge remains to identify strategies and tools to help make physical activity a lifelong habit for the majority of the population.

Selected Glossary Terms

adherence—Maintenance of a treatment or protocol.

adoption—Beginning a recommended treatment or protocol.

barriers—Real or perceived reasons affecting an individual's ability to engage in an activity or belief (e.g., lack of time can be a real or perceived barrier to participation in physical activity.)

behaviour change—A complex process of altering an observable activity, usually a lifestyle habit, influenced by both external and internal stimuli.

extrinsic reward—A prize or incentive external to the individual and activity, for example, social recognition.

intervention—Strategy or tool designed to help an individual or group achieve a recommended target or goal.

intrinsic reward—A prize or incentive inherent to the individual and activity, for example, enjoyment.

relapse prevention—An approach used to help anticipate and cope with situations that may inhibit behaviour change.

self-efficacy—Confidence in one's ability to perform a specific behaviour.

social norms—An individual's perception of positive and negative pressures from family, friends and cultural groups regarding a recommended behaviour change.

Student Activities and Study Questions

1. What other tools to measure self-efficacy have been validated? Have these tools been validated with an Australian population?

2. Determine stage of change for 10 individuals in each of the following groups:

   a. Under 18 years

   b. 18-25 years

   c. 25-55 years

   d. Over 55 years

   Discuss patterns of behaviour and intention to change for each group. Are these patterns expected? Why or why not? What interventions aimed at the community level would be suitable to address these patterns?

3. Develop a practical and easily implemented intervention for hypothetical clients in each of the five stages of change. Have these interventions been studied with Australian populations?

   a. Choose one subject and try each intervention. Discuss both the ease and difficulty of administration. Discuss the expected effectiveness with the subject based on his or her stage of change.

   b. Practice one intervention on yourself. What changes could be made to make it more effective?

4. Measure exercise-specific self-efficacy and general physical self-efficacy on a group of 10 physically inactive and 10 physically active individuals. Plot the scores and discuss the similarities and differences. Discuss possible interventions that may help increase self-efficacy.

CHAPTER 5

Maximising Pre-Activity Screening and Consultation

Before starting a physical activity test or program, each participant should provide specific information as part of a screening process. The purpose of pre-activity screening is to identify the risk of participation for a given individual in order to recommend direct inclusion, referral to a medical practitioner or exclusion. Additional information may be collected during this initial encounter for evaluation purposes and to help optimise activity programs, educate the client and maximise the likelihood of adoption and adherence. Written or oral screening tools are designed to identify an individual's physical, psychological and social readiness for physical activity. Information is gathered systematically, and the information collected is based on program and testing factors. This chapter provides an overview of recommendations for screening and initial consultation to ensure safe participation and to optimise programming, evaluation and education.

Pre-Activity Screening

Pre-activity screening is often the first step in writing an activity prescription or developing an activity program for an individual or group. The screening process maximises the safety of physical fitness assessments and exercise programs by identifying individuals who

▶ may proceed without further assessment,

▶ may require medical evaluation before participation because of certain risk factors or symptoms, and

▶ should be excluded because of medical considerations.

Generally, information is obtained on demographics (e.g., age, sex), current and past health, medical and physical activity status, and health behaviours. Screening tools are designed to routinely collect sufficient information yet remain cost-effective and time-efficient. An enormous amount of medical and personal information would need to be obtained to thoroughly assess physical and health status. Excessively long written screening tools may discourage potential clients, and comprehensive oral interviews are too costly for large community-based programs. A balance exists that considers client safety, program effectiveness, evaluation, education and adoption with time-efficiency and cost-effectiveness (see figure 5.1).

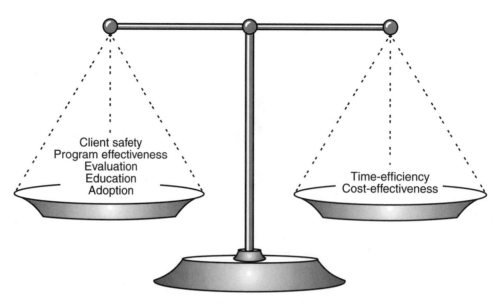

FIGURE 5.1   Screening assessments: A balancing act.

A number of screening models may be used or adapted for pre-activity screening. Which tool to use or what information to address depends on the program or test and the expected population. The Australian Association for Exercise and Sports Science (AAESS) and Sports Medicine Australia (SMA) endorse the American College of Sports Medicine (ACSM) guidelines. The ACSM guidelines are summarised in the following sections, along with additional recommendations for the design of pre-activity screening tools.

Safety

Although there are clear health benefits from participation in regular physical activity, there is some risk involved in physical fitness testing and physical activity programs. Inappropriate physical activity may cause cardiovascular events (e.g., heart attack), musculoskeletal injuries (e.g., muscle strains) and metabolic problems (e.g., hypoglycaemia). However, the risk of cardiovascular events is very low: the risk of death during a maximal exertion exercise test is approximated at ≤0.01%, and the risk of myocardial infarction is ≤0.04% (ACSM 2000). These risks are reduced significantly by using submaximal exercise tests and moderate physical activity programs. Musculoskeletal injuries are more likely to occur from high-impact activities or high volumes of repetitive activities such as running or fast bowling in cricket. Metabolic events

such as hypoglycaemia may result if individuals with diabetes participate in inappropriate activities or if the diabetes is not well controlled. Although these risks are real, the benefits of participation far outweigh the risks when appropriate precautions are taken.

For some, albeit a few, individuals, the risk of participating in physical activity is greater than the potential benefits. Exercise scientists must be able to identify individuals for whom exercise may be unsafe. ACSM (2000) provides guidelines for absolute and relative exclusion from any form of physical activity testing and programming. These recommendations are reviewed in table 5.1.

Screening Tool Design

To identify potential at-risk clients and ensure safety, specific information should be gathered. Implementation of a systematic scheme to routinely collect relevant information ensures that the correct information is obtained for all clients. Typically, this information is obtained via completion of a questionnaire. Before developing a questionnaire, the designer must consider the intended intensity of the physical activity test or program; intensity helps determine the extent of medical and health information required to maximise safety. Low- to moderate-intensity activities require minimal screening because they are generally safer and incur less risk than participation in high-intensity activities. Mod-

TABLE 5.1—Contraindications to Exercise Testing and Programming

Absolute	Relative
A recent significant change in the resting ECG, suggesting significant ischaemia, recent MI (within 2 days) or other acute cardiac event	Left main coronary stenosis
	Moderate stenotic valvular heart disease
Unstable angina	Electrolyte abnormalities (e.g., hypokalaemia, hypomagnesaemia)
Uncontrolled cardiac arrhythmias causing symptoms or haemodynamic compromise	Severe arterial hypertension (i.e., systolic BP >200 mmHg or diastolic BP >110 mmHg) at rest
Severe symptomatic aortic stenosis	Tachyarrhythmias or bradyarrhythmias
Uncontrolled symptomatic heart failure	Hypertrophic cardiomyopathy and other forms of outflow tract obstruction
Acute pulmonary embolus or pulmonary infarction	
Acute myocarditis or pericarditis	Neuromuscular, musculoskeletal or rheumatoid disorders that are exacerbated by exercise
Suspected or known dissecting aneurysm	High-degree atrioventricular block
Acute infections	Ventricular aneurysm
	Uncontrolled metabolic disease (e.g., diabetes, thyrotoxicosis, myxedema)
	Chronic infectious disease (e.g., mononucleosis, hepatitis, AIDS)

Abbreviations: ECG = electrocardiogram; MI = myocardial infarction; BP = blood pressure.

Reprinted, by permission, from American College of Sports Medicine, 2000, *ACSM's guidelines for exercise testing and prescription*, 6th ed. (Philadelphia: Lippincott Williams & Wilkins), 50.

erate- to high-intensity programs (which increase the risk of cardiovascular and musculoskeletal events) require additional information before participation begins.

As a minimum for entry into low- or moderate-intensity programs/tests, pre-activity screening questionnaires should be designed to collect the following information on each client:

▶ Age and sex

▶ Current heart disease/impairment

▶ Presence or absence of hypertension

▶ Signs and symptoms of CVD and musculoskeletal impairment

The **Physical Activity Readiness Questionnaire (PAR-Q)** is a pre-activity screening tool that has been validated with numerous populations and gathers the recommended client information.

PAR-Q

The Physical Activity Readiness Questionnaire (PAR-Q), the most widely used screening tool, is recommended by various groups including the ACSM and

AAESS as a minimal standard for entry into low- and moderate-intensity exercise programs. The PAR-Q was developed in the late 1970s in Canada by the British Columbia Ministry of Health to identify individuals who should consult a medical practitioner before participating in an exercise program. Studies evaluating the original PAR-Q found a high level of exclusion (i.e., apparently healthy adults were required to consult a medical practitioner); a revised edition was developed to correct this low specificity (i.e., percent of true negatives). Studies examining the revised edition have reported a higher specificity and generalisability (e.g., age, ethnicity). In other words, the revised edition appears less likely to require healthy adults of various ages and ethnic backgrounds to unnecessarily consult a doctor before beginning a low- to moderate-intensity physical activity program. The revised PAR-Q is shown in figure 5.2 (Canadian Society for Exercise Physiology 1994).

The PAR-Q requests a *yes* or *no* response to seven questions. A *yes* response to any of the questions recommends approval from a medical practitioner before initiating the program or test. This survey asks

PAR - Q & YOU

(A Questionnaire for People Aged 15 to 69)

Regular physical activity is fun and healthy, and increasingly more people are starting to become more active every day. Being more active is very safe for most people. However, some people should check with their doctor before they start becoming much more physically active.

If you are planning to become much more physically active than you are now, start by answering the seven questions in the box below. If you are between the ages of 15 and 69, the PAR-Q will tell you if you should check with your doctor before you start. If you are over 69 years of age, and you are not used to being very active, check with your doctor.

Common sense is your best guide when you answer these questions. Please read the questions carefully and answer each one honestly: check YES or NO.

YES	NO	
☐	☐	1. Has your doctor ever said that you have a heart condition <u>and</u> that you should only do physical activity recommended by a doctor?
☐	☐	2. Do you feel pain in your chest when you do physical activity?
☐	☐	3. In the past month, have you had chest pain when you were not doing physical activity?
☐	☐	4. Do you lose your balance because of dizziness or do you ever lose consciousness?
☐	☐	5. Do you have a bone or joint problem that could be made worse by a change in your physical activity?
☐	☐	6. Is your doctor currently prescribing drugs (for example, water pills) for your blood pressure or heart condition?
☐	☐	7. Do you know of <u>any other reason</u> why you should not do physical activity?

If you answered

YES to one or more questions

Talk with your doctor by phone or in person BEFORE you start becoming much more physically active or BEFORE you have a fitness appraisal. Tell your doctor about the PAR-Q and which questions you answered YES.

- You may be able to do any activity you want—as long as you start slowly and build up gradually. Or, you may need to restrict your activities to those which are safe for you. Talk with your doctor about the kinds of activities you wish to participate in and follow his/her advice.
- Find out which community programs are safe and helpful for you.

NO to all questions

If you answered NO honestly to <u>all</u> PAR-Q questions, you can be reasonably sure that you can:

- start becoming much more physically active—begin slowly and build up gradually. This is the safest and easiest way to go.
- take part in a fitness appraisal—this is an excellent way to determine your basic fitness so that you can plan the best way for you to live actively.

DELAY BECOMING MUCH MORE ACTIVE:

- if you are not feeling well because of a temporary illness such as a cold or a fever—wait until you feel better; or
- if you are or may be pregnant—talk to your doctor before you start becoming more active.

Please note: If your health changes so that you then answer YES to any of the above questions, tell your fitness or health professional. Ask whether you should change your physical activity plan.

<u>Informed Use of the PAR-Q:</u> The Canadian Society for Exercise Physiology, Health Canada, and their agents assume no liability for persons who undertake physical activity, and if in doubt after completing this questionnaire, consult your doctor prior to physical activity.

You are encouraged to copy the PAR-Q but only if you use the entire form

NOTE: If the PAR-Q is being given to a person before he or she participates in a physical activity program or a fitness appraisal, this section may be used for legal or administrative purposes.

I have read, understood and completed this questionnaire. Any questions I had were answered to my full satisfaction.

NAME _____

SIGNATURE _____ DATE _____

SIGNATURE OF PARENT _____ WITNESS _____
or GUARDIAN (for participants under the age of majority)

©Canadian Society for Exercise Physiology   *Supported by:* Health   Santé
  Société canadienne de physiologie de l'exercice   Canada Canada

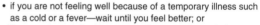

FIGURE 5.2   Revised Physical Activity Readiness Questionnaire (PAR-Q).

questions about some cardiovascular and musculoskeletal symptoms and suggests initial exclusion of individuals who may be at increased risk of these conditions through participation. It is important to reassure the client that the requirement to visit a doctor before participating is beneficial so that the client does not feel he or she "failed" before even beginning the program. Contacting the client within the next 2 weeks may help ensure the client remains positive about joining the program.

In appropriate settings, the PAR-Q is a time-efficient and inexpensive tool that may be suitable for screening low- to moderate-intensity exercise programs targeting apparently healthy individuals. For example, the PAR-Q is easily administered and can be used in geographically isolated areas for individuals who may have limited access to exercise scientists. From a public health perspective, the seven questions included on the PAR-Q encourage individuals to increase daily physical activity or regular moderate exercise without the need to seek professional assistance. However, the PAR-Q has some shortcomings. **Metabolic conditions** (e.g., diabetes, obesity) and other conditions (e.g., pregnancy) are not addressed, and extension of this document is needed for many people. The PAR-Q does not address risk factors for heart disease or the presence of some signs or symptoms that may indicate heart disease. Therefore, the PAR-Q is not suitable for screening individuals entering a high-intensity exercise program that may exacerbate known or unknown heart disease or for programs designed to target individuals with or at risk of diseases or conditions affected by exercise; additional information is needed. The following questions may help decide when the PAR-Q is suitable. A *no* response to each of the four questions indicates that the PAR-Q would be an acceptable tool to use.

1. Is the program/test high intensity?
2. Are the expected participants <15 years or >69 years?
3. Is **risk stratification** (see next section) desirable?
4. Are there specific groups (e.g., pregnant women, diabetics, obese individuals) to be targeted?

A *yes* response to any of the questions indicates a need for additional information on the screening document. In addition, if the intended program is likely to be moderate or high intensity, additional information on current and past health is necessary. Inclusion of a risk stratification procedure will help dictate what type of information is needed.

Risk stratification

Risk stratification uses additional client health information to categorise clients by risk of an adverse event occurring during participation. This process helps ensure the safety and efficacy of the proposed program. ACSM (2000) suggests that clients are categorised as either low risk, moderate risk or high risk (see table 5.2).

Individual risk is based on age, the presence or absence of risk factors for coronary artery disease (CAD), and signs and symptoms of cardiovascular disease (CVD), metabolic conditions and pulmonary disease. Risk factors for CAD are listed in table 5.3. Possible signs or symptoms (ACSM 2000) suggestive of cardiovascular or pulmonary disease include

► chest pain,
► shortness of breath,
► dizziness,
► dyspnoea,

Case Study 5.1

Roger is a 37-year-old accountant and has decided to join the yoga class at the church hall near his home. The yoga class is low intensity and generally attracts apparently healthy, middle-aged (e.g., 30-55 years) clients. The yoga instructor has all participants complete the PAR-Q prior to participating. Roger answered "no" to all seven questions. Would you recommend that Roger join the yoga class?

Key Issues

1. Is the PAR-Q an appropriate screening tool for this type of program? Why or why not?
2. What additional information may be important to obtain?
3. How can the information obtained from the PAR-Q guide activity prescription?

TABLE 5.2—Initial Risk Stratification

Low risk	Individuals who are asymptomatic, have no more than one major coronary risk factor or are younger (males <45 years, females <55 years)
Moderate risk	Individuals who have two or more major coronary risk factors or are older (males ≥45 years, females ≥55 years)
High risk	Individuals with known cardiovascular, pulmonary or metabolic disease or with one or more symptoms of CVD or pulmonary disease

Adapted, by permission, from ACSM, 2000, *ACSM's guidelines for exercise testing and prescription*, 6th ed. (Philadelphia: Lippincott Williams & Wilkins), 26.

TABLE 5.3—Risk Factors and Thresholds for Coronary Artery Disease

Risk factor	Threshold
Family history	Myocardial infarction, coronary revascularisation or sudden death before 55 years in a first-degree male relative (father, brother, son) or before 65 years in a first-degree female relative (mother, sister, daughter)
Cigarette smoking	Current cigarette smoker or quit within past 6 months
Hypertension	Systolic blood pressure ≥140 mmHg or diastolic blood pressure ≥90 mmHg measured on at least two separate occasions or on antihypertensive medication
Hypercholesterolaemia	Total serum cholesterol >5.2 mmol · L^{-1} or high-density lipoproteins <0.9mmol · L^{-1} or on lipid-lowering medication.
Impaired fasting glucose	Fasting blood glucose ≥6.2 mmol · L^{-1} measured on at least two separate occasions
Obesity	Body mass index ≥30 kg · m^{-2} or waist circumference >100 cm
Sedentary lifestyle	Persons not participating in a regular exercise program or meeting the minimal physical activity recommendations from the U.S. Surgeon General's report (accumulating ≥30 min of moderate physical activity on most days of the week)

Adapted, by permission, from ACSM, 2000, *ACSM's guidelines for exercise testing and prescription*, 6th ed. (Philadelphia: Lippincott Williams & Wilkins), 24.

▶ ankle oedema,

▶ palpitations,

▶ intermittent claudication,

▶ heart murmur, and

▶ unusual fatigue or shortness of breath with usual activities.

Adopting a risk stratification procedure such as ACSM's requires additional information to be gathered on the client; figure 5.3 presents additional health factors that may be included on a screening document. For risk stratification purposes, questions should be included that pertain to cardiovascular, pulmonary and metabolic disease, symptoms of CVD and risk factors of CAD. As shown in figure 5.4, many of the items within these three groups can be tabled together to minimise document length yet obtain relevant information. Accurate and detailed responses can be expected from individuals diagnosed with any of these conditions or who have experienced any of the symptoms. For example, a client with asthma is likely to be medically aware of the condition.

Information on factors that the client may be less aware of (e.g., high cholesterol levels, obesity and family history) may be better obtained from separate questions. Questions such as "What is your to-

RISK FACTORS FOR CVD

Cigarette smoking

Family history

Impaired fasting blood glucose

Hypercholesterolaemia

Hypertension

Obesity

Physical inactivity

Stress

PRESENCE OF

Heart disease

Cerebrovascular disease

Pulmonary disease

OTHER DISEASE STATES/CONDITIONS

Anaemia

Cancer

Diabetes mellitus

Eating disorders

Emotional disorders

Osteoporosis

Peripheral vascular disease

Phlebitis

HISTORY OF SYMPTOMS

Ankle oedema

Chest pain

Dizziness

Dyspnoea

Heart murmurs

Intermittent claudication

Palpitations

Unusual shortness of breath with usual activities

RECENT ILLNESS, HOSPITALISATIONS

ORTHOPAEDIC AND MUSCULOSKEL-ETAL PROBLEMS

MEDICATIONS

PREGNANCY

FIGURE 5.3   Additional health history factors to address in a screening document.

tal cholesterol level?" and "When was it last measured?" may be easier for a client to answer and may provide better information. An option to state *do not know* should be included. Similarly, more detailed information is obtained if clients are asked their body weight and height rather than requesting a *yes* or *no* response to "experiencing obesity".

Clients tend to know the medication they take regularly (or keep a list), so a question regarding medication is often beneficial to include. Details about medication can yield important information on current medical conditions. Questions about other conditions (e.g., pregnancy) and musculoskeletal problems or injuries are often useful to help optimise physical activity programming. This additional information enables the exercise scientist to appropriately modify physical fitness tests and programs.

After the categorisation of an individual as low, moderate or high risk, recommendations can be made for medical evaluation and physical fitness testing before participation or for the presence of a medical practitioner at submaximal and maximal

testing. These recommendations are based on the intended intensity of the physical activity program or test (see table 5.4). For individuals classified as low risk or moderate risk who are seeking to participate in low- to moderate-intensity activities (e.g., 3-6 METs), medical examination and testing are not needed to safely participate in exercise. For individuals classified as either moderate risk or high risk who are seeking to participate in vigorous activity (e.g., >6 METs, >60% $\dot{V}O_2$max), medical examination or testing may be recommended before prescribing activity.

The American Association of Cardiovascular and Pulmonary Rehabilitation and the American Heart Association have developed more comprehensive risk stratification procedures for individuals with known heart disease. Both of these risk stratification procedures classify clients as low, intermediate or high risk based on the likelihood of further cardiovascular events occurring during or after participation in exercise. These systems may be more appropriate for patients with known heart disease (AACVPR 1999; ACSM 2000).

Have you experienced any of the following conditions?

(Please √ the appropriate column and give details for a √ response)

Condition	No	Yes	Details
Rheumatic or scarlet fever			
Heart trouble			
High blood pressure			
Chest pain/angina			
Stroke			
Disease of arteries or veins			
Palpitations			
Heart murmur			
Unusual and intermittent leg pain			
Swelling in the ankles			
Undue limited shortness of breath with usual activities			
Dizziness, fainting or blackout			
Epilepsy			
Lung disorder			
Asthma			
Hay fever			
Anaemia			
Diabetes			
Thyroid disorder			
Cancer			
Osteoporosis			
Phlebitis			
Excessively high levels of stress or anxiety			

FIGURE 5.4   Sample questionnaire on personal medical history.

Medical Evaluation

Recommendations to consult a medical practitioner before participation result from a number of situations discussed previously. For example, referral to a medical practitioner is recommended if a client responds *yes* to any of the seven questions on the PAR-Q, if age may be a factor (men ≥45 years and women ≥55 years) and in the presence of signs or symptoms of cardiovascular or musculoskeletal conditions. The extent of the medical evaluation and testing is based on the client's disease status or risk of disease. At minimum, a medical history is assessed including identification of diseases or conditions, health history and previous evaluations, recent hospitalisations or illnesses, medications used, employment and family status, family history of disease and other health habits including diet and exercise.

For clients referred because of age with no known risk of CAD, evaluation may include CAD risk factors. A blood profile may be performed to measure

---

TABLE 5.4—ACSM Recommendations for Medical Examination and Supervision Before Participation

MEDICAL EXAMINATION AND TESTING

	Low risk	Moderate risk	High risk
Moderate exercise (3-6 METs)	Not necessary[a]	Not necessary[a]	Recommended
Vigorous exercise (>60% $\dot{V}O_2$max, >6 METs)	Not necessary[a]	Recommended	Recommended

MEDICAL PRACTITIONER SUPERVISION OF TEST

	Low risk	Moderate risk	High risk
Submaximal test	Not necessary[a]	Not necessary[a]	Recommended
Maximal test	Not necessary[a]	Recommended	Recommended

[a]The designation of "not necessary" reflects the notion that a medical examination, exercise test and physician supervision of exercise testing would not be essential in the pre-participation screening; however, they should not be viewed as inappropriate.

Adapted, by permission, from ACSM, 2000, *ACSM's guidelines for exercise testing and prescription*, 6th ed. (Philadelphia: Lippincott Williams & Wilkins), 27.

Case Study 5.2

Susan is a 54-year-old teacher and has not participated in regular physical activity for more than 15 years. She quit smoking two months ago and would like to participate in a university exercise study for people aged 50 to 75 years (moderate high-intensity resistance training). Her blood pressure is 145/90 mmHg and a maximal exercise test is required for entry into the study. Apply the ACSM risk stratification procedures and classify Susan as low, moderate, or high risk. In addition, make recommendations for pre-participation medical evaluation and the possible need for a medical practitioner to be present during the maximal exercise test.

Key Issues

1. Discuss possible risks of Susan participating in the study.

2. Consider the requirement to undertake a maximal exercise test prior to entry and consult table 5.4 for recommendations.

3. How would you justify these recommendations to Susan?

---

blood glucose, total cholesterol, high-density lipoproteins, low-density lipoproteins and **triglycerides.** Resting blood pressure and body weight are also determined to evaluate risk of CAD. For individuals with heart disease or who are high risk, the medical evaluation is more extensive and may include measurement of the above factors in addition to evaluation of the disease itself. Clinical testing to evaluate heart disease may include a **stress test** with 12-lead **electrocardiogram (ECG)** monitoring, **echocardiography** or **coronary angiography.** Individuals with pulmonary disease require additional tests, including **pulmonary function tests, oximetry** and extensive **blood gas analysis** (e.g., CO_2 levels).

Pre-Activity Consultation

Pre-activity screening is normally performed at a first encounter. For some clients, this may be a face-to-face meeting; for others, screening may be self-administered or via electronic media (e.g., the Internet). Pre-participation screening tools can be used to help optimise program design by providing a forum for valuable client consultation. Consultation is an ideal time to identify additional information that might enhance program adoption and maintenance. Information on current and past physical activity and environmental factors influencing physical activity and behaviour change can help guide effective program design. Pre-activity consultation also provides an ideal opportunity to educate the client and to gather relevant information for evaluation purposes.

Evaluation

Evaluation refers to the systematic gathering of information for a specific purpose. There are numerous reasons to evaluate physical activity programs, instructors or clients. To address some of these reasons, information is collected during an initial consultation, such as identification of client profile (e.g., demographics, health history) and readiness to change behaviour (e.g., stages of change; refer to chapter 4). It is important to decide the purpose for evaluation and, thus, what specific information should be collected. Published and validated tools should be used when available, and the same information should be gathered about each client. The reason for evaluation often drives the design of a pre-activity screening document. For example, an adapted screening document may be desirable for a proposed walking program that is to be added to an existing corporate fitness program. The program will be low to moderate intensity and open to employees (<65 years). It is decided that risk stratification is not necessary, and participants are likely to be apparently healthy. Thus, the PAR-Q is an acceptable screening tool to use. However, given the large percentage of female employees, a question regarding pregnancy (e.g., Are you currently pregnant?) will be necessary. In addition, the instructors would like to identify stage of readiness, so the stage of change question will also be added. For client profiling purposes, questions will be added regarding the length of time with the company and job description. The new screening document contains 11 questions (PAR-Q + pregnancy + stage of change + time with company + job description).

Effective Programming

Design of activity programs is often most effective using the results of a physical fitness assessment (discussed further in chapter 6). However, not all clients need or wish to undergo a fitness assessment before beginning a new physical activity regime. For example, a low- to moderate-intensity community

walking program would be considered safe for a 25-year-old with no known risk factors or signs and symptoms of CVD (low risk, table 5.2; moderate exercise, table 5.4); a physical fitness test is not needed before participation. Information obtained during an initial consultation can also help guide programming. Oral or written questions can be designed to generate discussion between the exercise scientist and the client.

Although research has shown that participation in physical activity or sports during youth does not correlate with activity in adulthood, an indication of the type of activities in which the individual has previously participated may assist with the exercise prescription. To generate information on past physical activity experiences, a written question might be "List the sports, exercise activities and physical leisure-time activities you have done in the past." Questions for discussion are generated, such as when the client was involved, at what level, for how long, whether the client enjoyed the activity and if he or she would like to participate in that activity again. The exercise scientist can determine through discussion whether or not the client would like to continue with current activities or re-start previous activities. For example, a client entering a company-based fitness program stated she participated in tennis for many years. During consultation, the exercise scientist learns that the client enjoyed tennis and would like to play again but feels too unfit and overweight. The exercise scientist can then design a specific program to help the client regain the fitness needed to play tennis once more.

Information on current participation in physical activity, exercise and sport can assist in designing programs to help clients achieve individual goals. For example, a client joins a commercial fitness club to lose weight. Examination of current physical activity reveals the client swims twice per week and plays squash twice per week. Modification so that she continues with some of her current activities and adds additional ones that may accelerate fat loss (refer to chapter 7) will help her attain her goals and help maximise adherence. Strategies to accelerate the adoption and maintenance of physical activity (discussed in chapter 4) often require clients to respond to specific questions. The initial consultation provides a good opportunity to gather responses needed to consolidate information on behaviour change and strategies to accelerate change. For example, identification of stage of change at the initial consultation allows specific interventions to be implemented for the individual.

Environmental factors such as access, available time and program convenience may also affect exercise adoption and maintenance. These factors, discussed in more detail in chapter 7, can either assist with program adoption and maintenance or be a barrier to participation. In terms of pre-activity information, environmental factors are often included at the initial consultation to help guide program recommendations. In Australia and worldwide, lack of time is the most frequently stated reason for not participating in physical activity and for dropping out of programs. It is critical to help each client examine available time for exercise and to suggest ways the client can incorporate exercise into a busy schedule. For some clients, it may be useful to review weekly schedules and select set times for physical activity; for other clients, it may be appropriate to suggest activities that he or she can easily access several times during the day whenever a free moment arises.

Screening As an Educational Tool

The screening process can be helpful for client education. Completion of screening documents, whether minimal or comprehensive, raises awareness of physical and health factors that may affect or be affected by participation in physical activity. For example, question 4 on the PAR-Q (refer to figure 5.2) asks "Do you lose your balance because of dizziness or do you ever lose consciousness?" Respondents become aware that these symptoms need to be discussed with a medical practitioner before participating in activity. Questions about risk factors for CAD can be used to educate each client about what he or she can do to alter particular risk factors.

Additional questions may be asked on a screening document to assess other health behaviours such as diet, alcohol consumption and stress. An overall view of health can be assessed, which may assist in setting realistic, specific and clear goals (discussed in chapter 4).

Questions regarding past and present physical activity can help educate the client about how to choose appropriate factors such as exercise frequency, intensity, duration and mode. There is often confusion in the general community about what is appropriate physical activity to improve health. Screening can help dispel myths and teach clients what physical activity is appropriate for achieving health goals. Finally, initial consultation documents that include questions on readiness to participate may increase awareness of the need to be psychologically as well as physically ready.

Cost-Effectiveness and Time-Efficiency

It is important to remember that a screening document must be time-efficient and cost-effective. A nine-page document that addresses health, physical and psychological factors may provide extremely useful information, but it is neither time-efficient nor cost-effective for an apparently healthy individual initiating a moderate exercise regime. In addition, a lengthy and wordy document may be daunting to non-English-speaking groups, individuals with low functional literacy or individuals with

Case Study 5.3

A group of fourth year, exercise science students would like to design and implement a walking program for university staff as part of their final year project. Course requirements for the project include outcome evaluation of an approved measure of behaviour change and ethical clearance. The program would be an eight-week, low- to moderate-intensity program and would target clients less than 69 years old. Select an appropriate measure of behaviour change and a suitable screening tool, and design an informed consent.

Key Issues

1. What would be appropriate measures of behaviour change? What validated tools exist to address these measures? Is the selected tool appropriate and efficient for the target population?

2. Is the PAR-Q an acceptable tool for this program? Why or why not?

3. What information needs to be included within an informed consent? How can this information be presented efficiently?

little time. The cost of producing a lengthy document for large groups may be excessive and may not be necessary for some organisations. Alternatively, a PAR-Q does not elicit sufficient information from individuals with known disease entering a cardiac rehabilitation program, which may lead to an unsafe program. Consideration of the clientele and the intended intensity of the program or tests helps the exercise scientist design a document that balances information needed for safety and programming with time and cost factors.

Informed Consent

For both ethical and legal reasons, all programs should require an informed consent, which notifies the participant of all procedures and potential risks of participation. It is imperative that participants understand the purposes and risks of participation in the physical activity program or test. An informed consent explains in written form

- the test or program itself,
- possible risks or discomforts,
- participant responsibilities,
- potential benefits to be gained, and
- confidentiality of results between the tester and participant.

An informed consent also gives participants the opportunity to ask questions. Freedom of consent is requested and a signature is witnessed; for participants under legal age, a signature is required from a legal guardian or parent. Figure 5.5 provides an example of an informed consent document designed

---

CENTRE FOR PHYSICAL ACTIVITY & SPORT EDUCATION

School of Human Movement Studies–The University of Queensland

UNIFIT CIRCUIT

MEMBERSHIP AGREEMENT

Indemnity form for exercise classes

Name: _____

Address: _____

Contact number: (day) _____ (evening) _____

I, _____, voluntarily join UNIFIT. I understand that I am free to withdraw from UNIFIT at any time and that any unused portion of my fees will not be refunded.

I understand that a qualified instructor will supervise all of the exercise sessions and these exercise sessions will use a variety of exercise equipment. I will inform the instructor if I feel any discomfort during any part of the exercise session since I understand that there is a slight possibility that submaximal exercise may induce abnormal changes such as a high blood pressure response.

If over 45 years, I have submitted a written clearance for exercise from my doctor. All medical, health and physical information will remain confidential.

I certify that I have read and understand the terms and conditions of consent.

Signed: _____ Date: _____

Supervisor's name: _____

Supervisor's signature: _____

FIGURE 5.5   Sample informed consent.

for entry to Unifit, a university-based circuit training program. Legal issues are explored further in chapter 13.

Summary

Screening is a process implemented before participation in physical activity. Pre-activity screening documents help identify whether participation is safe or whether further evaluation is needed before participating. Certain information should be obtained from all prospective participants in physical activity tests or programs regardless of the type of test or program. Entry into low- to moderate-intensity programs for apparently healthy individuals may require only a minimal standard screening document such as the PAR-Q, whereas entry into a vigorous program or test requires consideration of additional health information or risk stratification. Adoption of risk stratification procedures can help determine the type of additional information to routinely collect. Careful evaluation of a screening document helps the exercise scientist determine whether the client can safely proceed without further testing or if he or she must undergo physical fitness testing or consult a medical practitioner before proceeding; the program or test may even be contraindicated.

Screening can be self-administered (as in community-based programs or in geographically isolated areas) or can be administered by an exercise scientist at an initial consultation. This initial consultation is an ideal opportunity to gather additional information on current and past physical activity, environmental factors and behaviour change goals in order to optimise effective programming, education and adoption of the recommendations. Often, evaluation requirements guide the design of screening documents. Effective screening tools provide a balance of safety, effective programming, education and adoption with time-efficiency and cost-effectiveness. Client informed consent should be requested before participation in any physical activity test or program. Explanation of the test or program itself, possible risks and benefits, and confidentiality along with the opportunity to ask questions will help meet legal responsibilities and help the client understand the test or program.

Selected Glossary Terms

blood gas analysis—Measurement of arterial P_aO_2 and P_aCO_2.

blood glucose—The amount of the simple sugar glucose measured in the blood; normal postprandial blood glucose is <10.0 mmol $\cdot$ L^{-1}.

coronary angiography—An invasive technique used to fluoroscopically outline the coronary arteries; coronary angiography is used to diagnose coronary artery disease and help plan revascularisation if necessary.

echocardiography—Evaluation and interpretation of images of the heart, heart chambers, heart valves and myocardial blood flow using non-invasive ultrasound technology.

electrocardiogram (ECG)—A graphic recording of the electrical activity of the heart.

high-density lipoprotein (HDL)—A category of cholesterol transported on proteins that has a protective effect on the development of atherosclerosis; high levels of HDL are associated with a reduced risk of developing coronary artery disease.

low-density lipoprotein (LDL)—A category of cholesterol transported on proteins; most of the plasma cholesterol is transported as LDL, which may accelerate accumulation of lipoproteins on the artery wall; high levels of LDL are associated with an increased risk of coronary artery disease.

metabolic conditions—Impairments or disorders of the body system(s) used to convert nutrients to usable energy.

oximetry—Measurement of arterial oxygen saturation.

Physical Activity Readiness Questionnaire (PAR-Q)—A seven-question pre-activity questionnaire for people aged 15 to 69 years.

pulmonary function tests—Physical tests used to assess lung capacity and airflow such as spirometry and breathing patterns.

risk stratification—Part of the health risk screening process to classify individuals by age and risk factors or symptoms to determine the appropriate type of fitness testing and degree of medical supervision needed before beginning an exercise program.

stress test—An exercise test (either maximal or submaximal) performed under controlled conditions with selected parameters monitored such as haemodynamics, electrocardiography and echocardiography.

total cholesterol—The measured amount of cholesterol in the bloodstream; cholesterol is an essential lipid, but elevated levels of total cholesterol indicate an increased risk of coronary artery disease; cholesterol is transported through the blood on proteins (lipoproteins), and it is beneficial to measure the different categories of lipoproteins, particularly high-density lipoprotein and low-density lipoprotein.

triglyceride—A fat transported in the blood on a lipoprotein (often chylomicrons and very low-density lipoproteins); elevated triglyceride levels are associated with an increased risk of coronary artery disease if accompanied by low HDL or elevated LDL levels.

Student Activities and Study Questions

1. Collect a screening tool from organisations catering to the following groups:
   a. A running club for all age groups
   b. An aqua exercise program for pregnant women
   c. A community walking program
   d. An over-60 circuit training class

   How are these tools similar? Different? And why? Discuss the balance of cost-effectiveness and time-efficiency with safety, effective programming, education and activity adoption.

2. Discuss the advantages and disadvantages of utilising the PAR-Q as a screening tool for the following situations:
   a. Just Walk It, a community walking program
   b. An on-site corporate health and fitness program for a manufacturing company with >1,500 employees
   c. A new commercial fitness facility based in a metropolitan city centre
   d. A Web-based tool for individuals in remote areas without direct access to activity centres

3. Administer the PAR-Q to 10 to 20 adults of different ages. How many would be required to consult a medical practitioner before participating in physical activity? Discuss the implications in terms of cost, adoption of physical activity and client education.

4. Review the research literature on the use of risk stratification procedures for participation in physical activity. What populations would benefit from the use of risk stratification procedures? How will stratifying clients, within these populations, by risk assist with physical activity prescriptions?

CHAPTER 6

▪ ▪ ▪ ▪ ▪ ▪ ▪ ▪ ▪ ▪

Assessing Physical Fitness

Physical fitness is a set of attributes people have or achieve that relate to the ability to perform physical activity (USDHHS et al. 1996). These attributes include **cardiorespiratory fitness, gait, balance, agility, muscular endurance, strength** and **flexibility.** Generally, physical fitness is defined in terms of health, performance or condition. Health-related fitness is associated with a reduced risk of prematurely developing **hypokinetic diseases** or disabilities. Performance-related fitness is activity specific and refers to attributes that enhance sport- or occupation-specific skill and movement. Condition-related fitness encompasses both health-related fitness and the ability to perform daily activities with vigour. The physical attributes associated with health- and condition-related fitness are similar. This chapter presents information on tests developed to assess health- and condition-related physical fitness. Some of these tests are used within specific sport-related performance tests and are described briefly; suggested readings listed at the end of the book give more detailed sport-specific testing information.

Generally, testing of physical fitness provides baseline and subsequent data to optimise exercise prescription, monitor progress, help motivate and set goals, educate the participant, provide a more accurate risk stratification and evaluate the program and clientele.

Often included in physical fitness assessments are measures of

> ▶ *body composition:* body mass, fat and fat-free mass;
> ▶ *cardiorespiratory fitness:* ability to sustain dynamic activity;
> ▶ *muscular strength and endurance:* development of muscle force and ability to sustain force; and
> ▶ *some parameters of joint flexibility:* joint range of motion and muscle flexibility.

Tests to assess gait (walking pattern), balance (ability to maintain stability) and agility (ability to change direction) are sometimes included with specific populations such as the aged.

Numerous textbooks are devoted to physical fitness assessment. The aim of this chapter is to provide a general overview of the physical fitness assessment, to discuss the relative merits of specific tests and to make recommendations for inclusion of such tests in health- and condition-related physical fitness assessments. Consequently, this chapter contains technical information regarding test procedures in addition to practical information for application of these procedures.

Factor Selection

Two steps are involved in developing a physical fitness assessment:

Step 1: Selection of physical fitness attributes (e.g., cardiorespiratory fitness, body composition, muscular strength, endurance, flexibility)

Step 2: Selection of specific tests and protocols to measure the attributes selected in step 1

The choice of attributes to be assessed (step 1) depends on evaluation needs (client profiling, progress), client goals (health-, performance- or condition-related) and client needs (outcomes of screening). The selection of specific tests and protocols (step 2) is guided by consideration of accuracy needs, cost, validity for the intended population, equipment availability and client acceptability.

Step 1

Evaluation needs, client needs and client goals help determine what type of tests to include in a physical fitness assessment. Evaluation is discussed in more detail in chapter 13; briefly, evaluation needs often include identifying who is attending a program (client profiling) and monitoring progress (reassessment results). Identification of the clients to be targeted (e.g., young and healthy, older) and the expected benefits to be achieved from participation in the program (e.g., increased strength, reduced body fat) helps guide decision making. For example, a program designed for overweight and obese clients must include assessment and reassessment measures of body composition to determine if the targeted population is in fact attending and if body composition has changed as a result of the program.

Potential client goals and needs should also be considered when developing a physical fitness assessment. Different attributes are tested depending on the individual's goals: to improve health, cardiorespiratory fitness or sport performance. Health-related tests include assessment of body composition, cardiovascular fitness and other factors such as balance and gait. To assess level of body fat or to monitor weight loss, body composition may be required. Assessment of cardiovascular fitness can be used for diagnosis of disease in a clinical setting or to assess functional capacity in either clinical or non-clinical settings. Tests to assess body composition, cardiorespiratory fitness and muscular strength, endurance and flexibility are often included in a condition-related fitness assessment. Athletes and individuals with goals to improve sport performance benefit

from specific tests that may not be suitable for the general public. Sport-specific testing and testing for athletes is complex and beyond the scope of this book. Refer to other textbooks such as Gore (Gore and ASC 2000) for further information on this topic.

Client needs can be identified through pre-activity screening (refer to chapter 5). Some clients may require a medical evaluation and physical fitness testing before participating in a physical activity program. Usually, if the client needs physical fitness testing, it is because of health-related reasons, and health-related tests are therefore recommended. Risk stratification (refer to chapter 5) helps determine if a medical practitioner should be present for functional testing.

Step 2

After deciding which attributes to assess, the specific tests and protocols must be selected; the selection process is guided by accuracy needs, cost, validity for the intended population, equipment availability and client acceptability. Some tests and protocols designed to measure a certain attribute of physical fitness are more accurate than others. For example, a maximal effort treadmill test with measurement of expired gases yields a more accurate measure of $\dot{V}O_2$max than a submaximal step test that uses heart rate to estimate $\dot{V}O_2$max. The exercise scientist must decide the level of accuracy needed for the individual or group. Athletes tend to require tests that provide more accurate results, whereas individuals participating in a fun activity class may find tests that are not as accurate equally beneficial.

Some tests and protocols are more costly than others. Staff costs and cost of consumables (e.g., expired gas, electrodes) should be considered along with equipment availability, which often directs test selection.

Finally, the tests selected must be valid, reliable and relevant to the client or program. Many protocols have been validated for specific populations; when choosing specific protocols, it is important to consider the population for which the protocol has been validated. For example, the Balke-Ware treadmill protocol (refer to table 6.7) has been validated for sedentary adults and those with average cardiorespiratory fitness. This protocol may be too time consuming and thus inefficient for trained athletes.

Systematic consideration of the issues addressed in step 1 and step 2 helps guide the development of an appropriate physical fitness assessment. The following sections outline the attributes to consider during step 1 and information on protocols to guide step 2.

Body Composition and Anthropometry

It is well accepted that excess body fat is detrimental to health. Excess fat has been linked to an increased risk of hypertension, type 2 diabetes, coronary artery disease (CAD), osteoarthritis and certain forms of cancer. Many community and commercial physical activity programs offer specific programs for overweight and obese clients. Furthermore, reduction of body fat has been associated with performance improvements in specific sports. Hence, body composition analysis is frequently included in physical fitness assessments.

Body composition is assessed to evaluate individual body mass and the proportion of body fat and fat-free mass. Chemical analysis of specific tissues and dissection of cadavers provide direct evidence of body composition, and data obtained from these direct studies yield critical information for the development of indirect models. Indirect methods range from expensive and time-consuming laboratory techniques to simple and inexpensive field tests.

Laboratory techniques include the following:

▶ Hydrostatic weighing—Underwater submersion of the body, and the weight of water displaced allows calculation of body volume (Archimedes' Principle). Calculation of body density accounts for the volume of air in the lungs and assumes a constant density for fat (0.900 g · ml^{-1}) and fat-free mass (1.100 g · ml^{-1}).

▶ Dual energy x-ray absorpiometry (DEXA)—A partial or whole body scanner that uses x-ray to measure bone density and to estimate fat and fat-free mass.

▶ Near-infrared interactance (NIR)—Provides evaluation of the chemical composition of the body based on the principles of light absorption and reflection.

Compared with field tests, laboratory techniques are generally more expensive, require specialised equipment, may involve complicated and time-consuming calculations, require subject compliance with pre-test recommendations (e.g., abstain from eating, drinking; void completely before test) and may be anxiety-provoking for some clients. As a result, field testing, using anthropometry to assess body composition, is used more frequently in health and fitness settings.

Anthropometry is the scientific measurement of the human body and its skeleton through measurement of body size, mass and proportions. Anthropometric measures such as circumferences, body diameters, skinfold fat thickness and body mass are used to predict body density and percentage of body fat. To ensure validity and reliability, anthropometric measurements must be standardised; the International Society for the Advancement of Kinanthropometry (ISAK) has established standardised procedures for anthropometric measurements. *Kinanthropometry* refers to the technical measurement of the human body, hence ISAK is concerned with measurement technique. To minimise error, ISAK recommends that testers are trained and accredited, the time of day is recorded to account for diurnal variations (e.g., people are taller in the morning) and standard procedures are utilised. The ISAK accreditation is endorsed by the AAESS and the Australian Sports Commission Laboratory Standards Assistance Scheme (LSAS).

Height, weight, girths and skinfold thicknesses are typically included in an anthropometric assessment. Height, weight and girth measurements reflect total body measures, and skinfold measures allow an estimation of fat versus fat-free mass. Table 6.1 presents commonly used forms of anthropometric measurements and the relative merits of each. A similar table will be presented for cardiorespiratory endurance tests and tests of muscular strength and endurance. These tables are intended to help guide protocol selection (step 2). Exercise scientists first review the advantages and disadvantages of each test and consider the issues of accuracy, cost, validity, equipment and client acceptability, then they select the most appropriate tests and protocols. A community-based program with a minimal budget and a variety of health professionals referring clients may choose to include body mass index (BMI) and waist to hip ratio as measures of body composition (inexpensive, valid, no special equipment, not threatening). On the other hand, a corporate program with a full-time exercise scientist may choose to include a sum of skinfold measures (better accuracy, relatively inexpensive, valid, calipers available, client choice).

Body Mass Index

Height and weight have been used for decades to identify overweight individuals. **Body mass index (BMI)** is weight in kilograms divided by height in

> ### TABLE 6.1—Types of Body Composition Assessment and Their Advantages and Disadvantages

Type	Advantages	Disadvantages
Body mass index (BMI)	Easy Inexpensive Self-monitor Indicator of health risk Least intrusive	No indication of overfat Norms may be irrelevant Not a sensitive indicator of individual body composition changes
Girths	Inexpensive Self-monitor Not intrusive	No indication of fat vs. fat-free mass Limited indication of health risk
Waist to hip ratio	Inexpensive Indicator of health risk	No indication of fat vs. fat-free mass
Skinfolds, sum	Measure of subcutaneous fat Monitor increases and decreases in fat	Trained tester needed Norm data limited Difficult to determine goals for fat loss Most intrusive
Skinfolds, regression equations	Easily understood Measure of subcutaneous fat	Trained tester needed Questionable validity of assumptions underlying regression equations Population specific May not be sensitive enough for athletes Most intrusive

metres squared ($kg \cdot m^{-2}$). Although BMI does not differentiate fat mass from fat-free mass, a high BMI ($\geq 30 \ kg \cdot m^{-2}$) is associated with an increased risk of CAD, insulin resistance, high triglyceride levels, gallbladder disease and overall mortality. BMI is not an accurate tool to monitor changes at the individual level; however, it is useful for assessing "heaviness" of a population because it is easily measured, inexpensive and time-efficient. Health professionals not accredited in anthropometry can determine BMI easily and accurately. Furthermore, measurement of height and weight are the least threatening of any of the measures of body composition; it is therefore useful for large groups and for clients who appear anxious about more intrusive measures. BMI is not appropriate for athletes or those with a history of heavy strength training because an increase in BMI after an exercise training program may be associated with an increase in muscle rather than fat mass.

Girths

A standard tape measure is used to determine specific **girths** by measuring the circumference of a given site. Standard anthropometric tape should be used and held with constant tension perpendicular to the body. ISAK provides standardised procedures for girth measurement, and typical sites measured are upper arm, thigh, chest, waist and hip. Three measurements should be taken at each site and an average recorded. Girth measures do not differentiate between fat and fat-free mass and are typically used to evaluate pre- to post-program changes in body shape.

One measurement involving girths, the waist to hip ratio (WHR), is advocated by a number of groups as a predictor of health risk. WHR is the circumference of the waist divided by the circumference of the hips (see table 6.2). It is recognised that excess over-

TABLE 6.2—Measurement Sites for the Waist to Hip Ratio	
Site	**Location**
Waist girth	Approximately half way between the costal border and the iliac crest at the level of noticeable waist narrowing
Hip girth	At the level of greatest gluteal protrusion (subject should stand erect, relaxed and with feet together)

Adapted, by permission, from K. Norton and T. Olds, 1996, *Anthropometrica*. (Sydney: UNSW Press), 58.

all fat is unhealthy, but fat distribution is also an important indicator of health risk. A WHR >1.0 in men and >0.9 in women has been shown to increase risk of CAD morbidity and mortality, stroke and type 2 diabetes for both sexes. Over the short term, changes in WHR are usually small, so evaluating progress of an individual is not effective; its main use is to identify overweight/obese individuals with elevated risk of CAD and type 2 diabetes. WHR can be easily and accurately measured by a range of clinicians in a variety of settings (e.g., GP office, hospital ward) and may be less intimidating than skinfold measures.

Skinfold Measurements

Skinfold measurements are performed with calipers that measure the thickness of subcutaneous fat. Equations using skinfold measures determine if a client is within a healthy or unhealthy weight range. The assumptions used to develop these equations are that

▶ subcutaneous fat is proportional to total body fat,

▶ the compressibility of skin and subcutaneous fat is constant,

▶ fat distribution among the population is constant, and

▶ the composition and density of fat-free mass is constant.

Each of these assumptions has a degree of error associated with it because of differences between sexes, ethnic groups and age groups. However, skinfold measurements do give an indication of fat versus fat-free mass, and they are safe, relatively time-efficient and inexpensive.

To minimise error, testers should be trained and preferably accredited, calipers should have a pressure of $10 \text{ gm} \cdot \text{mm}^{-2}$ and be calibrated regularly, and standardised procedures should be followed. The right side of the body should always be used, the measurement should be taken 2 s after full pressure is applied (to standardise timing for the compressibility of fat), two to three measurements should be taken at each site and averaged, and standardised sites should be used (see table 6.3). The greatest source of error is the inaccurate location of skinfold sites. Table 6.3 presents the ISAK standardised locations for nine skinfold sites, and figure 6.1 depicts the anterior and posterior locations of these sites.

Skinfold measurements are the most intrusive of the anthropometric measures, and some clients may feel intimidated with skinfold procedures. The exercise scientist needs to determine if skinfold measures are acceptable and useful for the client. If the client appears uneasy, the benefits of both skinfolds and girths can be explained to the client, who can then choose which method he or she prefers.

Percentage Body Fat

Historically, skinfold measures have been used to estimate percentage body fat by regression equations that use skinfold thickness to calculate body density and then percentage of whole body fat. Regression equations are based on information obtained from direct measures of body composition and hydrostatic weighing; these equations convert skinfold measurements of subcutaneous fat to an estimate of whole body fat, including internal fat. Typically, 15 to 20% body fat is considered healthy for men and 20 to 28% for women. It is usually easy for a client to understand percentage body fat. For example, a client can easily comprehend that he is

TABLE 6.3—Measurement Locations for Skinfold Sites

Site	Location
Biceps	Anterior mid-acromiale-radiale line: half way between the acromion (posterior point of the scapula) and the radiale (proximal and lateral border of the head of the radius); vertical measure
Triceps	Posterior mid-acromiale-radiale line; vertical measure
Subscapular	2 cm below the inferior angle of the scapula; approximately 45° measure[a]
Mid-abdominal	5 cm to the right of the omphalion (midpoint of the navel) at the midline; vertical measure[b]
Supraspinale	Intersection of the line from the anterior axillary border of the iliac spine and the horizontal line from the superior border of the ilium; approximately 5-7 cm above the iliospinale (insertion of sartorius muscle at anterior superior iliac spine); approximately 45° measure
Mid-axilla	Vertical fold on the ilio-axilla line at the level of the xiphoidale of the sternum
Medial calf	Medial side at the greatest calf circumference; vertical fold with right leg non-weight-bearing and knee at 90°
Iliac crest	Immediately superior to the iliac crest on the ilio-axilla line (vertical line from the armpit to the lateral superior edge of the ilium); slightly downward measure
Front thigh	Midway between the inguinal fold and the superior border of the patella (with knee bent); vertical measure

[a]The Australian Fitness Norms[c] define the site as a 45° measure, 1 cm below the inferior angle of the scapula.

[b]The Australian Fitness Norms use the same site 5 cm to the left of the navel.

Adapted, by permission, from K. Norton and T. Olds, 1996, *Anthropometrica*. (Sydney: UNSW Press), 47-53.

[c]Adapted, by permission, from C. Gore and D. Edwards, 1992, *Australian fitness norms*. (South Australia: Children's Health Development Foundation), 12-13.

slightly over desirable weight if his percentage body fat is 21%. However, the substantial error involved in the prediction equations makes it difficult to standardise results.

There are numerous equations for predicting body density and thus percentage body fat (refer to suggested readings [Heyward 1991; Norton and Olds 1996; Schell and Leelarthaepin 1994] at the end of the book). Figure 6.2 presents two commonly used regression equations and the difference in predicted body fat from each equation. Equation 1 (Durnin and Womersley 1974) is a commonly used and recommended equation, and equation 2 (Withers et al. 1987) is one of the few equations based on assessment of Australian males. As shown in figure 6.2 the results from equation 1 show the client to be at the top of the healthy range (and recommendations may be to monitor body fat to ensure it does not increase), whereas the results from equation 2 show the client

at the low end of healthy (and therefore should not need to lose body fat). This discrepancy emphasises the difficulty in interpreting data from regression equations. Equation error can be minimised by selecting an appropriate equation based on sex, age, level of physical activity (e.g., athletic population) and ethnic or racial group. In addition, equation error can be eliminated by using a sum of skinfold measures rather than converting to a percentage body fat.

Sum of Skinfolds

A sum of skinfolds merely totals selected skinfold site measures to provide a number in millimetres of subcutaneous fat. Numerous norm tables are available for specific populations, but differences exist between these tables because of the number of skinfold sites, population assessed, age and sex. It is therefore important to refer to appropriate tables. Compared with percentage body fat methods, changes over time are more accurately monitored with this method. The disadvantage of using a sum of skinfolds measure is that it is more difficult for many clients to understand and to set measurable targets. In addition, ideal sums of skinfold measures have not yet been determined. Large epidemiological studies are needed that relate sum of skinfolds to risk of disease.

Numerous sites that include central measures (on the torso: abdominal, iliac crest, subscapular, supraspinale) and peripheral measures (on the arms and legs: triceps, biceps, front thigh, medial calf) should be used so that changes in fat patterning can be observed after interventions. Table 6.4 presents the Australian fitness norms for the sum of six skinfolds for the general Australian population.

Summary of Body Composition

Anthropometric tests indirectly assess body composition. Measurements of height, weight and girths are inexpensive, easy to perform and do not require trained personnel; however, they do not give an indication of fat versus fat-free mass. An advantage of girths is that they can be self-monitored. BMI provides general population-based data and gives an indication of health risk; the more specific WHR also offers an indication of health risk. Although skinfold measures are relatively inexpensive to perform and provide an indication of fat versus fat-free mass, they require specific equipment and trained personnel and are difficult to perform on a population basis.

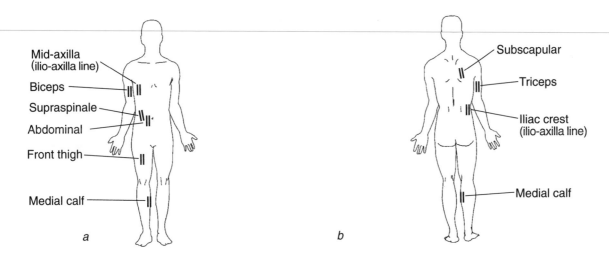

FIGURE 6.1   Skinfold site locations for skinfold measures presented in table 6.3. *(a)* Anterior view. *(b)* Posterior view.

Case Study 6.1

FITHEALTH is a community physical activity organisation with various group programs located throughout the city. Samantha is employed by FITHEALTH to design and implement an after–hours activity program for overweight and obese adults at a primary school. She needs to recruit local GPs to help with referral and she will need to monitor the program's progress. In addition, the clients are likely to want to monitor their progress. Consider the two-step process for physical fitness factor and protocol selection. What would be an appropriate fitness assessment for Samantha to recommend as part of the program?

Key Issues

1. What protocols could be performed by GPs?
2. What protocols are valid for the target population?
3. What protocols will provide useful information to the clients?

Subject: Male, 35 years old, with the following skinfold measurements (mm):

Triceps: 7.2	Iliac crest: 15.4	Front thigh: 12.8
Biceps: 5.8	Supraspinale: 18.2	Medial calf: 7.0
Subscapula: 14.2	Abdominal: 20.4	

Equation 1: Developed from 209 males in Scotland for males 17-72 years old (Durnin and Womersley 1974).

$$X_1 = \Sigma \text{ triceps, biceps, subscapula, iliac crest}$$

$$\text{Body density [BD]} = 1.1765 - 0.0744 \,(\log_{10} X_1)$$

$$\text{Subject: } X_1 = 42.6$$

$$BD = 1.0565$$

$$\text{\% body fat [\%BF]} = 495/BD - 450 \text{ (Siri equation)}$$

$$\%BF = 18.5\%$$

Equation 2: Developed from 207 males in Australia for males 15-39 years old (Withers, Craig, Bourdon and Norton 1987).

$$X_2 = \Sigma \text{ triceps, biceps, subscapula, supraspinale,} \\ \text{abdominal, front thigh, medial calf}$$

$$BD = 1.0988 - 0.0004(X_2)$$

$$\text{Subject: } X_2 = 85.6$$

$$BD = 1.06456$$

$$\%BF = 495/BD - 450$$

$$\%BF = 14.98\%$$

FIGURE 6.2   Example of two regression equations developed to estimate percentage body fat and the corresponding results for one subject.

Skinfold measures are useful for determining whether or not there is excess fat, where that fat is located and whether fat has been lost after an intervention (e.g., diet or exercise). Selection of the most appropriate tool is guided by accuracy needs (e.g., general, BMI vs. specific, sum of skinfolds), cost (most are considered relatively inexpensive), validity (e.g., the appropriate equation or norm table for the intended population), equipment availability (e.g., skinfold calipers) and client acceptability (e.g., least intrusive, BMI vs. more intrusive, skinfolds).

Cardiorespiratory Fitness

Cardiorespiratory fitness (CRF) is the ability to perform sustained dynamic activity using large muscle groups. The most commonly accepted measure of CRF is maximal oxygen uptake ($\dot{V}O_2$max). Maximal oxygen uptake is expressed in three forms: (1) an absolute value measured in $L \cdot min^{-1}$; (2) a relative value that accounts for body mass in $ml \cdot kg^{-1} \cdot min^{-1}$; and (3) a relative value that accounts for fat-free body mass in $ml \cdot kgFFM^{-1} \cdot min^{-1}$. Measurement of cardiorespiratory fitness is important for health-, condition- and sport-related testing and may be desirable for evaluation needs.

▶ *Health-related testing:* low $\dot{V}O_2$max is associated with increased risk of cardiovascular events and all-cause mortality; high $\dot{V}O_2$max is associated with higher levels of regular physical activity and exercise and a reduced risk of morbidity and mortality from numerous conditions (refer to chapter 2).

TABLE 6.4—Australian Fitness Norms for the Sum of Six Skinfolds

Percentiles	Age					
	18-29	30-39	40-49	50-59	60-69	70-78
MALES						
5	30.3	31.7	49.1	42.8	46.5	34.3
25	41.5	64.1	69.1	68.7	66.4	53.5
50	62.8	80.6	88.5	88.5	80.6	73.5
75	89.6	102.9	106.9	106.4	101.9	87.2
95	140.2	146.6	156.1	138.7	144.6	109.0
Mean	71.7	84.4	92.2	89.3	86.4	72.0
Standard deviation	37.8	32.0	32.2	28.8	27.9	20.9
Number of subjects	92	120	137	110	108	32
FEMALES						
5	51.6	49.5	66.1	60.7	67.1	65.8
25	79.1	74.7	91.1	105.9	106.5	98.4
50	103.2	100.3	129.8	141.5	134.7	129.1
75	141.9	140.7	168.2	174.1	160.3	149.2
95	204.2	201.4	222.3	211.0	201.4	193.4
Mean	112.5	110.1	133.3	139.7	134.6	127.8
Standard deviation	45.7	45.7	48.0	43.8	38.6	34.7
Number of subjects	85	130	139	125	87	26

The skinfolds assessed were biceps, triceps, subscapula, mid-abdominal, supraspinale and medial calf measured in mm.

Reprinted, by permission, from C. Gore and D. Edwards, 1992, *Australian fitness norms*. (South Australia: Children's Health Development Foundation), 31.

▶ *Condition-related testing:* regular endurance activity increases $\dot{V}O_2$max; hence measurement of $\dot{V}O_2$max can be used to assist with the development of initial exercise programs, to help set individual goals, to monitor improvements and as a motivational tool.

▶ *Sport-related testing:* elite endurance athletes typically have very high $\dot{V}O_2$max values. As a single value, $\dot{V}O_2$max is not the best predictor of performance, although it may be useful with other more specific measures to help with training and testing regimes (refer to chapter 11).

▶ *Evaluation needs:* specific programs can be designed to target specific groups (e.g., inactive, low fitness). Profiling clients can address whether or not the target population is in fact attending. Reassessment of clients can help provide valuable information on whether the program is indeed helping clients achieve goals.

Many factors affect $\dot{V}O_2$max, and approximately 20 to 50% of the value is thought to be related to genetic determinants. Females typically have a 15 to 30% lower $\dot{V}O_2$max compared with males of the same age; this difference decreases to 9% when $\dot{V}O_2$max is expressed relative to fat-free body mass. The mode of exercise testing also affects the $\dot{V}O_2$max value because the amount and efficiency of muscle mass recruited varies with the activity. For example, $\dot{V}O_2$max obtained from a treadmill test is approximately 5 to 7% higher than that achieved on a cycle **ergometer** test. Finally, it is estimated that $\dot{V}O_2$max is reduced by 1% per year after the age of 25; however, recent research has suggested that lifetime activity that promotes maintenance of lean muscle mass may slow this reduction (refer to chapter 9).

There are numerous published and validated protocols to measure $\dot{V}O_2$max. Most involve the client exercising either maximally or submaximally while specific variables are measured (e.g., oxygen consumed, heart rate, workload); $\dot{V}O_2$max can also be estimated using a validated questionnaire. Maximal effort testing requires the client to exercise to the highest possible level, whereas submaximal effort testing requires less than maximal effort. Direct measurement of oxygen consumption is the most accurate method of determining gas exchange during exercise. Expired gases (O_2 and CO_2) and ventilation are collected and analysed using a variety of gas-analysis systems. Direct measurement requires

▶ expensive calibrated equipment,

▶ trained supervision,

▶ a controlled laboratory environment, and

▶ a high level of motivation from the subject.

Because of these factors, direct measurement of $\dot{V}O_2$max is usually performed during maximal effort tests (see next section). Submaximal effort tests may be used for clients with pulmonary disease to directly assess oxygen exchange capacity.

Mathematical equations have been developed from direct measures of $\dot{V}O_2$max to indirectly estimate $\dot{V}O_2$max through the measurement of heart rate or workload. Expensive gas-analysis equipment is not necessary, and maximal and submaximal effort protocols for indirect measurement can be used. These protocols involve various exercise modes such as ergometry, step tests and field tests. Common modes of testing include the treadmill, bicycle ergometer, arm crank ergometer, bench stepping, sport-specific ergometers (e.g., rowing, kayaking) and field tests; table 6.5 presents advantages and disadvantages of these modes of exercise testing. Bicycle ergometers and treadmills are the most common types of testing equipment used for maximal effort testing and for programs with appropriate facilities and trained personnel. For groups and in transient settings, field tests and bench stepping are effective. Sport-specific ergometers are usually reserved for athletes, and arm crank ergometers tend to be used with individuals who require substantial upper body strength (e.g., paraplegics). Selection of the appro-

priate test mode can be assisted by referring to the recommendations for step 2 (e.g., accuracy needed, cost, validity, equipment, client acceptability) and reviewing the advantages and disadvantages of the test modalities. Maximal and submaximal effort protocols have been developed and validated for each of these modes and are discussed in the following sections.

Maximal Effort Testing

Maximal effort testing requires the client to exercise to the highest level possible (volitional fatigue). Exercise begins at a low workload, and workload increases according to the specific protocol until volitional fatigue occurs. Workload (and thus exercise intensity) is increased by increasing the pace (treadmill or ergometer), resistance (ergometer) or inclination (treadmill). $\dot{V}O_2$max is defined as the highest oxygen consumption achieved during the test. Several criteria are used to determine if a measure of $\dot{V}O_2$max has been achieved:

▶ A plateau in oxygen uptake or a progressively reduced increase in oxygen consumption with increasing exercise intensity

▶ A **respiratory exchange ratio** ≥1.1 (**RER** = $\dot{V}CO_2/\dot{V}O_2$)

▶ An exercise heart rate within 10 beats · min^{-1} of age-predicted maximum heart rate (age-predicted maximum heart rate = 220 – age)

A test that requires maximal effort provides the most accurate measure of $\dot{V}O_2$max. An overview of a common maximal treadmill, bicycle ergometer and field test is presented in table 6.6. The Bruce protocol is a common treadmill test in which workload increases by large increments every 3 min. A general bicycle ergometer protocol common in Australia begins at 40 W (females) or 50 W (males) and increases workload every 2 min until volitional fatigue. The most widely used maximal effort field test is the multi-stage 20-m shuttle run, or the "beep test". Subjects are required to run back and forth between two lines spaced 20 m apart while an audio cassette provides a "beep" sound to set the pace. There are 21 stages of increasing pace, and the client continues until he or she can no longer maintain the intensity. Tables have been developed from regression equations to estimate $\dot{V}O_2$max. Refer to the suggested readings (Gore and ASC 2000; Heyward 1991; Schell and Leelarthaepin 1994) for section 2 at the end of the book for additional protocols.

TABLE 6.5—Exercise Test Modalities and Their Advantages and Disadvantages

Test	Advantages	Disadvantages
Treadmill	Constant pace (motor driven) Largest muscle mass used, therefore highest $\dot{V}O_2$ achieved Common form of activity (walking), therefore may be more comfortable for some Able to monitor haemodynamics	Expensive Requires a large amount of space Client may feel imbalance, dizziness if unaccustomed to treadmill walking Weight bearing, which may be inappropriate for some clients (e.g., obese, gait problems)
Bicycle ergometer	Relatively small Less expensive than a treadmill Weight supported Easily calibrated Relatively portable Easier than treadmill to measure haemodynamics	Moderately expensive Difficult to compare client results with population norms because of the large differences in mechanical efficiency between clients, which is assumed to be constant within test protocols $\dot{V}O_2$max achieved is typically 10-15% lower than that on a treadmill Requires frequent adjustment and calibration More likely to have localised leg fatigue, which prohibits completion May be less comfortable than the treadmill because of unfamiliarity
Arm crank ergometer	Beneficial for individuals unable to perform leg exercise Assists with prescription and monitoring of dynamic upper body exercise Relatively small Portable	Small muscle group used, so estimated $\dot{V}O_2$max is about 20-30% lower than that on a treadmill Difficult to monitor haemodynamics Used infrequently, so difficult to find population norms and standardised protocols
Sport-specific ergometers (e.g., rowers, kayaks)	Provides skill-specific data for athletes Assists with athletes' training regimes Generally portable	Expensive Requires validation and testing for reliability Developed for specific group of athletes: differences in mechanical efficiency within the general public limit its use
Step tests	Inexpensive Portable Relatively easy to administer to large groups	Estimates $\dot{V}O_2$max from post-exercise heart rate, which has a 10-15% error Difficult to standardise protocols and adjust step height for clients of varying heights and weights Difficult to compare with population norms because of the large differences in mechanical efficiency between clients Some clients have difficulties maintaining a constant step rate Slight inaccuracies in post-exercise heart rate will result in large inaccuracies in $\dot{V}O_2$max prediction Difficult to monitor haemodynamics

(continued)

	TABLE 6.5 (continued)	
Test	**Advantages**	**Disadvantages**
Field tests	Inexpensive	Difficult to monitor haemodynamics
	Easy to administer to large groups	Requires client to self-select pace
	Less time consuming	Difficult to standardise because of changes in weather and testing place
		Error due to differences in mechanical efficiency

Clinical Exercise Testing

Maximal exercise testing is used in the clinical setting as a diagnostic and prognostic tool for coronary artery disease (CAD). Typically, clinical exercise tests are performed under the supervision of a medical practitioner with the assistance of an exercise scientist or other trained health professional. Clinical exercise testing is beneficial for individuals

- classified as moderate or high risk (refer to chapter 5),
- beginning a vigorous exercise program,
- with CAD to monitor disease progression, and
- employed in occupations where public safety may be affected by the individual experiencing a cardiovascular event.

Electrocardiography (evaluation of the electrical activity of the heart) is often used during the clinical exercise test to monitor electrical activity changes of the heart. Careful examination of the electrocardiogram yields information about heart rhythm, existing ischaemia (insufficient supply of oxygen) and evidence of previous or recent myocardial infarction (blockage of oxygen supply). Monitoring blood pressure response and symptoms also provides important information about the haemodynamic response to exercise. Functional capacity can be determined through test end-points (e.g., initiation of ischaemia or onset of symptoms) and can be used to help prescribe exercise.

Maximal effort tests are the most accurate way to determine $\dot{V}O_2max$ and to help with diagnosis and prognosis of CAD. In addition, they can also provide the most accurate indication of the presence or absence of ischaemia in a clinical exercise test. However, maximal effort tests are time consuming, require a high level of motivation from the client, can

be intimidating and may be inappropriate for certain individuals. To motivate the client to attain a $\dot{V}O_2max$, the exercise scientist must continually encourage the client verbally. Encouragement such as "keep it up", "you are almost there" and "you are doing great" will help keep the client motivated.

Submaximal Estimation of $\dot{V}O_2max$

Because of the difficulties associated with maximal exercise testing, it may be preferable to use submaximal exercise tests. Typically, exercise or post-exercise heart rate is measured and extrapolated to age-predicted maximum heart rate (predicted maximum heart rate = 220 – age). Several assumptions allow for the prediction of $\dot{V}O_2max$ from submaximal workloads; submaximal effort tests assume

- a linear relationship between heart rate, oxygen uptake and workload;
- a constant mechanical efficiency between individuals; and
- a maximum heart rate similar for all individuals of a given age.

There are some errors in these assumptions, leading to a degree of inaccuracy in estimation of $\dot{V}O_2max$ from submaximal exercise tests. For example,

- the relationship between heart rate and oxygen consumption is linear until higher workloads, where it becomes curvilinear;
- a variance between individuals in mechanical efficiency of approximately 6% exists for walking and cycling and 10% for stepping; and
- maximum heart rate varies by approximately ±10 beats · min^{-1} for a given age group.

TABLE 6.6—Advantages and Disadvantages of Cardiorespiratory Fitness Test Protocols for Maximal Effort Testing

Test	Protocol				Advantages	Disadvantages
Bruce treadmill test[1]	ST	TM	SP	GR	Valid	Large increments not suitable for older or deconditioned individuals
	1		2.7	10	Reliable	
	2	3	4.0	12	Quick	Overestimation of $\dot{V}O_2$max when plateau fails to occur because of large increments
	3	6	5.5	14	Most commonly used treadmill protocol	
	4	9	6.7	16		
	5	12	8.0	18		
	6	15	8.8	20		
	7	18	9.6	22		
	8	21	10.4	24		
Bicycle protocol[2]	*Females:* Begin at 40 W and increase 40 W every 2 min *Males:* Begin at 50 W and increase 50 W every 2 min				Cycle at desired rate on air-braked ergometers Relatively small workload increments	Bicycle protocols not standardised because of differences in ergometers May be difficult for individuals not accustomed to cycling
Multi-stage 20-m shuttle run[3]	Mark two parallel lines 20 m apart After a warm-up, begin the tape[a] The tape emits "beeps" to instruct subjects on pace Subjects start at one line and reach the other line in pace with the beep Three beeps together signals an increase in pace The test is stopped when the subject is 2 or more steps from the line on two consecutive laps				Easy to perform with large groups Quick	Subjects must be able to run Requires a level of agility, and some subjects may have difficulties with turning around at the end of a lap

[a]Cassette tape can be purchased from the Australian Sports Commission.

Abbreviations: ST = stage; TM = time in min; SP = speed in km · h^{-1}; GR = percent grade.

[1]Adapted from J. Schell and B. Leelarthaepin, 1994, *Physical fitness assessment in exercise and sport science,* 2nd ed. (New South Wales: Leelar Biomediscience Services), 140; [2]as above, 142-143; [3]as above, 205-207.

When combined, these result in a 10 to 20% error in estimation of $\dot{V}O_2$max from submaximal testing. Although an error in estimation exists, submaximal testing is less stressful, less time consuming, more cost-effective and requires less sophisticated equipment. Consequently, submaximal testing may be the method of choice for many clients and programs.

Submaximal tests have been developed for various modalities (refer to table 6.5) and are typically either single stage (one workload) or multi-stage (two or more workloads). Equations, nomograms or graphs are used to estimate $\dot{V}O_2$max from submaximal or post-exercise heart rates. Table 6.7 presents two validated submaximal protocols for the

	Protocol				Advantages	Disadvantages
TREADMILL						
Bruce	Refer to table 6.6 Predicted $\dot{V}O_2$max (ml · kg^{-1} · min^{-1}) = 4.326 × (time in min) – 4.66				Valid and reliable Quick	Large increments Not suitable for all populations
Balke-Ware	ST	TM	SP	GR	Valid and reliable	Time consuming
	1	0	5.3	0	Small increments	Not suitable for all populations (young, physically fit)
	2	2	5.3	2	Constant speed is useful with older adults	
	3	4	5.3	3		
	4	6	5.3	4		
	5	8	5.3	5		
	6	10	5.3	6		
	7	12	5.3	7		
	8	14	5.3	8		
	Predicted $\dot{V}O_2$max (ml · kg^{-1} · min^{-1}) = 1.444 × (time in min) + 14.99					
BICYCLE						
Åstrand-Rhyming	See appendix				Valid and reliable Widely used	Does not observe an incremental change in HR Needs to use age correction factor
YMCA	See appendix				Valid and reliable Heart rate response to ↑ intensity	Needs two exercise heart rates within 110-140 range
STEP						
Queens College	Bench height: 41.3 cm *Males:* step rate = 24 steps · min^{-1} *Females:* step rate = 22 steps · min^{-1} Set metronome, step for 3 min, palpate pulse from 5-20 s post-testing *Males:* $\dot{V}O_2$max = 111.33 – 0.42 × HR *Females:* $\dot{V}O_2$max = 65.81 – 0.1847 × HR				Single step needed Predicts $\dot{V}O_2$ Short duration	Step height the same for males and females Cannot test males and females together because of different rates

	Protocol	Advantages	Disadvantages
STEP			
Harvard	Bench height	Uses same step rate	Does not predict $\dot{V}O_2$
	Males: 50 cm	Different step height for males and females	Fitness norms the same across sex and age
	Females: 43 cm		Longer duration
	Step rate: 30 steps · min^{-1}		
	Set metronome at 120, step for up to 5 min, sit down and palpate pulse from 1 to 1 1/2 min Post-testing		
	Physical Fitness Index = duration of exercise(s) × 100/(5.5 × pulse count)		
	PFI <50 Poor		
	50-80 Average		
	>80 Good		

Abbreviations: ST = stage; TM = time in min; SP = speed in km · h^{-1}; GR = percent grade.

Adapted from J. Schell and B. Leelarthaepin, 1994, *Physical fitness assessment in exercise and sport science,* 2nd ed. (New South Wales: Leelar Biomediscience Services), 188-194, 140.

treadmill, the bicycle ergometer and bench stepping. The protocols and norms for the bicycle ergometer tests are presented in the appendix. Again, the factors in step 2 come into play when considering the advantages and disadvantages of these tests for specific groups. For example, a program targeting older, less fit clients with a treadmill available may choose the Balke-Ware protocol; a program targeting the same population with a bicycle available may choose the Åstrand-Rhyming protocol, which does not require an increase in resistance that may be difficult for some participants. On the other hand, a program targeting young people may choose the Bruce protocol because it is quick or the YMCA protocol because it gives an indication of change in heart rate response to increasing workload.

Estimation of $\dot{V}O_2$max by Questionnaire

In population studies and public health programs, it may not be feasible to physically test all participants. Regression equations have therefore been developed that estimate individual functional capac-

ity based on non-exercise factors; some of these tools have been shown to be valid indicators of functional capacity. Factors such as age, age^2, gender, physical activity status (on a 0 to 7 scale), body mass and height have been used in such regression equations (Matthews et al. 1999). However, individual improvements over time are difficult to assess with these tools. If assessing motivation or monitoring progress is the reason to assess the cardiorespiratory fitness of a client, other methods may be more useful. In addition, because of limitations of activity scales, these tools tend to underestimate $\dot{V}O_2$max in very fit subjects. Improvements in the CRF of a population can be estimated from questionnaire responses, which may be useful in health promotion. Population-based physical activity projects can be developed based on population-based questionnaire results of CRF.

Monitoring

Objective and subjective factors are measured during exercise tests to ensure client safety, provide data for monitoring during physical activity and, in some cases, to estimate $\dot{V}O_2$max. Heart rate, blood pressure, electrical activity of the heart (electrocardiography, ECG) and subjective **rating of perceived exertion,** pain or breathlessness are some of the factors commonly monitored during a cardiorespiratory fitness test. Selection of factors to be monitored depends on client needs, client risk and equipment availability.

Heart Rate

Measurement of heart rate is required for most indirect tests used to estimate $\dot{V}O_2$max. Heart rate can be measured through palpation, ECG or automated heart rate monitors; an ECG monitors both heart rate and rhythm. Automated heart rate monitors are relatively inexpensive and have been shown to be reliable and accurate. Heart rate can be palpated (see figure 6.3) at the

▶ brachial artery: behind the biceps brachii and below the axilla on the inside of the arm,

▶ radial artery: at the base of the thumb on the anterolateral side of the wrist, or

▶ carotid artery: on the neck lateral to the larynx.

The exercise scientist should be competent in all three measurements of heart rate. Because palpation at the radial artery is the least intrusive, it should be attempted first. Carotid artery pulse is usually the easiest to palpate, though care should be taken not to press too hard and occlude the vessel. Palpation

of the brachial artery is useful before measuring blood pressure.

To ensure an accurate palpation of heart rate and to maximise safety, the tip of the middle and index fingers should be used with a light pressure, and the count should begin with "0" at the first pulse beat. Beats can be counted for 10 s (and multiplied by 6) or for 15 s (and multiplied by 4) to provide heart rate in beats $\cdot$ min^{-1}.

Blood Pressure

Measurement and monitoring of blood pressure is also common to ensure client safety (e.g., drop in systolic blood pressure $\geq$10 mmHg indicates the test should be stopped). Systolic blood pressure is the pressure against the arteries during contraction (i.e., systole) of the heart, and diastolic blood pressure is the pressure against the arteries while the heart is in between contractions (i.e., diastole). To measure blood pressure, an anaeroid or mercury column sphygmomanometer (see figure 6.4) is used with a stethoscope. The anaeroid sphygmomanometer is more portable; however, because of increased movement of the dial, additional practice is often required. The sphygmomanometer is attached to a cuff with an inflatable bladder, which is placed around the upper arm in line with the brachial artery. The following procedure is recommended for blood pressure measurement:

1. Palpate brachial pulse and place the cuff over the brachial artery above the antecubital space.

Case Study 6.2

Warren is a 34-year-old sales rep for a health care company and is to undertake a fitness assessment with the company's health and fitness centre. He is moderately active (plays tennis once a week and walks the dog three mornings each week). The fitness assessment includes pre-activity screening, assessment of body composition and cardiorespiratory fitness. Following measurement of BMI, WHR and sum of six skinfolds (weight = 82 kg), Warren participates in a cardiorespiratory fitness test. Suggest an appropriate protocol to assess cardiorespiratory fitness and recommend the initial workload.

Key Issues

1. Would a maximal or submaximal exercise test be most appropriate for Warren?

2. What protocols will provide useful information to Warren?

3. What protocol(s) would be appropriate for most of the company's employees?

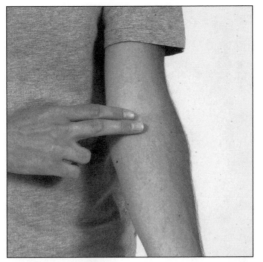

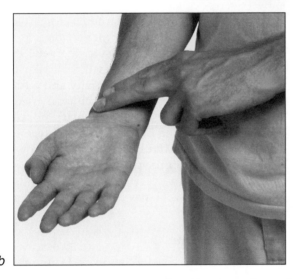

a

b

c

FIGURE 6.3　Correct position for palpating pulse at the *(a)* brachial artery, *(b)* radial artery and *(c)* carotid artery.

2. Palpate radial artery and inflate the cuff until the pulse is occluded; note the value and deflate the cuff.

3. Place the stethoscope over the brachial artery and inflate the cuff to the level recorded in step 2 + 20 mmHg.

4. Slowly deflate the cuff, noting the change in sounds; systolic blood pressure is indicated by the first sound as blood flow returns (1st Korotkoff sound), and the diastolic pressure is indicated with a muffled sound (4th Korotkoff sound) or no sound (5th Korotkoff sound).

5. Remove the cuff and re-measure 5-10 min later (for resting values).

The World Heath Organization defines normal resting blood pressure as systolic blood pressure <140 mmHg and diastolic blood pressure <90 mmHg. Elevated blood pressure (i.e., hypertension) is described as systolic or diastolic blood pressure equal or greater to these values measured on at least two separate occasions. Measurement of blood pressure is not usually intimidating for clients, and a client should be referred to a medical practitioner,

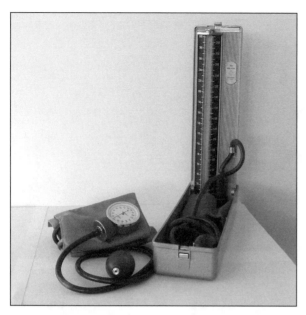

FIGURE 6.4   An anaeroid and a mercury column sphygmomanometer.

before testing, if his or her resting blood pressure is above normal values.

During a maximal or submaximal cardiorespiratory exercise test, systolic blood pressure should increase with increasing heart rate (from increased cardiac output), and diastolic blood pressure should stay the same or reduce slightly (from vasodilation) (see figure 6.5). An abnormal blood pressure response to exercise (e.g., failure of systolic blood pressure to increase, a decrease ≥10 mmHg in systolic blood pressure, an increase in systolic blood pressure to >260 mmHg or an increase in diastolic blood pressure to >155 mmHg) may indicate the presence of cardiovascular disease and warrants test termination and referral to appropriate medical practitioners. It is imperative to make sure the client understands the reason for stopping the test, the importance of following up with the referral and the possibility that return to exercise and perhaps the exercise test remain important.

Electrocardiogram (ECG)

An ECG, which measures the electrical conductivity of the heart, may be used during specific cardiorespiratory tests, particularly for individuals with, or at risk of, cardiovascular disease. The heart is paced with its own electrical conduction system that begins in the sino-atrial (SA) node and creates a wave

that depolarises through a specific pathway, resulting in contraction of the atrial and ventricular chambers of the heart. This wave of depolarisation follows a path through the SA node to the atrial-ventricular node (contraction of the right and left atrium), through the bundle of His to the left and right bundle branches and to the Purkinje fibres (ventricular contraction). The ECG presents this electrical conduction in graph form (see figure 6.6) and allows identification of normal and abnormal rhythms, underlying ischaemia and other conditions.

To prepare for an electrocardiogram, electrodes are placed at specific points on the body. A "lead" represents the deflections caused by a difference in polarity between two electrodes. Figure 6.7 shows electrode placement for a 12-lead ECG, and figure 6.8 shows electrode placement for a 3-lead ECG (see suggested readings for section 2 at the end of the book: ACSM 2000; Goldberger 1999). A 12-lead ECG, which presents 12 different pictures of the heart's electrical activity and a fuller picture of the heart's electrical ability, is used to help diagnose CAD and to identify possible arrhythmias. A 3-lead ECG allows for determination of normal rhythm but does not provide adequate information for the diagnosis of disease. In clinical settings, a 12-lead ECG is normally used, whereas a 3-lead ECG may be used in health and fitness programs.

Subjective Measures

Indicators of perceived exertion and discomfort (chest pain, difficult or laboured breathing, leg discomfort/pain) provide a subjective assessment of exercise tolerance. The rating of perceived exertion (RPE) scale is a validated scale that has demonstrated a high correlation with exercise heart rate and workload (Borg 1998). The RPE scale rates exercise intensity on a 6 to 20 scale, and another scale, the CR10, uses a 0 to 11 scale (see figure 6.9); either version can be used. A client is asked to rate how hard the exercise feels according to the scale provided. To help the client use the RPE scale initially, the client's heart rate is monitored and related to his or her perception of effort. It is important for the client to understand that the rating should be related to overall exertion and not exertion of a particular body part. For example, a client unaccustomed to cycling may feel leg soreness and state a high RPE; if instructed to provide a rating of overall exertion, the client may suggest a lower number.

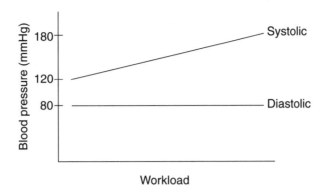

FIGURE 6.5   Changes in systolic and diastolic blood pressure with increased workload.

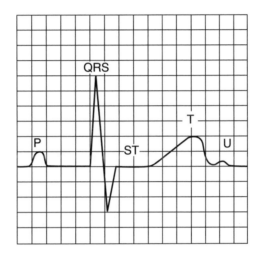

FIGURE 6.6   ECG recording of a single contraction of the heart. The P wave represents atrial contraction; the QRS complex, ventricular contraction; and the T and U waves, ventricular repolarisation.

Some medications, particularly for hypertension, cause a change in the haemodynamic response to exercise, thus exercise heart rate cannot be used to estimate $\dot{V}O_2$max. Monitoring RPE during the test provides useful data to ensure safe test end-points and to safely prescribe exercise.

During a clinical exercise test, some clients may become symptomatic (e.g., chest pain, difficult or laboured breathing), and subjective scales relating to the specific symptoms are used to assess discomfort. Subjective rating of discomfort is generally given on a 4-point scale, with a "1" indicating minimal discomfort and a "4" most severe discomfort. Figure 6.10 shows a generic example of a 4-point scale used to assess subjective symptoms. A specific symptom (chest pain, leg pain, breathlessness) can be inserted individually, and tests are ceased when a patient rates his or her symptoms at "3", or moderately severe.

Summary of Cardiorespiratory Fitness

Measurement of cardiorespiratory fitness can provide information about an individual's physical health and functional capacity, physical condition and, in some cases, sporting ability and improvement. Oxygen consumption is the most widely accepted indicator of CRF and can be determined through direct and indirect techniques. Although direct measurement of oxygen consumption provides the best measure of $\dot{V}O_2$max, direct measures

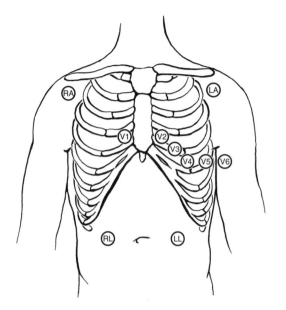

FIGURE 6.7   Electrode placement for a 12-lead ECG.

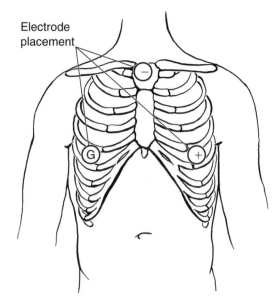

FIGURE 6.8   Electrode placement for a 3-lead ECG.

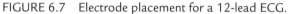

6	No exertion at all		0	Nothing at all	"No P"
7			0.3		
8	Extremely light		0.5	Extrememly weak	Just noticeable
9	Very light		1	Very weak	
10			1.5		
11	Light		2	Weak	Light
12			2.5		
13	Somewhat hard		3	Moderate	
14			4		
15	Hard (heavy)		5	Strong	Heavy
16			6		
17	Very hard		7	Very strong	
18			8		
19	Extremely hard		9		
20	Maximal exertion		**10**	Extremely strong	"Max P"
			11		

Borg RPE scale
© Gunnar Borg, 1970, 1985, 1994, 1998

● Absolute maximum   Highest possible

Borg CR10 scale
© Gunnar Borg, 1981, 1982, 1998

FIGURE 6.9   The Borg RPE scale and Borg CR10 rating of perceived exertion scales.

are time consuming, expensive and require calibrated equipment and supervision by trained personnel. Hence, inclusion of direct measures are generally limited to laboratory settings. Indirect measures, which estimate $\dot{V}O_2$max, are used more frequently in commercial, corporate and community programs. Both maximal and submaximal ef-

fort tests can be used. In health and fitness settings, submaximal estimation of $\dot{V}O_2$max is normally preferred, whereas clinical and sporting settings may benefit from information obtained through maximal tests. To guide protocol selection, it is necessary to identify the accuracy needed (direct vs. indirect, maximal vs. submaximal), cost (expired gases,

1	Light, slight discomfort
2	Moderate, uncomfortable
3	Moderately severe, very uncomfortable
4	Most intense pain experienced

FIGURE 6.10 Example of a 4-point scale to subjectively assess clinical symptoms during an exercise test or program.

trained personnel), validity (protocols with norms validated for the intended population should be chosen), equipment availability (treadmill, bicycle ergometer, steps) and client acceptability (maximal vs. submaximal, mode). Results from any of these tests and from factors monitored (e.g., HR, BP, RPE) provide information that can help guide physical activity prescription, motivate a client to continue, set specific and individualised goals for participation, and provide useful information for program evaluation.

Muscular Strength and Endurance

Muscular strength is defined as the maximal force that can be exerted by a muscle or muscle group in a single contraction. Muscular endurance is the ability of a muscle or muscle group to sustain repeated contractions. Both muscular strength and muscular endurance are important factors for health, fitness and sporting performance. Adequate muscular strength and endurance are important for

▶ maintenance of activities of daily living in the elderly and in individuals with musculoskeletal or neuromuscular impairment,

▶ healthy development of children,

▶ reducing the risk of developing low back and other musculoskeletal injuries,

▶ specific occupational groups (e.g., emergency services, law enforcement agencies),

▶ performance of many sports, and

▶ prevention of falls in the elderly.

Numerous tests measure individual muscular strength and endurance. These tests can be described as either

▶ *static:* measuring **isometric contraction** (force applied with no muscle shortening or lengthening) using tools such as dynamometers and cable tensiometers or

▶ *dynamic:* measuring concentric (force exerted as muscle shortens) and eccentric (force exerted as muscle lengthens) movements such as (1) **isotonic contraction** (force measured during shortening and lengthening of the muscle) with tools such as free weights and pin weights or (2) **isokinetic contraction** (force measured during constant speed and variable force) using Kin-Kom or Cybex.

Dynamometers and cable tensiometers measure static strength and 1 repetition maximum (RM); multiple RM and isokinetic tests assess dynamic strength. Muscular endurance can also be assessed with static and dynamic tests. Table 6.8 presents some of the common tests, along with advantages and disadvantages, and each test is described further in the next two sections. Similar to protocol selection for body composition and cardiorespiratory fitness, the advantages and disadvantages of each test must be reviewed with consideration to accuracy, cost, validity, equipment and client acceptability.

Regardless of the method of testing, test results will be relevant only for the muscle or muscle group assessed (principle of specificity). For example, 1 repetition maximum (1 RM) on the bench press provides information on upper body strength only and gives no information on lower body strength. To gather more useful information on whole body muscular strength, it is recommended that at least three areas are assessed—upper body, lower body and abdominal region. In addition, training to improve a test measure (e.g., 1 RM on the bench press) must mimic the test itself for improvements to be seen. Finally, norm tables have been developed separately for select populations, so it is important to refer to appropriate norms for a particular client.

Assessing Static Strength

Dynamometers and **cable tensiometers,** designed to measure isometric strength of one contraction, are both used to measure static strength. These tools are useful for some athletes (e.g., grip strength dynamometer for tennis players) and individuals rehabilitating from injury (e.g., leg extension cable tensiometers after knee reconstruction).

TABLE 6.8—Types of Muscular Strength and Endurance Assessments and Their Advantages and Disadvantages		

Type	Advantages	Disadvantages
Dynamometer	Easy to perform Time-efficient Inexpensive Portable Can determine imbalance	Not likely to mimic ADLs or sporting performance Improves only with specific isometric training
Cable tensiometer	Easy to perform Time-efficient Inexpensive Portable	Not likely to mimic ADLs or sporting performance Improves only with specific isometric training
1 RM (1 repetition maximum)	Most accurate measure of dynamic strength	Time consuming Need to do multiple tests to develop prescription Requires specific equipment Not appropriate for all (e.g., children, people who are hypertensive, pregnant, arthritic) Intimidating for some Need to continually assess for program to progress
Multiple RM	Safer Not as intimidating Time-efficient Easy to monitor and change with improvements	May not be as specific for some athletes Need to do multiple tests to develop prescription
Isokinetic (Cybex, Kin-Kom)	Measures peak torque Measures change in force throughout range of movement Best measure of muscular imbalance	Very expensive equipment Requires large amount of space Requires maximal effort
Static endurance tests	Measures ability to sustain maximal contraction Easy to perform Time-efficient Inexpensive Portable	Requires sustained maximal effort Improves only with specific isometric training
Timed tests (e.g., 60-s push-up test)	Measures muscular endurance Equipment not necessary	Intimidating to client Induces muscle soreness Requires sustained effort that may become maximal at the end Differences in body size, weight and mechanical efficiency make it difficult to develop population norms for timed field tests (e.g., sit-ups, push-ups)

Abbreviation: ADLs = activities of daily living.

Static muscular endurance tests require the subject to maintain a near maximum force for a set period of time. For example, to assess abdominal endurance, maximal trunk flexion is first measured with a cable tensiometer, and then the client is encouraged to try to maintain that maximal force for 30 s. The force is recorded every 6 s and a percentage of maximum force is calculated. For all of these tests, adjustments to body size and correct body alignment ensure valid measurement. Because most activities requiring muscular strength involve movement (i.e., are dynamic), other uses for static testing are limited and data from dynamic testing may provide more useful information.

Testing Dynamic Strength

Most applications of muscular strength and endurance involve dynamic movement. The best method of determining dynamic muscular strength is con-

sidered to be the **1 repetition maximum (1 RM),** the greatest amount of weight that can be lifted in 1 repetition. The following steps are followed to assess 1 RM:

1. Teach the client the correct technique, then instruct the client to stretch the muscle/ muscle groups and practice without resistance.

2. Add resistance equivalent to 30 to 50% of body weight and have the client perform 1 repetition.

3. Let the client rest 1 to 5 min, then increase the resistance by a small amount of weight and have the client perform 1 repetition.

4. Repeat step 3 until the client fails to perform 1 repetition.

5. Divide the weight lifted on the last full repetition by body weight and compare to norms (see table 6.9, a and b).

TABLE 6.9A—1 RM Norms for the Bench Press

| Rating | Age | | | | | |
	<20	20-29	30-39	40-49	50-59	60+
MALES						
Superior	≥1.34	≥1.32	≥1.12	≥1.00	≥0.90	≥0.82
Excellent	1.20-1.33	1.15-1.31	0.99-1.11	0.89-0.99	0.80-0.89	0.72-0.81
Good	1.07-1.19	1.00-1.14	0.89-0.98	0.81-0.88	0.72-0.79	0.67-0.71
Fair	0.90-1.06	0.89-0.99	0.79-0.88	0.73-0.80	0.64-0.71	0.58-0.66
Poor	≤0.89	≤0.88	≤0.78	≤0.72	≤0.63	≤0.57
FEMALES						
Superior	≥0.78	≥0.81	≥0.71	≥0.63	≥0.56	≥0.55
Excellent	0.66-0.77	0.71-0.80	0.61-0.70	0.55-0.62	0.49-0.55	0.48-0.54
Good	0.59-0.65	0.60-0.70	0.54-0.60	0.51-0.54	0.44-0.48	0.43-0.47
Fair	0.54-0.58	0.52-0.59	0.48-0.53	0.44-0.50	0.40-0.43	0.39-0.42
Poor	≤0.53	≤0.51	≤0.47	≤0.43	≤0.39	≤0.38

Reprinted, by permission, from The Cooper Institute for Aerobics Research, revised 2001, *The Physical Fitness Specialist Certification Manual.* (Dallas, TX: The Cooper Institute for Aerobics Research).

TABLE 6.9B—1 RM Norms for the Leg Press

Rating	Age					
	<20	20-29	30-39	40-49	50-59	60+
MALES						
Superior	≥2.28	≥2.13	≥1.93	≥1.82	≥1.71	≥1.62
Excellent	2.05-2.27	1.98-2.12	1.78-1.92	1.69-1.81	1.59-1.70	1.50-1.61
Good	1.91-2.04	1.84-1.97	1.66-1.77	1.58-1.68	1.47-1.58	1.39-1.49
Fair	1.71-1.90	1.64-1.83	1.53-1.65	1.45-1.57	1.33-1.46	1.26-1.38
Poor	≤1.70	≤1.63	≤1.52	≤1.44	≤1.32	≤1.25
FEMALES						
Superior	≥1.71	≥1.68	≥1.47	≥1.37	≥1.25	≥1.18
Excellent	1.60-1.70	1.51-1.67	1.34-1.46	1.24-1.36	1.11-1.24	1.05-1.17
Good	1.39-1.59	1.38-1.50	1.22-1.33	1.14-1.23	1.00-1.10	0.94-1.04
Fair	1.23-1.38	1.23-1.37	1.10-1.21	1.03-1.13	0.89-0.99	0.86-0.93
Poor	≤1.22	≤1.22	≤1.09	≤1.02	≤0.88	≤0.85

Reprinted, by permission, from The Cooper Institute for Aerobics Research, revised 2001, *The Physical Fitness Specialist Certification Manual.* (Dallas, TX: The Cooper Institute for Aerobics Research).

Case Study 6.3

Angela is instructing a 23-year-old client (body weight = 65 kg) in a 1 RM bench press. First she demonstrates the action to the client emphasising to breathe out with the "upward lift" and breathe in on the downward phase. The client then practices the lift without weight. Suggest an initial weight for the test and the procedure for the 1 RM test. The client's 1 RM for the bench press is 35 kg. Provide appropriate information for Angela to give her client.

Key Issues

1. Is the 1 RM bench press an appropriate test for this client?

2. How is initial weight determined? How are the increments determined?

3. How can the client be encouraged to continue?

4. What information do norm tables suggest about the client's upper body strength? How can this information be reported to the client and how can it be used to prescribe exercise?

It can be intimidating, difficult and even unsafe for some groups of people to perform a maximum exercise. Maximal strength testing is not recommended for

▶ hypertensives, because of the possible excessive increase in blood pressure;

▶ diabetics with diagnosed retinopathy, because of the risk of eye damage;

▶ children, because of possible damage to the epiphyseal growth plates;

▶ pregnant women;

▶ individuals with musculoskeletal injuries; and

▶ individuals with arthritis in stages of pain or inflammation.

Contraindicated groups and people unaccustomed to resistance training may prefer a less strenuous test. A multiple RM test is one method of submaximally assessing muscular strength. A process similar to that used for a 1 RM is employed, except clients perform a set number of repetitions and lift until only that number (selected from 2-10) of lifts. For example, a 3 RM (the maximum weight that can be lifted three times) on the bench press and leg press may be used to assess upper and lower body strength. Performing tests such as a 10 RM can be useful for monitoring the progress of a resistance training program, and clients can learn to self-progress (increase resistance to maintain a 10 RM).

RM testing is generally useful for most individuals and groups who have access to equipment with increasing resistance. However, sometimes resistance equipment is not available, or there is a need for more specialised testing measuring isokinetic strength. Body weight testing and isokinetic testing may be beneficial in these respective situations.

Body weight exercises can be performed to assess dynamic muscular strength and endurance. Chin-ups (with added ankle weights if needed) can be used to assess upper body strength, and timed tests such as a 60-s push-up test (perform as many push-ups as possible in 60 s) can be used to assess muscular endurance. This type of assessment is advantageous for many groups because it does not require equipment and can be performed anywhere. Ensuring client safety is paramount during all of these tests.

Isokinetic strength can be assessed using specialised equipment. The speed of movement is preselected and kept constant (0° to 300°) and muscular torque is measured. Muscular strength is typically assessed with low velocity (30° to 60°), muscular endurance assessed with medium veloc-ity (120° to 180°) and power assessed with high velocity (240° to 300°). Because of the high cost of the equipment, most isokinetic testing is performed in either rehabilitation settings after musculoskeletal injury or for specific athletic testing.

Safety

Safety is an important issue with muscular strength and endurance testing. Musculoskeletal injury and inappropriate haemodynamic responses can occur without control of specific safety items. Because there are enormous variations in the equipment that can be used for strength testing, the tester should be familiar with the equipment, testing space, testing procedures and movement technique. Clients should perform a cardiovascular warm-up before testing; they should also be taught the correct movement technique and posture and be familiarised with the movement without resistance. Correct breathing technique—breathing out with exertion and breathing in with relaxation—should be taught (to avoid the **Valsalva manoeuvre**). Inappropriate equipment settings, inadequate warm-up and incorrect client technique can increase the risk of musculoskeletal injury and reduce the effectiveness of the tests.

Flexibility

The ability of a joint to move through its complete range of motion (ROM), or flexibility, is important for most sports and for general health. Adequate flexibility is important for

▶ preventing musculoskeletal injury,

▶ maintaining functional independence,

▶ executing daily activities that require a certain amount of flexibility (bending down, twisting), and

▶ performing most sporting activities.

Flexibility is related to age, gender, body type and physical activity. Flexibility decreases with age because of reduced compliance of connective tissue, and females generally have greater joint flexibility than males (because of different pelvic structure and sex hormones). Compared with individuals with low body fat, individuals with high body fat can have limited mobility around joints. Physically inactive individuals are less flexible, although regular physical activity has been shown to increase flexibility.

Sport performance may be limited by poor flexibility, and some sporting injuries can be prevented with adequate flexibility and stretching activities. Some groups of athletes (e.g., gymnasts, swimmers) are at risk of joint laxity and hypermobility of joints; care must be taken when testing flexibility and prescribing flexibility exercises.

As with testing for muscular strength and endurance, measurement of flexibility is joint specific; that is, one single test does not accurately assess flexibility of the entire body. Depending on client goals and needs, flexibility tests may have to be performed at multiple sites. Clients should be instructed in the correct technique, and the stretch should be stopped if painful. Flexibility increases by up to 20% after a warm-up, so muscles should be warmed up before testing. For example, the client should perform repetitive activity before flexibility tests, such as a test of CRF or 5 to 10 min of low-intensity cycling or walking. Multiple trials should be carried out during a test and the best value recorded.

Flexibility of specific joints can be measured directly with goniometers (a protractor-type instrument with arms to measure degree of rotation) or indirectly with tape measures. A goniometer measures range of motion as a degree of movement that can be assessed in most joints and compared with average values (see Schell & Leelarthaepin 1994). Testers must be trained for results to be accurate.

Indirect assessment of joint ROM and muscle flexibility using tape measures is more common in health and fitness settings. Because of the incidence of low back pain and the subsequent risk of injury, tests to assess lower body, and particularly lower back, flexibility are included more frequently than tests to assess upper body flexibility. The sit-and-reach test is a common measure of lower back and hamstring muscle flexibility. The client sits on the floor with a metre stick between his or her legs, both legs straight and heels positioned at the 35-cm mark or against the edge of the box (if using a standard sit-and-reach box). The client slowly leans forward along the stick as far as possible. Measurement from the fingertips is taken and the process is repeated three times, with the best result recorded. Australian fitness norms for the sit-and-reach test are shown in table 6.10.

It is sometimes difficult to find appropriate norms for upper body flexibility tests because of the reduced use of indirect tests to assess upper body flexibility. The "arm over/under" is an example of one indirect measure of upper body flexibility, with norms developed for Australian University students (Schell and Leelarthaepin 1994). The testing procedure, shown in figure 6.11, is as follows:

1. Mark the 7th cervical vertebra.

2. Testing the left side of the body first, have the subject reach over the left shoulder and down the spine as far as possible.

3. Measure the difference between the tip of the longest finger and the mark; record the value as positive if the finger is below the mark and negative if the finger is above the mark.

4. Repeat the procedure.

5. Have the subject reach behind and up the back with the back of the left hand against the spine.

6. Measure the difference between the tip of the longest finger and the mark; record the value as positive if the finger reaches higher than the mark and negative if the finger is below the mark.

Case Study 6.4

Fiona and Marcus are in the process of opening a commercial health club. Consider the two-step process to help design the fitness assessment that will be offered to all clients.

Key Issues

1. Why is it important to profile clients? What factors should be measured?

2. What protocols will provide valid and appropriate results? Should several protocol options be available for specific fitness parameters?

3. What is the most appropriate test order?

4. Approximately how long will the assessment take? Will this amount of time be acceptable to most clients?

Percentiles	Age					
	18-29	**30-39**	**40-49**	**50-59**	**60-69**	**70-78**
			MALES			
5	25.4	28.1	25.6	21.0	16.5	—
25	38.1	38.5	35.0	32.0	29.0	22.0
50	44.1	43.0	41.3	38.0	35.5	32.5
75	49.9	48.1	45.8	45.2	42.5	37.7
95	57.3	54.7	53.4	55.0	51.3	56.6
Mean	43.4	42.7	40.5	37.8	35.0	30.0
Standard deviation	9.0	7.7	7.9	9.9	10.8	13.3
Number of subjects	85	110	127	95	91	24
			FEMALES			
5	36.6	32.9	26.5	25.1	14.4	—
25	43.6	39.9	39.4	36.2	37.1	37.0
50	48.4	44.4	45.0	42.9	43.5	45.0
75	52.5	50.5	50.9	47.7	46.9	52.0
95	59.9	57.6	57.3	54.2	53.9	56.7
Mean	47.8	44.7	44.1	41.5	40.2	41.1
Standard deviation	6.5	8.2	10.1	8.9	11.4	15.2
Number of subjects	81	125	125	106	73	24

TABLE 6.10—Australian Fitness Norms for the Sit-and-Reach Test

Measurements in cm. Reaching one's toes equals 35 cm.

Reprinted, by permission, from C. Gore and D. Edwards, 1992, *Australian fitness norms.* (South Australia: Children's Health Development Foundation), 32.

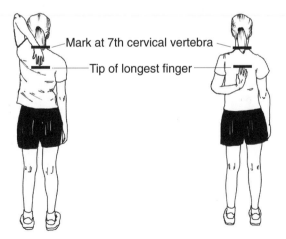

FIGURE 6.11   The "arm over/under" test assesses upper body flexibility.

Mark at 7th cervical vertebra

Tip of longest finger

7. Perform the same procedure twice with the right arm.

8. Add the best over and under scores for the left and the right arms together and compare with norms (see table 6.11).

Gait Analysis

Clinical gait analysis is the study of an individual's walking pattern. Gait assessment is used with information from other sources, such as medical diagnostic reports, to develop intervention programs to improve walking efficiency and reduce the risk of injury. This information may be useful for athletes,

TABLE 6.11—Norms for the Arm Over/Under Test of Upper Body Flexibility

Rating	Male	Female
Superior	30.0	31.8
Good	16.8	25.0
Satisfactory	10.2	19.4
Fair	3.7	11.6
Poor	–9.0	3.9

From tests with Australian university students.

Adapted, by permission, from J. Schell and B. Leelarthaepin, 1994, *Physical fitness assessment in exercise and sport science*, 2nd ed. (New South Wales: Leelar Biomediscience Services), 287-288.

individuals with neurological or musculoskeletal disorders, or individuals at risk of falls and fractures. Gait assessment is also a useful tool to help individuals with type 1 and type 2 diabetes identify pressure points that may eventually lead to foot ulcerations. Interventions can be implemented to correct gait and reduce these pressure points, thus decreasing the risk of ulceration. In addition, gait analysis provides an objective assessment for individuals with prescribed orthotics and prosthetics.

Sophisticated techniques such as force platforms (measures ground reaction force) and EMG (measures the electrical activity of the contracting muscle) are used in motion analysis laboratories to assess gait (Whittle 1996). In field situations, general gait parameters can be observed and used to assist gait assessment. Typically, the client is instructed to walk a specified distance (3-20 m) and is observed visually, and possibly videotaped, for future reference and analysis. Common gait parameters include

▶ *cadence:* the steps taken per minute [steps counted × 60/time (s)];

▶ *cycle time:* the time in seconds to complete one walking cycle [time (s) × 2/steps counted];

▶ *stride length:* the length of one full stride, measured in metres [speed (m/s) × cycle time (s)]; and

▶ *speed:* a measurement of how fast the specified distance was completed, measured in metres per second [stride length (m)/cycle time (s) or measured with a stop watch].

Table 6.12 presents norms for each of these parameters for males and females of different ages.

Pre-Test Preparation

To ensure test accuracy and validity, participants should be given careful and thorough instructions. In general, participants are requested to refrain from food, alcohol, caffeine and tobacco for at least 3 h before physical fitness testing. Ingestion of these items can cause an increase in heart rate and blood pressure, leading to inaccurate results. In addition, test validity is improved if participants do not exercise on the day of the test, get adequate sleep the night before and wear appropriate clothing. Test order should be standardised. Because of the dehydration effect of cardiorespiratory exercise and the subsequent effect on skinfold measures, body composition should be tested before CRF. Fatigue can affect gait, so gait analysis should occur before cardiorespiratory and muscular strength and endurance testing. Muscles and muscle groups should be warmed up before muscular strength and endurance testing and flexibility testing; consequently, these tests are often performed after a cardiorespiratory test. Although a physical fitness assessment does not need to include all of the factors discussed in this chapter, the test order for a full physical fitness assessment is

1. resting haemodynamics,
2. body composition,
3. gait analysis,
4. CRF,
5. muscular strength and endurance, and
6. flexibility.

TABLE 6.12—Normal Ranges for Gait Parameters

FEMALES

Age	Cadence (steps/min)	Cycle time (s)	Stride length (m)	Speed (m/s)
13-14	103-150	0.80-1.17	0.99-1.55	0.90-1.62
15-17	100-144	0.83-1.20	1.03-1.57	0.92-1.64
18-49	98-138	0.87-1.22	1.06-1.58	0.94-1.66
50-64	97-137	0.88-1.24	1.04-1.56	0.91-1.63
65-80	96-136	0.88-1.25	0.94-1.46	0.80-1.52

MALES

Age	Cadence (steps/min)	Cycle time (s)	Stride length (m)	Speed (m/s)
13-14	100-149	0.81-1.20	1.06-1.64	0.95-1.67
15-17	96-142	0.85-1.25	1.15-1.75	1.03-1.75
18-49	91-135	0.89-1.32	1.25-1.85	1.10-1.82
50-64	82-126	0.95-1.46	1.22-1.82	0.96-1.68
65-80	81-125	0.96-1.48	1.11-1.71	0.81-1.61

Approximate range (95% limits) for general gait parameters in free-speed walking by normal subjects of different ages.

Reprinted, by permission, from M.W. Whittle, 1996, *Gait analysis.* (Oxford: Butterworth, Heinemann), appendix 1.

A standardised lab environment helps ensure cardiorespiratory test results are accurate. Room temperature should be maintained between 20 and 22° C and humidity should equal <60%. Higher temperatures or humidity causes an increase in heart rate, which results in an underestimation of $\dot{V}O_2$max. As well, it is expected that personnel who provide fitness assessments are either tertiary qualified in exercise or sport science or are experienced medical practitioners.

Summary

Physical fitness assessments provide useful data for individuals who, for a range of reasons, are adopting or changing a physical activity program. A host of factors can be evaluated through physical fitness assessments to help with subsequent exercise and physical activity prescription or to help motivate an individual to adopt and maintain an exercise program. For the majority of the population, the most commonly measured factors include body composition, cardiorespiratory fitness and muscular strength, endurance and flexibility. Assessment of body composition is important for individuals wishing to reduce or maintain body weight and for athletes seeking to enhance performance. Assessment of cardiorespiratory fitness is helpful for prescription of physical activity and exercise. Muscular strength and endurance are important across all age groups and populations, and muscle flexibility and joint ROM are measured to assess risk of injury. Additional measures such as gait assessment can be useful with some populations.

A two-step process can help guide the design of a physical fitness assessment. Factor selection (step 1) is based on evaluation requirements (client profiling, progress) and intended client goals (health, condition, performance) and needs (pre-activity screening). There are many tests to assess each of these factors. Test and protocol selection (step 2) depends on accuracy needed, cost, validity, available equipment and client acceptability. Results from these tests can help optimise physical activity prescription, monitor progress and motivate clients.

Selected Glossary Terms

agility—The ability to change direction while maintaining balance.

anthropometry—The scientific measurement of the human body and its skeleton, including measures of circumferences, body diameters, skinfold fat thickness and body mass.

balance—The ability to control physical movement of the body and maintain stability.

body mass index (BMI)—The ratio of body mass (in kg) to height (in metres squared), expressed as $kg \cdot m^{-2}$; a simple method to determine an optimal body weight range.

cable tensiometer—A device used to measure isometric strength at a specific angle.

cardiorespiratory fitness (CRF)—The ability to perform prolonged exercise, quantified in a test of maximum oxygen consumption ($\dot{V}O_2max$) or time to fatigue at a certain work rate.

dynamometer—A device used to measure isometric strength.

ergometer—A device used to measure muscular work performance and able to be calibrated, for example, the Monark bicycle ergometer.

flexibility—The ability of a specific joint to move through its full range of motion.

gait—Walking pattern.

girth—The circumference value of a given site using a standard tape measure.

hypokinetic diseases—Chronic diseases associated with low levels of physical activity and movement.

muscular endurance—The ability of a muscle or muscle group to generate force repeatedly or continuously over time; an important component of sports requiring repetitive application of force, such as swimming, rowing or cycling.

muscular strength—The maximum force a muscle or muscle group can generate in a single maximal contraction or movement.

rating of perceived exertion (RPE)—A participant's estimation of the level of effort undertaken during a specific physical activity; valid and reliable scales exist to help participants rate level of physical exertion (refer to figure 6.9).

repetition maximum (RM)—The greatest amount of weight lifted in a specified number of repetitions; for example, a 1 RM is the greatest amount of weight lifted once, whereas a 3 RM is the greatest amount of weight lifted in three consecutive motions.

respiratory exchange ratio (RER)—The ratio of expired carbon dioxide to consumed oxygen.

skinfold measurement—A measure of subcutaneous fat at a given site using specialised calipers.

Valsalva manoeuvre—Forced exhalation against a closed glottis, which causes increased intrathoracic pressure, thus reducing venous return and possibly leading to excessively elevated systolic and diastolic blood pressure.

Student Activities and Study Questions

1. List three tests to indirectly estimate $\dot{V}O_2$max. State two advantages and two disadvantages of each. Give one situation in which each test would be the most appropriate to use. Why?

2. Which of the tests in question 1 have been studied with older populations (>60 years) and which with younger (<40 years)? What were the justifications for using the selected tests? What other test(s) could have been useful? Why?

3. Develop a battery of tests for a public health physical activity program aimed at reducing the risk of falls in the elderly. Describe the specific tests, test order and expected time to complete the tests. Who would/could administer these tests? What results do you expect?

4. Have three or four subjects participate in three different submaximal cardiorespiratory tests. Compare the norm values calculated for each. Discuss the implications of test results.

5. Measure BMI, WHR and sum of six skinfolds on 10 subjects. Discuss the results obtained. How are the results similar? Different?

6. Observe comprehensive physical fitness tests in several locations such as commercial fitness facilities, community-based physical activity programs, elite sporting associations, club sporting teams or clinical programs for individuals with special needs. Briefly explain each of the tests observed. Why were each of the tests included? What benefits would subjects receive from the results of each of these tests? How and why are the battery of tests similar and different between each of the locations?

CHAPTER 7

Developing Prescriptions for Physical Activity

A prescription for physical activity is a guide that describes the recommendations for participation. Physical activity prescription depends on the needs and goals of the client and is designed to help the client achieve these benefits effectively and safely. Although there are many goals for participating in physical activity, most of these goals can be grouped into one of four categories: health, fitness, weight or sport performance. The health benefits associated with participation in physical activity are numerous. For example, an individual may wish to participate in physical activity to improve psychological health, to follow physician recommendations or to reduce the risk of cardiovascular disease. Many individuals begin an exercise or physical activity program to increase physical fitness, including aerobic fitness, muscular strength or flexibility. Weight control is another common reason for exercising, and clients may wish to exercise to maintain weight, lose weight or gain weight. Recreational and elite athletes exercise to improve sport performance; the prescription details for athletes are included in chapter 11.

One of the basic functions of exercise management is to consider the desired benefits and then prescribe appropriate and effective programs. Program design has changed significantly over the past few decades. Thirty years ago, people interested in improving health and fitness were told to join an exercise group or simply jog. Research then showed that a more individualised approach to exercise prescriptions was safer and more effective for helping clients meet physical fitness goals. Recommendations were refined (3-5 days per week at 40-85% HRR) to target the individual, and this required a specific approach to prescription. It has been recently demonstrated that moderate amounts of regular physical activity yield many health benefits. The USSG and ACSM currently recommend a more general approach to prescription: accumulation of 30 min of physical activity on at least five days per week. Thus, exercise prescription and programming have again changed to now include promotion of daily physical activity in addition to individualised weekly exercise. This variety widens the possibilities for the individual to remain physically active and for exercise managers to develop appropriate exercise and physical activity regimes for different needs and goals.

Daily and weekly physical activity prescriptions yield physical, health, social and psychological benefits. The challenge is to design a program that maximises adoption and encourages the maintenance of lifelong physical activity. Individuals with goals to improve health may benefit from a more general prescription, whereas a specific traditional prescription may be more appropriate for individuals who want to increase cardiorespiratory fitness or reduce body weight. Goals for individual sports require an even more specific approach to prescription.

Activity training follows the **principle of specificity,** which states that specific types of physical fitness (e.g., cardiorespiratory endurance, muscular strength, flexibility) improve with specific types of training. For example, an individual whose goal is to increase cardiorespiratory fitness (CRF) requires an exercise prescription based on aerobic activities; an individual whose goal is to increase muscular strength requires a prescription that concentrates on resistance training. The purposes of physical activity prescriptions are to

- provide guidance to the client,
- ensure client's needs and goals are met,
- ensure physical activity is within the limits of specific health concerns (e.g., does not raise blood pressure excessively),
- provide a balanced program of various aspects of fitness,
- recommend variety to avoid boredom, and
- enhance the maintenance of lifelong activity.

To develop safe and effective physical activity prescriptions, a certain amount of information is required from the client: at minimum, health status, risk of participation, needs, goals and choice of activity. As described in the previous chapter, it is usually optimal for prescriptions to be based on the results of a comprehensive physical fitness assessment. However, performance of physical fitness tests is not always possible or feasible, and appropriate physical activity prescriptions can be based on other information, such as the results of screening or consultation. This chapter presents the basic components of physical activity prescriptions and the manipulation of these variables to meet various goals and needs of individual clients and groups. Specifically, information is presented on the prescription process for CRF, muscular strength and endurance, and flexibility. Underpinning the prescription process is the careful consideration of issues associated with program adoption and maintenance. Section 3 presents more specific information on exercise prescription for those with special health concerns and for athletes.

Components of Physical Activity Prescriptions

Prescriptions of all types, both for individuals and groups, follow a similar recommended format. That is, most activity sessions should include a warm-up,

a physical activity component and a cool-down. The warm-up is performed immediately before the activity component. Typically, a warm-up is 5 to 10 min in duration, includes stretches of the muscle groups to be exercised, may include light calisthenics and consists of an activity that gradually increases in intensity. A warm-up

- reduces the risk of musculoskeletal injury (particularly before high-intensity activity),
- increases body temperature,
- gradually increases heart rate and systolic blood pressure,
- reduces the risk of cardiac arrhythmias,
- enhances psychological readiness for activity, and
- improves muscular performance.

The physical activity component is the basis of the physical activity prescription and may include endurance, muscular strength, flexibility and recreational activities. Each of these is discussed in detail in subsequent sections. A cool-down performed immediately after the conditioning part of a workout consists of 5 to 15 min of activity at a reduced intensity and repeated stretches. A cool-down

- enhances venous return, reducing the risk of venous pooling and post-exercise hypotension and cardiovascular complications,
- promotes heat dissipation,
- increases flexibility,
- increases removal of lactic acid,
- may reduce muscle soreness, and
- promotes return of heart rate and blood pressure to pre-exercise levels.

Prescription Variables

Several common variables are found in all types of physical activity prescriptions. These variables include

- frequency: number of sessions per week,
- intensity: force or difficulty of the prescription,
- duration: length of the session,
- mode: type of activity, and
- progression: increases over time.

Each of these variables can be manipulated to help meet individual or group needs and goals. More important, there are many combinations that provide equally effective activity prescriptions. The challenge for the exercise manager is to develop a physical activity prescription that enhances health and performance while encouraging continued participation. Figure 7.1 presents a flow chart to assist with selection of each of the variables.

To determine mode at the individual level, the client's choice, accessibility, health constraints and previous experience must be addressed. Once the mode or modes have been determined, time constraints need to be examined so that duration of each session can be recommended. With the mode and duration identified, client goals and needs should then be addressed. As well, with consideration given to the prescribed duration, exercise intensity can be suggested. Recognition of the client's past experience with physical activity and readiness to become active or change activity levels can help when recommending activity frequency. Finally, the exercise prescription should include strategies to help the client maintain lifelong activity (refer to chapter 4).

A similar flow chart can be used to design group prescriptions. Rather than consider these issues with individual clients, the targeted group is examined. A needs assessment identifies group choice, goals, needs and experience, and thus can direct program development. If a needs analysis is not available, relevant normative data and results for studies with similar populations can be used to estimate group choice, goals and needs.

Mode

An enormous range of activities can be performed to gain health-, fitness- or sport-related benefits. Activities are grouped according to what components of physical fitness they help improve—cardiorespiratory, musculoskeletal or flexibility. To maximise activity adoption and maintenance, it is necessary to consider client goals, choice of activity, access to activities, health constraints, and skills and experience when recommending mode of activity (refer to figure 7.1).

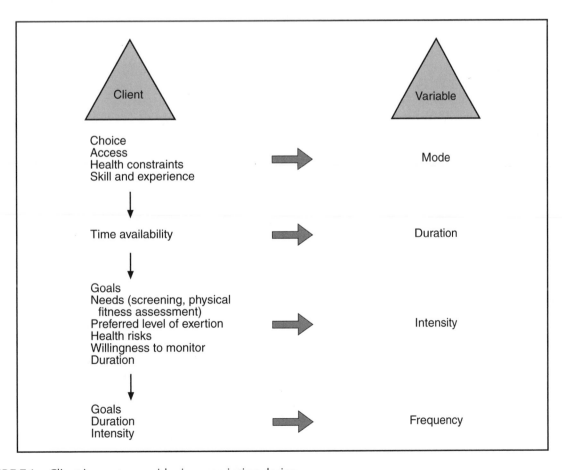

FIGURE 7.1 Client issues to consider in prescription design.

Although many modes of activity are appropriate for general health, fitness and weight control goals, the selected mode must be available to the client and considered enjoyable by the client. Other factors must also be taken into consideration. An individual is likely to drop out of a program if swimming or aquaexercise is recommended but the client is unable to pay the sessional cost. However, adherence may be enhanced if walking is prescribed and the client lives near a large park with a walking track considered to be accessible and safe. Walking is a preferred activity for many because it is familiar, easily accessible and can be performed anywhere. Even so, a client is unlikely to maintain a walking regime if he or she lives in an inner-city suburb deemed unsafe. Hence, it is critical that exercise modality is chosen carefully, based on client preference, accessibility, time availability, past experience and skill level.

Activity selection is more restricted when the goal is to increase muscular strength. Types of activities prescribed to increase muscular strength are described in the following sections and shown in table 7.6. Sport-specific goals may result in an even greater restriction of choices. Selected mode for group programs targets the expected interest of the group—dance, stretching, team sports and circuit training will be attractive to different groups.

Health constraints may prohibit recommendations for some activities. For example, musculoskeletal and orthopaedic injuries may preclude participation in some weight-bearing activities and resistance training exercises. Certain groups, such as the obese, have a higher risk of musculoskeletal injuries and may benefit from non-weight-bearing activities such as swimming and cycling. At the same time, specific resistance training exercises may assist rehabilitation from musculoskeletal injuries. Specific modes of training may be recommended for athletes, and these are described in chapter 11.

Duration

The duration of a particular activity session is clearly related to both the intensity and frequency of the activity. At the individual level, the client's time constraints need to be considered. To maximise adoption and maintenance of exercise, the time factor in exercise prescription needs to be flexible and adaptable to meet individual client needs, goals and time constraints. Research has shown that sessions of longer duration at lower intensity yield similar health benefits, improvements in fitness and improvements in body composition as those of shorter duration and higher intensity. Consideration of time available for participation guides the recommendations for intensity and frequency. For example, a client may state she has 1 to 2 h on three afternoons available for exercise, but availability is limited during other parts of the week. It is decided to prescribe activity for 30 to 60 min three times per week. Alternatively, a client may state that he has no time for activity; assessment of his weekly schedule reveals long work hours and family commitments. A prescription of two 15-min daily walking sessions (to and from a distant bus stop) is recommended.

Group programs tend to be scheduled several times during the week for approximately 45 to 60 min duration. Because of the reduced frequency (two to three times per week), duration is increased. The selected duration is guided by mode of activity and anticipated goals of the group.

Intensity

Activity intensity is the most complex factor of a physical activity prescription. Some evidence suggests that exercising at a preferred level of exertion may help improve adherence and that, for many, the preferred level of exertion is lower than traditional recommendations. Not only should activity intensity be prescribed to help meet the individual goals of the client, it also must take into account individual needs, preferred level of exertion, health risks, willingness to monitor intensity, and duration of activity. For example, a client with the goal to reduce body fat prefers low-intensity activities with a rating of perceived exertion (RPE) of 10 to 11. It is recommended she walk at this exertion for 45 to 60 min on most days. She has difficulty with this time commitment, so it is decided that she will walk at her preferred intensity for 60 min, 3 days per week and at a higher intensity (RPE of 11-13) for 30 min, 3 days per week. For some clients, particularly those with hypertension or coronary artery disease, participation in high-intensity activity (RPE ≥14) may be considered unsafe. Examination of health risks helps guide recommendations for activity intensity.

Intensity of physical activity can be recommended, measured and monitored in several ways. The most efficient method is based on data obtained from fitness tests before the prescription. Table 7.1 presents a range of methods used to monitor exercise intensity and the recommended ranges to improve CRF; advantages and disadvantages must be considered when selecting the most appropriate method for the individual or group. Group and community programs consider group goals and prescribe activity based on anticipated intensity for the group. The recent recommendations to accumulate 30 min of daily moderate physical activity minimise the importance of monitoring intensity. However, intensity level is important for prescription of CRF; many of the methods to monitor intensity are thus relevant only to CRF prescription.

Heart Rate Methods

A range of heart rate (HR) is often prescribed to gauge intensity of cardiorespiratory prescriptions. HR methods are based on the linear relationship between cardiorespiratory exercise HR and oxygen uptake ($\dot{V}O_2$), work rate and energy expenditure in a given activity. This linear relationship is not as reliable during muscular strength training because of the pressor response. The pressor response occurs because resistance exercises, prescribed to build

TABLE 7.1—Methods to Monitor Exercise Intensity, Recommendations, Advantages and Disadvantages

Method	Description	Recommendations	Advantages	Disadvantages
Target heart rate	Percentage of maximum heart rate or APMHR	Cardiorespiratory 55-90%	Range of intensity Specific Prescriptive	Need to palpate pulse
Heart rate reserve (HRR)	Resisting heart rate is considered and a percentage is prescribed	Cardiorespiratory 40/50-85%	Correlates to $\dot{V}O_2$ Specific Prescriptive	Need to palpate pulse
$\dot{V}O_2$max	Direct plot of HR vs. O_2 uptake from maximal exercise test	Cardiorespiratory 40/50-85%	Criterion measure	Must undergo maximal exercise test
RPE	Perceived level of exercise exertion using a scale (figure 6.9)	Cardiorespiratory Daily activity Muscular strength 12-16	No need to palpate pulse Individual Self-control	Training time needed Individual levels of exertion
MET	MET levels for various activities have been determined (table 7.3)	Cardiorespiratory Daily activity Muscular strength	Allows for prescription of activity	Non-specific Individual variances not accounted for in figures
Talk test	Exercise in a range you are able to continue to talk	Daily activity	Self-control	Non-specific No data

Abbreviations: APMHR = age-predicted maximum heart rate; HR = heart rate.

muscular strength, can create an increase in intramuscular and intrathoracic pressure. These pressure increases lead to an increase in blood pressure and a reduction in stroke volume, which may then lead to a disproportionately high heart rate (e.g., not linear with $\dot{V}O_2$).

Heart rate is a simple and useful tool for monitoring exercise intensity. Typically, a percentage of maximum heart rate is prescribed. Maximum heart rate (HRmax) can be measured either directly through a maximum exercise test or predicted with an equation (predicted maximum heart rate = 220 – age); a 10 to 15% error exists in estimating age-predicted maximum heart rate (APMHR). A percentage of APMHR is prescribed with low-, moderate- and high-intensity ranges (see table 7.2). Moderate-intensity physical activity would be equivalent to 55 to 70% of APMHR, 40 to 60% of HRR and an RPE of 12 to 13. Each of these methods is described in detail as the chapter progresses.

Heart rate reserve (HRR) is another method of utilising heart rate as an indicator of exercise intensity. HRR uses resting heart rate as a measure of current fitness level, and this has been shown to correlate better with oxygen uptake. Compared with percentage of HRmax, HRR is more accurate for older individuals and those with cardiovascular disease. To calculate HRR,

1. measure resting heart rate (HRrest),
2. determine maximum heart rate (HRmax), and
3. use the following equation: HRR = (HRmax – HRrest).

Target heart rate range is then determined by multiplying a selected percentage by HRR and adding HRrest (Target HR = (selected percentage) (HRR) + HRrest). For example, a 64-year-old subject with a resting heart rate of 68 bpm would like to exercise at 40 to 60% of his HRR. His predicted HRmax is 156 bpm (220-64); HRR = 88 bpm (156-68); and target HR is 103 (0.4 × 88 + 68) to 121 bpm (0.6 × 88 + 68). A percentage of HRR is recommended to meet client needs and goals (refer to table 7.2).

Clearly, a client must be capable and willing to monitor pulse rate if methods based on heart rate are to be useful. The use of a heart rate range to prescribe intensity may therefore be appropriate for only some clients. Other methods, such as rating of perceived exertion or metabolic equivalent, discussed in the following sections, may be more appropriate for those who are uninterested or are incapable of palpating pulse.

Rating of Perceived Exertion

Rating of perceived exertion (RPE) is a measure of an individual's perception of how hard an activity is. Borg (1998) formalised this concept into a scale. The Borg RPE scale ranges from 6 to 20, and the CR10 scale, a subsequent 1 to 10 scale, has been devised (refer to figure 6.9). Clients subjectively assign a number in the scale to their perceived level of exertion. On the RPE scale, low levels of exertion correspond to a rating of 10 or 11, moderate is 12 or 13 and high-intensity is 14 to 16 (refer to table 7.2).

A strong correlation exists between RPE and intensity of exercise as measured by heart rate. For example, Dishman and colleagues (1994) initially classified subjects as either high or low active and asked subjects to cycle at a self-selected intensity. Both groups chose to cycle at similar relative intensities (although the absolute intensity was higher for the high active group) and expressed similar RPE values, which ranged from 11 to 14 (on the Borg RPE scale) for the 20-min exercise sessions. The results of this study suggest that encouraging individuals to exercise at preferred intensities using the RPE concept may not only assist in improving adherence, but it appears that individuals choose an intensity that may elicit beneficial health and fitness effects.

TABLE 7.2—Low-, Moderate- and High-Intensity Ranges for Measures of Activity Intensity

	HRmax (%)	HRR (%)	RPE (6-20 scale)
Low	35-55	20-40	10-11
Moderate	55-70	40-60	12-13
High	70-90	60-85	14-16

Adapted, by permission, from ACSM, 2000, *ACSM's guidelines for exercise testing and prescription*, 6th ed. (Philadelphia: Lippincott Williams & Wilkins), 150.

Clients must be taught to use the scale and allowed to practice with the scale; it has been suggested that at least three training days are needed to reduce errors. RPE reflects local factors at lower intensities and central factors at higher intensities. For example, leg fatigue while cycling at lower intensities may influence RPE, whereas shortness of breath may influence RPE at higher intensities. This tool may therefore be inappropriate for some individuals, but it is the method of choice for many clients and groups. RPE is one method that may help clients monitor intensity without the need to palpate pulse or measure $\dot{V}O_2$max. In addition, this is often the method of choice for clients taking medication that affects exercise heart rate (e.g., beta-blockers). RPE is often used if heart rate data is not available from CRF tests.

Maximum Oxygen Uptake

Intensity can also be prescribed as a percentage of maximum oxygen uptake ($\dot{V}O_2$max). Current ACSM (2000) recommendations suggest the use of $\dot{V}O_2$reserve ($\dot{V}O_2$R). The concept of $\dot{V}O_2$R is similar to HRR ($\dot{V}O_2$R = $\dot{V}O_2$max − $\dot{V}O_2$rest). Resting oxygen consumption is accounted for in the following equation:

$$\dot{V}O_2\text{rest} = 3.5 \text{ ml} \cdot \text{kg}^{-1} \cdot \text{min}^{-1} \text{ and target } \dot{V}O_2 =$$
$$(\text{exercise intensity}) \times (\dot{V}O_2\text{max} - \dot{V}O_2\text{rest}) + \dot{V}O_2\text{rest}$$

Heart rate is plotted against $\dot{V}O_2$, or work rate, during an exercise test, and target heart rates are determined by finding the heart rates that correspond to the recommended percentages of $\dot{V}O_2$ max.

Oxygen consumption may also be determined to correspond with specific lactate levels, which can be a useful tool for some athletes (see chapter 11). Although $\dot{V}O_2$max is the most accurate measure of intensity, a maximal exercise test is usually necessary, and disadvantages such as safety, cost, time and comfort for the client must be considered. Calculation of target $\dot{V}O_2$ using $\dot{V}O_2$R or a percentage of $\dot{V}O_2$max can be useful for specifying METs (metabolic equivalents).

MET Method

Another way to prescribe intensity is the MET method. The metabolic equivalent (MET) reflects multiples of resting metabolic rate. One MET is defined as $3.5 \text{ ml} \cdot \text{kg}^{-1} \cdot \text{min}^{-1}$. MET values have been calculated for various activities (see table 7.3), and activities within a certain MET range may be prescribed. For example, activities in the 4 MET to 6 MET range may be prescribed for an inactive client; the client is able to choose to walk on flat ground at about $6 \text{ km} \cdot \text{h}^{-1}$ (4 mph) or cycle at 75 W.

Obviously, there are inaccuracies with this method because of individual differences in mechanical efficiency. To reduce the variability of

TABLE 7.3—Approximate MET Values for Various Activities

MET value	Activity
5.0	Stationary cycling, 75 W
7.0	Stationary cycling, 150 W
8.0	Circuit training
4.0	Aquaerobics
5.0	Low impact aerobic dance
7.0	Rowing, moderate effort
6.0	Leisure bicycling, low effort
5.0-6.5	Dancing, (line-dancing, ballroom, Latin)
5.0	Golf, pulling clubs
6.0-8.0	Tennis
8.0	Touch football
4.0	Lawn bowling
4.0	Walking, flat at 4 km · hr^{-1}
6.0	Walking, 5% grade at 5.5 km · hr^{-1}
8.5	Jogging, flat at 8 km · hr^{-1}
8.0-11.0	Swimming laps

estimating METs, intensity should be prescribed by this method in environments with controlled equipment (e.g., treadmill, ergometers). MET levels are often used in clinical settings to recommend types of activities. MET levels can also be used with metabolic equations to estimate energy expenditure and identify specific ranges (e.g., treadmill speed and grade) to exercise within (ACSM 2000).

Other Methods

The "talk test" is often suggested as a monitor of exercise intensity (the National Heart Foundation of Australia advocates the talk test). The premise is that exertion should not exceed a level where normal conversation can be maintained. Although there is little scientific evidence concerning the use of the talk test, there may be a place for this type of monitoring with a select group of clients, given the recent recommendations for moderate-intensity daily activity. For example, individuals who do not want to measure heart rate and lack consistency in reporting RPE may find the talk test an easier monitoring tool.

Finally, each of these tools may be appropriate for some clients yet inappropriate for others. The ability to effectively prescribe activity requires careful observation and the capacity to select appropriate tools for individual clients.

Frequency

Frequency, or how often activity is recommended, can vary from daily to only a few sessions per week depending on the individual's goals and intended duration and intensity. Frequency of exercise is not an isolated factor: intensity, duration and mode must also be considered when prescribing activity. Table 7.4 provides several examples of recommendations for activity frequency.

A recommendation to participate in multiple daily physical activity sessions is appropriate for many individuals and groups. The current recommendation to accumulate 30 min of moderate-intensity physical activity daily clearly states that three sessions of 10-min duration may provide health benefits. Individuals in acute recovery phases from disease may be unable to maintain activity for more than a couple of minutes, and multiple daily sessions of short duration may accelerate the rehabilitation process. Individuals with time constraints may find it easier to be active for short periods of time several times during the day. In addition, athletes prescribed cross-training regimes (i.e., different modes of activity) might participate in two or more training sessions each day, though different modes of activity are usually performed to reduce the risk of overuse injury.

TABLE 7.4—Examples of Recommendations for Frequency of Participation in Physical Activity

Recommendation	Situation
Multiple bouts per day	Accumulation of daily physical activity
	Rehabilitation from acute and chronic disease or medical procedures
	Time limitations
	Athletic training
Daily	Physical activity for health
	Metabolic (e.g., type 1 and type 2 diabetes) or other chronic medical conditions
	Weight management
	Athletic training
Multiple sessions per week	Physical activity for fitness
	To coincide with group exercise class times
	Specific fitness parameters (e.g., strength, flexibility)

Individuals who are able (physically or with time available) to maintain longer bouts of activity may find a daily physical activity prescription useful. Health benefits can be gained from daily moderate activity, although daily vigorous activity increases the risk of injury. Individuals with some chronic diseases and conditions such as obesity and type 1 and type 2 diabetes benefit metabolically from participating in the same volume of activity every day. Furthermore, many athletes participate in some form of activity daily.

Some individuals who find it too difficult to be active every day may wish to participate in a group class that meets several times each week, or they may wish to participate in vigorous activity. Improvements and maintenance of muscular strength and flexibility can still occur with three to five sessions per week. Prescriptions that include multiple sessions per week may be more suitable for these individuals.

Progression

Over time an individual will adapt to a specific activity prescription. Once a particular program has been maintained, the client achieves a given level of fitness (or weight loss or muscle strength). Maintenance of physical and health benefits will continue if the same prescription is adhered to. To improve further, increases in frequency, duration or intensity need to occur; that is, the program must be progressed. For many individuals, maintenance of current levels is sufficient. However, others may wish to improve, and additional physical and health ben-

efits are not likely to occur unless the program changes.

The rate of program **progression** is dependent on health and fitness status, age, goals and the social and cultural environment. There are times when progression is not needed or desired, and the initial program could be considered a maintenance prescription. For example, a healthy young client who regularly plays tennis, plays touch football and swims and has a goal to maintain body weight and fitness may be happy to begin and then maintain the initial program. In contrast, goals of weight loss, increased CRF and muscle strength may require a client to progress intensity, duration or frequency. Program progression can also involve participation in new modes of activities to provide variety. Typically, progression occurs through three phases:

1. Initial conditioning: establishes individual goals and comprises a low- to moderate-intensity exercise program to minimise muscle soreness, fatigue and injury. Individuals progress at varying rates, and this stage typically lasts 4 to 6 weeks.

2. Improvement phase: aims to gradually increase the prescription so that goals can be achieved; may last 4 to 5 months.

3. Maintenance phase: aims to enhance lifelong adherence to the exercise prescription.

Progression occurs with all modes of activity. Case study 7.1 shows progression for a cardiorespiratory activity prescription; the same progression steps are recommended for muscular strength and flexibility

---

Case Study 7.1

Richard is a previously inactive 55-year-old who wishes to complete a 10K road race. The basic program design includes: (1) the initial conditioning program: a low-intensity, short-duration program; walking is prescribed 3 days per week for 12 to 20 min at an intensity of 40 to 60% HRR for the first 3 to 4 weeks; (2) improvement phase: during the next phase, intensity is increased to 50 to 85% HRR (walking and jogging) for 20 to 30 min and on 3 to 5 days per week for weeks 5 to 20; and (3) maintenance phase: finally, the prescription progresses to jogging for 30 to 60 min at 70 to 85% HRR with the intention that this prescription can be maintained indefinitely. What additional components should be included to complement and enhance this program?

Key Issues

1. What safety issues should be considered at each phase? How will these affect the prescription?

2. What strategies would help promote adoption and adherence?

prescriptions. For example, muscle strength testing revealed a client was in the 20th percentile for upper body strength. A low-volume resistance training program was prescribed for the first 4 to 6 weeks (initial phase). The same exercises were prescribed at a higher volume (e.g., increased resistance, increased repetitions) during the improvement phase. After 6 months at the improvement stage, additional exercises were introduced, and the client was taught to self-monitor intensity to increase and maintain as needed.

Caloric Threshold/Total Caloric Expenditure

Activity may also be prescribed to meet a threshold of caloric expenditure, and total caloric expenditure has recently been recommended as an alternative to prescribing activity by frequency. Frequency, intensity and duration of physical activity are combined to yield caloric expenditure. A minimal physical activity threshold of 630 kJ[150 kcal] to 1680 kJ[400 kcal]/day or 4200kJ [1,000 kcal]/wk is recommended by ACSM (2000) for health and fitness benefits. Calculation of optimal expenditure depends on the goals of the individual client. For example, ACSM recommends an optimal weekly energy expenditure of 8400kJ [2,000 kcal]/wk to assist with weight reduction. Long-term maintenance has been shown to occur with daily prescription of low- to moderate-intensity activity that expends at least 1260 kJ [300 kcal]/day (e.g., 40 to 60 min of walking at 4-5 km · h^{-1}).

Although there are inaccuracies in estimating caloric expenditure because of differences in individual energy expenditure, mechanical efficiency and skill, the caloric cost of exercise can be estimated using the equation

$$METs \times 3.5 \times body\ weight\ (kg)/48 = kJ \cdot min^{-1}$$

This method of prescribing exercise can be useful for clients who have specific fitness or weight loss targets and desire quantifiable structure. For example, a 20-year-old student would like to increase his fitness. His $\dot{V}O_2$max was estimated at 40 ml · kg^{-1} · min^{-1} (11 METs), his weight is 80 kg (176 lb), and he would like to walk or jog four times per week. The recommended initial prescription is 60% $\dot{V}O_2$max. Duration of activity is calculated as follows:

$$0.6 \times 11 = 6.6\ METs\ (brisk\ walk)$$

$$6.6\ METs \times 3.5 \times 80\ kg/48 = 38.5kJ\ k \cdot min^{-1}$$

To meet the minimum recommendation of 4200 kJ [1,000 kcal]/wk, he would have to walk briskly for 109 min/week, or four 27-min sessions per week.

The following sections discuss the prescription variables as they relate to the prescription process for specific physical fitness attributes: CRF, muscular strength and endurance, and muscular flexibility.

Cardiorespiratory Activity Prescription

Cardiorespiratory activity prescriptions are used to improve aerobic capacity (e.g., CRF), health and body composition. Aerobic activity includes longer duration, lower intensity activity relying primarily on the oxidative (aerobic) energy system. Aerobic exercise includes activities that utilise a large muscle mass and can be continued for a prolonged duration such as walking, running, swimming, cycling, some forms of dancing, and rowing. Health benefits include a reduced risk of hypertension, type 2 diabetes, cardiovascular disease and osteoporosis and improvements in blood lipids. In addition, cardiorespiratory activities are often the first mode of choice for prescriptions for body fat loss and body weight maintenance.

Mode, duration, intensity and frequency are combined to form a cardiorespiratory prescription. Historically, a specific amount of continuous exercise was suggested as a threshold to improve CRF and health. Recent research indicates that some health benefits, including improvements in CRF and body composition and the reduction of risk of cardiovascular disease and stress, can occur with several short daily physical activity sessions. Benefits have been shown to occur with 10-min bouts of activity; it is not yet known if shorter bouts yield similar benefits. Chapter 2 discusses the health continuum, which postulates that health and fitness benefits begin to accrue with minimum activity, progressing to greater benefits sustained with increased volumes of activity. As discussed in chapters 2 and 3, this is essentially the public health message behind recent recommendations and campaigns to increase participation in physical activity. Given the small percentage of adults participating in regular exercise, it may be that emphasis on more frequent, shorter and moderate physical activity may be more attractive to a larger percentage of the population. Table 7.5 presents general recommendations for cardio-

---

TABLE 7.5—General Recommendations for Frequency, Intensity, Duration and Type of Activity for Cardiorespiratory Prescriptions

Goal	Frequency	Intensity	Duration	Type
Improve health	Daily	Moderate 40-60% HRR 12-14 RPE	≥30 min of activity in up to three sessions	Any activity that can be continued for ≥10 min Weight bearing for bone health
Increase CRF	3-5 d/wk	40-85% HRR or $\dot{V}O_2$max 55-90% HRmax	20-60 min continuous	Aerobic activity using large muscle groups
Weight control	On most, preferably all, days	40-60% HRR 12-14 RPE	To yield 4200-8400 kJ [1,000-2,000 kcal] per week	Aerobic activity using large muscle groups

Adapted, by permission, from ACSM, 2000, *ACSM'S guidelines for exercise testing and prescription,* 6th ed. (Philadelphia: Lippincott, Williams & Wilkins), chapter 7.

---

respiratory prescriptions to improve health, increase CRF and control weight. These variables are manipulated to maximise adoption and adherence for the individual and for group aerobic programs.

Mode

Aerobic activity can be classified as non-weight-bearing (e.g., cycling, swimming, rowing) or weight-bearing (e.g., walking, running, dancing). Compared with weight-bearing activities, some non-weight-bearing activities may elicit a higher RPE at a given $\dot{V}O_2$max. This increased RPE may be due to localised fatigue. Obese clients or clients with musculoskeletal injuries may prefer non-weight-bearing or low-impact activities (e.g., cycling, water activities, rowing), whereas individuals without these impairments may prefer weight-bearing activities because of the benefits to weight loss and bone health—weight-bearing activities are the mode of choice when the goal is to increase or maintain bone mass. Regular participation and total energy expenditure are more critical than type of activity. The type of activity selected depends on choice, accessibility, health constraints and skill.

Ability to maintain a consistent exercise intensity can also be used to classify aerobic activities. Individuals are able to maintain a specific intensity during activities such as walking, running, rowing and ergometry. Activities such as outdoor cycling, aerobic dance, circuit training, swimming and gardening usually involve a range of exercise intensities during a given activity. Finally, sports such as netball, touch football, basketball and racquet sports are variable in exercise intensity and dependent on the individual's skill level. Activities that require skill (e.g., squash, netball, basketball) may be enjoyable, but may need to be supplemented with other types of activities. Because of differences in skill and mechanical efficiency, some clients may be able to sustain these activities while others may not.

Consider client choice and access to activities before recommending activity. The mode of activity for a group program is usually selected to target the interests of a specific population. Group aerobic activities such as walking, line dancing, Latin dancing, cycling and team sports will be attractive to different people. Identification of group choices can help guide development of these programs.

Duration

The recommendation for duration of an activity session is based on client time constraints. Intensity of activity is adjusted to provide a prescription that meets health, CRF and weight control goals. For example, a prescription to increase CRF may be 20 to 30 min at 60 to 80% HRR or 40 to 60 min at 40 to

60% HRR. A previously inactive client without time constraints may prefer the latter prescription. Moreover, dependent on the desired outcomes, a prescription of 40 to 60 min may be accumulated in two to three 15- to 20-min bouts of activity, which may be preferable for clients with busy schedules. Activity duration is not as flexible with group programs. The duration is usually constant, so variables such as intensity need to be adjustable to meet the varied needs of all participants.

Intensity

Activity intensity influences the extent of improvements in CRF (refer to table 7.5). To improve CRF, the recommended optimal HR range is between 55 to 90% of HRmax or 40 to 85% of $\dot{V}O_2$max or HRR. Studies have reported that low to moderate intensities (40 to 60% HRR) improve aerobic capacity in untrained and older individuals, whereas young and aerobically fit individuals may require a higher intensity program (60 to 85% HRR). In addition, there is some speculation that reductions in mortality resulting from lifelong physical activity may be associated with participation in higher intensity activity. A study of Harvard University alumni reported that men must participate in physical activities greater than 6 METs or 7.5 kcal · min^{-1} (e.g., jogging on flat ground at about 8 km · h^{-1}) to achieve a reduction in mortality and an increase in longevity (Lee, Hsieh and Paffenbarger 1995). Alumni who reported regular participation in less intense physical activity did not show these benefits.

It is important to note that the heart rate determined from a given percentage of APMHR does not equal the heart rate from the same percentage of HRR. For example, a target heart rate at 60% HRR will be greater than a target heart rate at 60% APMHR. Traditionally, 50 to 85% of $\dot{V}O_2$max was the recommended exercise intensity; current ACSM recommendations suggest 40 to 85% of $\dot{V}O_2$R.

Activity intensity is as important as frequency and duration when prescribing exercise for health benefits. Intensity is prescribed by balancing health needs, risks and factors influencing adherence. Although higher intensity exercise might be best for increasing fitness and altering blood lipids, it is not attractive to most adults. Lower intensity exercise may promote activity maintenance and has been shown to have many health benefits. Most health organisations (e.g., ACSM, USSG, NHFA, Active Australia) recommend participation in moderate-intensity exercise on most if not all days. Addition of more vigorous activities may provide additional health benefits (e.g., reduced blood lipids). ACSM (2000) continues to recommend moderate- to high-intensity activity to improve CRF. However, it is important to remember that the risk of cardiovascular and musculoskeletal injury and fatigue increases with intensity prescriptions greater than 85% HRR.

Activities at given MET levels can target specific groups. For example, a water aerobics class (about 4 METs) might be suitable for groups with lower levels of fitness (e.g., 6-8 METs). A circuit training class (about 8 METs) may target individuals with higher levels of fitness.

Frequency

Frequency recommendations range from multiple sessions daily (health and weight control) to multiple sessions per week. Prescription of activity frequency needs to consider intensity and duration of activity. Multiple short-duration sessions may be

Case Study 7.2

Diane is 35 years old, BMI = 28.6 and would like to lose weight. Diane would like to swim or walk and can only exercise when her partner is home to take care of the children, that is after 5:30 P.M. or before 7:00 A.M. Refer to figure 7.1 to guide the design of a cardiorespiratory prescription.

Key Issues

1. What additional considerations should be addressed before walking and swimming are prescribed?
2. How can duration, intensity and frequency be manipulated to help Diane meet her goals?
3. What strategies would help promote adoption and adherence?
4. Would you recommend a fitness assessment? Why or why not?

recommended to improve health, whereas daily sessions of longer duration are more likely to help with body fat reduction and weight control. Three to five sessions per week are recommended if the activity is going to be performed at higher intensities (refer to table 7.5). Participation in more than five sessions per week of high-intensity activity may increase the risk of injury in some clients.

Muscular Strength and Endurance

Muscular strength is the ability of a muscle group to produce force against a resistance. Muscular endurance is the ability of a muscle group to maintain force over an extended period of time. Physical activities that improve and then maintain muscular strength and endurance are called muscular conditioning activities; they are a critical component of a comprehensive fitness program. Activities of daily living (e.g., carrying groceries, gardening) require a minimal level of muscular strength and endurance. It is known that muscular strength declines with age because of reduced muscle mass. Supplemental exercises to maintain muscle mass and to increase muscular strength and endurance should therefore be included in most exercise programs. Resistance training increases bone mass, maintains fat-free mass, increases strength of connective tissue, enhances sporting performance, and helps glucose tolerance in overweight individuals when combined with aerobic activity.

Furthermore, there is some evidence to suggest that resistance training, in addition to cardiorespiratory activity, helps reduce the risk of coronary heart disease, type 2 diabetes, and certain types of cancer and helps decrease the probability of falls in the elderly. Resistance training is also beneficial in the treatment of some conditions such as arthritis and low back pain (discussed in chapter 9).

The USSG and ACSM recommend that muscle conditioning exercises be performed at least twice per week (refer to chapter 2 for more details). Mode (type of resistance exercise), duration (number of repetitions, number of sets), intensity (resistance) and frequency of training can be manipulated to produce an optimal resistance program that maximises adoption and maintenance. These factors may be manipulated in many possible variations to achieve goals of increasing or maintaining muscular strength, power, endurance or muscle mass.

Mode

There are three main types of muscle movement: isometric, dynamic (concentric and eccentric) and isokinetic. An isometric contraction is a static muscular contraction in which the muscle exerts a force against an immovable object without a change in length. Concentric (shortening) and eccentric (lengthening) contractions involve exerting force against a constant resistance through a range of movement. An isokinetic contraction involves exerting force against variable resistance through a range of movement at a fixed rate.

The type of resistance training incorporated into a program is based on client goals and access to equipment. Isokinetic training involves the use of specific equipment that is often costly and bulky. Isometric training, sometimes prescribed for rehabilitation of muscle injury, results in strength gains but only at the specific angle trained. Significant increases in diastolic blood pressure have been shown to occur with isometric training, which may be contraindicated for some clients.

Dynamic training is usually the mode of choice for the general public. Dynamic resistance activities tend to be adaptable, accessible and more likely to mimic movements needed for everyday activities; there are also many types of equipment available. Speed of movement and range of motion (ROM) can be varied to meet individual needs.

Types of equipment used for dynamic resistance training include free weights (dumbbells, barbells) and machine weights (including pin weights); body-weight activities are also performed. Table 7.6 presents a brief overview of the advantages and disadvantages of using these types of exercises. Although free weights allow full range of movement, machine-weight exercises are often prescribed for beginners. Clients are able to learn the movement with the benefit of safety mechanisms such as brakes and supports. Body weight and household items may be used in resistance training for individuals and groups. These have been shown to provide similar benefits to using specific resistance training equipment. It is important to determine if the client's body weight is appropriate for the exercise. For example, an individual's body weight may be too high to allow for a prescription of 10 to 12 push-ups. An alternative is to have the client perform wall push-ups, starting with the feet close to the wall and gradually increasing the resistance by moving the feet farther from the wall, eventually progressing to knee push-ups (see figure 7.2). It should be emphasised to the client that expensive equipment is not necessary for

TABLE 7.6—Advantages and Disadvantages of Types of Equipment for Resistance Training

Equipment	Advantages	Disadvantages
Free weights	Adaptable to ROM	Clear instructions needed to ensure full ROM
	Portable	Can require a spotter
	Can mimic most movements, ADLs	
	Inexpensive	
	Barbells enhance balance (contralateral)	
	Need to use stabilising muscles	
Machine weights	Most include safety mechanisms	Expensive
	Action guided	Immovable
	Accessory muscles supported	Designed for average size person—may be incorrect ROM for some
	Easy to teach	
	Can support weaker side with stronger	
Body weight	Free	Set resistance
	Range of activities: plyometrics, partner exercises	
	Easily implemented with groups	

Abbreviations: ROM = range of motion; ADLs = activities of daily living.

a well-designed and appropriate resistance training regime.

Duration

Duration of resistance activity is typically prescribed using a number of repetitions and a number of sets rather than by time. The number of repetitions prescribed is dependent on the client's goals and the resistance selected; table 7.7 presents recommendations for selection of the number of repetitions. For example, developing maximum strength requires a high resistance and a low number of repetitions (e.g., 6-8 for novice and 4-8 for advanced). For hypertrophy, 10 to 12 repetitions are recommended, whereas 15 to 20 repetitions are recommended to improve muscular endurance.

Goals for resistance training, time available and training status must be considered before prescribing a number of sets for each resistance exercise. To improve adherence to resistance training, it is recommended that a single set be prescribed for beginners. Significant health and fitness benefits can be achieved from a single set and less time is needed. Optimal improvements in strength occur with multiple sets (e.g., 2 to 3). Prescription of multiple sets can involve repetition of the exercise at the same resistance or may use sets of varying resistance, that is, either progressively lighter or heavier. Multiple set programs with varying resistance are usually prescribed for clients experienced in resistance training.

When multiple sets are recommended, the amount of rest between sets is also important to allow recovery. For example, goals to improve lactate tolerance require a short rest period (e.g., <1 min) to allow the body to adapt to altered pH levels and the presence of lactic acid. Short rest periods (<1 min) are also prescribed for improving muscular endurance. In contrast, rest periods are lengthened (e.g., 3-5 min) when the goal is to increase strength, thereby allowing the body to replenish fuel stores and work at high intensity (see table 7.7).

Intensity

The intensity component of muscular conditioning is prescribed by resistance. Selection of resistance depends on a number of factors including goals, functional ability, health status and duration. Ideally, an individual should first perform 1 repetition maximum (1 RM) for all included exercises (refer to recommended for improving muscular endurance.

Use of 1 RM is not always the most appropriate method for selecting resistance. For many clients, performing 1 RM is unrealistic in that it is time consuming, physically stressful, can lead to muscular soreness and requires qualified supervision. A multiple of 1 RM may be more appropriate for some clients and produces similar benefits without the need to re-test 1 RM repetitively. For example, a 6 RM refers to the maximum amount of weight that can be lifted in 6 consecutive repetitions. A 4 to 8 RM is recommended to increase strength, whereas a 15 to 20 RM is recommended to increase muscular endurance (refer to table 7.7).

For body-weight exercises, innovative and safe techniques are needed to adjust intensity. Typically, the longer the lever, the higher the intensity. For example, the intensity of a triceps dip using a chair is lowest when the edge of the seat is used as a brake and the feet are positioned close to the chair. The intensity can be increased by moving the feet away from the chair, thereby lengthening the lever of the body.

Frequency

To prevent overtraining and soreness, the muscles need time to recuperate. Research shows that up to 72 h may be needed for full recovery after high-intensity resistance training. Significant gains in muscular strength and endurance may occur with two to three resistance training sessions per week, and ACSM and USSG recommend resistance training two to three times per week for health benefits. Athletes requiring maximum strength or power development may train more frequently using various techniques such as split routines or alternating upper and lower body training to permit higher frequency of training while maintaining adequate recovery (discussed in chapter 11).

Program Development and Progression

Beginners are generally prescribed 8 to 10 exercises that use major muscle groups. **Compound exercises** (i.e., structural) utilise multiple muscles and joints and are more likely to mimic activities of daily living; examples include squats, rows and shoulder presses. Compound exercises are usually the mode of choice for the beginner, with graduation to isolated exercises as muscular strength increases and the client becomes familiar with resistance training. **Isolated exercises** (i.e., body part) utilise a single muscle mass or muscle group and

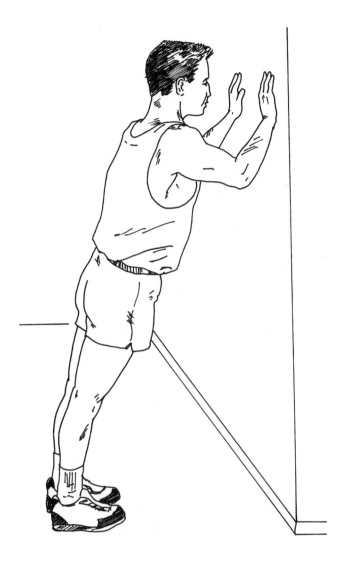

FIGURE 7.2 A wall push-up: intensity is lower with the feet close to the wall and increases as the feet move away from the wall.

chapter 6). One RM represents the maximum amount of weight an individual is able to lift once. A percentage of 1 RM for each exercise is then used to set the resistance. Varying percentages of 1 RM are prescribed for goals of improving strength, power, endurance and hypertrophy; table 7.7 presents definitions and recommendations for selection of resistance for each of these goals. If the goal is hypertrophy, a moderate resistance (e.g., 70-75%) is selected; to improve power, a low to moderate resistance (e.g., <80%) is prescribed. A higher resistance (80-95% 1 RM) is recommended for increasing strength, whereas a lower resistance (<60% 1 RM) is

TABLE 7.7—General Recommendations for Prescribing Resistance Training

Goal and definition	Resistance (multiple RM)	Resistance (% 1 RM)	Sets	Repetitions	Rest period if multiple sets
Strength: maximal amount of force muscle(s) can generate	Novice 6-8 RM Advanced 4-8 RM	80-85% 80-95%	3 5-6	Novice 6-8 Trained 4-6	3-5 min
Power: rate of work performance	Varied	<80%	4-10	Varied, usually <5	>2min
Hypertrophy: gains in muscle size	10-12 RM	70-75%	3	10-12	1 min
Muscular endurance: ability to sustain contraction	15-20 RM	<60%	3	15+	<1 min

may result in soreness. Biceps curls, leg extensions and abdominal curl-ups are examples of isolated exercises.

Compound and isolated exercises can be used in the design of circuit training programs, which typically incorporate multiple stations of resistance and aerobic activity, each performed for about 30 s to 1 min with 10- to 20-s rest in between. Circuit training programs are often marketed to groups as a means of increasing muscular strength and CRP. Although not the best mode to garner improvements in these areas, circuit weight training may indeed provide small improvements in muscular strength, endurance and CRF.

Maintenance of abdominal muscle strength and endurance is suggested to help prevent low back pain. A small amount of research supports this suggestion, although anecdotal evidence clearly endorses the use of exercises to improve and maintain abdominal muscle condition. Body-weight exercises (e.g., regular and oblique curl-ups) are often prescribed to increase the strength of the rectus abdominis and oblique muscle groups, and activities using the "fit ball" (or "Swiss Ball" as it was originally called when first introduced) have become popular as a means of increasing the endurance of stabilising muscles (e.g., transverse abdominis).

Development of muscular strength and endurance occurs according to the principle of overload, that is, increasing the resistance, either by load, duration or frequency, to above normally experienced levels. To promote further strength and endurance gains, progression must occur by periodically increasing training volume. In addition, muscular strength and endurance training is specific to the muscle groups trained and the actions performed. It is important to prescribe a balanced program, ensuring that opposing muscle groups (agonist and

Case Study 7.3

Tony is 46 years old and would like to do "some weights" to increase strength after the walking program at the gym. He is inexperienced with resistance training. Design an initial resistance training program for Tony.

Key Issues

1. Are compound or isolated exercises most appropriate for beginners? What type of equipment is recommended for beginners?

2. What needs to be considered to ensure a balanced program?

3. How will safety issues be addressed?

antagonist), contralateral (right and left) movements, and upper and lower body exercises are included in the program.

Safety

To avoid injury, it is important that the client is taught to use correct technique. Each exercise should be executed through a full range of movement with both the concentric (i.e., lifting) and eccentric (i.e., lowering) phases performed in a controlled manner. Ideally, a qualified instructor should coach the client on the appropriate technique and ensure that the client is able to perform each exercise correctly. All prescriptions for resistance training should include a warm-up and a cool-down, incorporating stretching exercises to maintain flexibility.

Clients should also be taught how to breathe when exercising; the recommendation is to exhale during the lifting phase of the exercise and inhale during the lowering phase. It is common for an individual to hold his or her breath while performing resistance training exercises. This practice is dangerous because of the possibility of initiating a Valsalva manoeuvre (forced exhalation against a closed glottis). A Valsalva manoeuvre leads to an excessive increase in systolic and diastolic blood pressure, which may be harmful for hypertensives.

Musculoskeletal Flexibility

An adequate range of motion through all joints is necessary for efficient movement and to reduce the risk of injury. In addition, adequate flexibility improves skill and ensures that maximum power can be achieved throughout the range of movement. Musculoskeletal flexibility declines with age, and lack of flexibility may limit some activities of daily living. For example, bending down to pick up something off the ground can be problematic for individuals with reduced lower back and hamstring flexibility. Stretching exercises are an important part of any physical activity program. However, care needs to be taken with individuals at increased risk of dislocation such as pregnant women, who release a hormone (relaxant) that can increase the hypermobility of joints, and other individuals with hypermobile joints.

Developing and then maintaining a good level of flexibility has been shown to increase ROM, reduce stress, improve posture, reduce the severity of low back pain, help prevent injuries and enhance physical and athletic skills. Thus, it is important for all physical activity regimes to include activities that improve and then maintain musculoskeletal flexibility. Stretching a muscle or group of muscles is joint and muscle specific; it is recommended that several stretches targeting major muscle groups (and joints) are performed. There are three main types of stretching exercises to help improve flexibility: static, ballistic and proprioceptive neuromuscular facilitation (PNF).

Static Stretching

Static stretches are executed slowly to the point of mild discomfort and then sustained for a specified length of time, typically 10 to 30 s. ROM has been shown to improve significantly after regular static stretching, and it is recommended for most individuals. Additional benefits include a low risk of injury and muscle soreness, no need for assistance, and time efficiency. Figure 7.3 shows several examples of stretches for the upper body (chest, triceps, spinal extension) and lower body (quadriceps, hamstrings, calves).

For the majority of the population, static stretching is the mode of choice because of ease, simplicity and low risk of injury. Static stretching should be incorporated into most physical activity regimes for individuals of all age groups, functional abilities and disease states. A general warm-up, preferably aerobic, that increases body temperature is recommended before all stretching activities because warm muscle tissue is more responsive to a stretch than cold. Stretches should also be included in general cool-downs for all activities. After activity at a reduced intensity, stretching should be performed to increase joint range of motion and help reduce muscle soreness.

It is recommended that a static stretch be held for 10 to 30 s and that three to five repetitions of each stretch be performed before and after an exercise session. The number of specific stretches depends on the type of activity and should include exercises to stretch the muscles just used. Because of the high incidence of low back pain, stretches that concentrate on the lower back and thigh (e.g., hip flexor, extensors, abductors, adductors) should also be emphasised for most individuals. It is important to note that a static stretch should not be painful; if pain is experienced, the client is stretching too far, too fast.

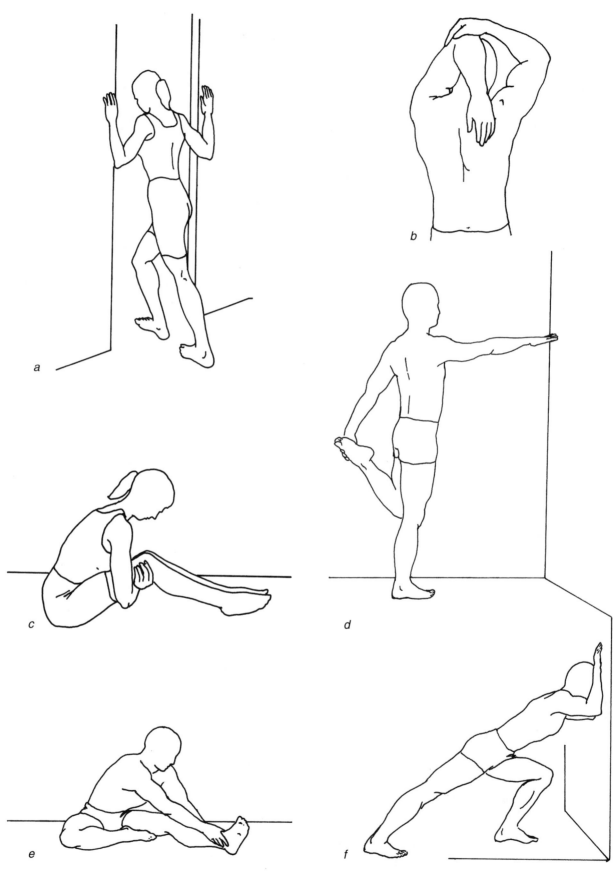

FIGURE 7.3   Sample stretches for *(a)* chest, *(b)* triceps, *(c)* lower back, *(d)* quadriceps, *(e)* hamstring and *(f)* calf.

Reprinted, by permission, from M.J. Alter, 1998, *Sport stretch,* 2nd ed. (Champaign, IL: Human Kinetics), 251, 180; figures 7.3 *b, d, e,* and *f* © Michael Richardson.

Ballistic Stretching

Ballistic stretching refers to bouncing through the stretch rather than slowly stretching and then holding the position. Although improvements in flexibility may result from regular ballistic stretching, there is a higher risk of injury and soreness. Thus, prescription of ballistic stretching is restricted to athletes and others who may need to regularly perform movements involving a ballistic stretch (e.g., kicking a football on the run, many dance and gymnastics movements). Typically, an athlete performs static stretches before ballistic stretches.

Proprioceptive Neuromuscular Facilitation (PNF)

The third type of stretching, PNF, has demonstrated the largest improvements in flexibility. PNF involves stretching after an isometric contraction. It is thought that stretching is facilitated by a reflex relaxation of the antagonist muscle group (muscle group stretched) after an isometric contraction of the same muscle group. This reflex action suppresses the contractile activity of the muscle and enhances the range of motion in a slow static stretch. PNF stretching can sometimes be performed alone, though it is often performed with a partner (see figure 7.4). The procedure involves the following steps:

1. Perform a static stretch of the antagonist muscle group.
2. Isometrically contract the muscle group.
3. Perform another slow static stretch.

PNF stretching may be recommended for some athletes and those needing extreme flexibility (e.g.,

gymnasts, dancers). Although significant improvements in flexibility occur with this type of stretching, it is time consuming, often requires a partner and may result in muscular soreness.

Environmental Factors to Consider

Recognising specific social and cultural constraints and incorporating them into the exercise program is likely to enhance the chances of compliance, especially in older, less fit individuals or those from groups with traditionally low rates of adherence (e.g., non-English-speaking background).

The workplace and home environments must be considered when designing an exercise program. Influential factors include physical intensity of the job and hobbies as well as location and availability of other facilities. A bricklayer who is likely to expend about 12,200 kJ [2,900 kcal]/day [(8 METs × 3.5 × 70 kg/48) × 300 min] may not achieve or be interested in additional cardiovascular benefits from walking three times per week for 30 min at a moderate intensity. However, if the goal is to improve cardiovascular health, other factors such as diet, smoking habits and stress may need to be examined before suggesting an increase in physical activity.

The physical location of the workplace and home also influences the exercise prescription. Availability of an on-site corporate fitness facility may be more convenient and thus encourage participation, providing the client is eager to participate in a company-based program. Nearby parks and walking and cycling tracks may provide easily accessible areas to exercise; however, time of day must be considered

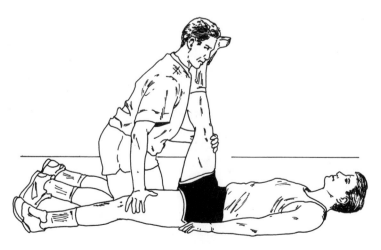

FIGURE 7.4   Partner-assisted PNF hamstring stretch.

because individuals are unlikely to participate if they deem the physical environment to be unsafe at night or early in the morning. Supervised group sessions (e.g., walks through parks or in shopping centres) may provide safe alternatives.

The client's social support and socio-economic status dictate to some degree the mode of exercise prescribed. Willingness of family and friends to participate may influence the mode and frequency of exercise. For many individuals, an exercise partner helps maintain exercise. Inclusion of active interests and hobbies such as bushwalking, surfing or golf also need to be taken into account when developing an exercise regime. Finally, the economic status of the client may need to be broached in specific circumstances for accessibility to facilities. It is pointless to prescribe exercise at a venue that charges an admission fee if the client feels it is unaffordable. Admission fee may not be a concern for some; however, because of long work hours and home responsibilities, the client may deem an external facility inaccessible.

An individual's cultural group can provide benefits or create limitations when prescribing exercise. Individuals of specific ethnic origin often reside in similar physical localities. A ready-made cultural group can provide the support needed to maintain exercise; alternatively, cultural dress and social norms may limit exercise prescription. It is critical that these issues are considered out of respect for the culture and to maximise compliance.

Summary

Designing the most appropriate and effective physical activity prescription for a given individual or group is a basic function of exercise management. Individualised exercise prescriptions may maximise adoption and maintenance of physical activity. For the physical activity prescription to be effective, critical factors that must be considered include client goals, needs, wants, access, and time constraints. Goals of improvement in health, cardiorespiratory fitness and weight control are best met with cardiorespiratory exercise prescriptions. Frequency, exercise intensity, session duration, mode of activity and progression can all be adjusted and manipulated to meet individual needs and goals. Resistance training will help a client meet goals of improving muscular strength and endurance. Type of resistance training, resistance, repetitions, sets and rest are factors to consider in this type of prescription. Finally, muscular flexibility is an important physical attribute that diminishes with age; stretching exercises should therefore be incorporated into all programs.

There are many approaches to prescribing safe and effective activity programs. Often, there is no single correct prescription for a given individual. With the number of variables that can be manipulated, there are many possible ways to develop activity prescriptions that meet client needs and goals.

Selected Glossary Terms

compound exercise—An exercise movement using multiple muscles and joints, for example, a squat.

isolated exercise—An exercise movement using a sinlge joint and muscle or muscle group, for example, a biceps curl.

principle of specificity—A principle stating that specific types of physical fitness (e.g., cardiorespiratory, muscular strength, flexibility) will optimally improve with specific types of training; the basis for prescribing exercise.

progression—Changes to program intensity, duration, or frequency (e.g., workload) to continue to improve a specific component of fitness.

Student Activities and Study Questions

1. What group physical activity programs are offered to older adults in your area? What is the type of prescription (e.g., cardiorespiratory, muscular strength)? Describe the mode, duration, intensity and frequency. What benefits could the participants expect to gain?

2. Perform a maximal exercise test with gas analysis on one subject. Plot HR vs. O_2 and answer the following questions:

   a. How does the measured HRmax compare with a predicted HRmax? Discuss the comparison.

   b. What HR range corresponds to 60 to 80% of $\dot{V}O_2$max? to 60 to 80% of HRR? To 60 to 80% HRmax? Discuss the comparisons. What are the implications for exercise prescription?

3. Visit a commercial or corporate fitness facility and ask to see five individual prescriptions for a variety of clients. Discuss the similarities and differences between these programs based on client needs, goals, health, skill and experience.

4. Design a group physical activity program for the following client groups:

   a. GP-based community physical activity program for GP-referred clients of all ages

   b. Under-14 club soccer team during the off-season

   c. Pregnant women

   d. Employees in a medium-sized law firm situated in an inner city with no on-site facility

5. Design a general resistance training program for the three groups, considering factors presented in tables 7.6 and 7.7. Explain the similarities and differences between these general programs.

   a. Retirement village

   b. Masters swim club

   c. Obese children

Section 3

PHYSICAL ACTIVITY PRESCRIPTION FOR SPECIAL POPULATIONS

In the previous section, the basic principles of exercise prescription and programming for healthy individuals were discussed. Also included were methods for pre-participation screening, physical fitness assessment and enhancing long-term compliance to physical activity. We now turn our attention to extending these basic principles to the wider community—to the currently sedentary, to the elderly and children, to athletes and to those with impairments or conditions that may influence exercise capacity.

In the practice of exercise management, it is rare to encounter only young, healthy and fit clients to whom the basic principles of exercise prescription apply without modification (even among elite athletes). With the recent recognition that regular physical activity helps prevent or manage a number of diseases, more and more people will be seeking these health benefits through exercise. As public health campaigns such as Active Australia gain momentum, an increasing number of older people and individuals with disease or impairment will be seeking services and venues to enhance their participation in physical activity.

Those at risk of or with known disease need individualised exercise prescription aimed at optimising the health benefits while reducing any risk associated with exercise (e.g., injury or heart attack). These individuals also tend to be currently inactive and possibly not attracted to physical activity. There are many situations in which the basic exercise prescription will need at least some alteration(s), as illustrated by the following examples:

▶ Exercise for the obese individual needs to be low impact to prevent injury but of appropriate intensity and duration to influence body composition.

▶ The recreational athlete who becomes pregnant will need to temporarily modify her program to ensure she can safely maintain her fitness during pregnancy; she can resume her former program after the birth of her baby.

▶ The athlete with physical disability will need to modify modes of exercise to optimally train cardiovascular endurance, muscular strength or sports skills.

▶ Muscular strength training specifically tailored to the elderly can do much to prevent the age-related declines in muscle function and ability to live independently.

▶ As many as 10% of all elite athletes may have asthma, and even at this level, training must be adapted to avoid triggering an attack while still optimising performance.

The same general principles of exercise prescription, as discussed in the previous section, apply to special populations but with some extra considerations, such as

▶ medical limitations or contraindications to exercise,
▶ specific exercises to encourage and those to avoid,
▶ the generally low initial fitness level,
▶ the focus on health rather than performance or fitness, and
▶ issues of long-term compliance in normally sedentary individuals.

Adapting the basic principles of exercise prescription to the specific needs of those at risk of or with disease or impairment is a particular challenge to the exercise manager. Indeed, much of the recent growth in exercise management services (hence employment) in Australia is within the fields of exercise rehabilitation or secondary prevention. Given the high prevalence of risk factors for certain diseases (e.g., heart disease) or other less serious conditions (e.g., asthma, low back pain, arthritis), however, it is likely that the exercise manager will encounter clients with special needs in virtually any practice. It is particularly gratifying in the practice of exercise management to be able to use our skills to help all clients achieve a physically active lifestyle.

CHAPTER 8

Exercise Prescription for People With Cardiovascular, Respiratory and Metabolic Impairment

As described in the first section of this book, cardiovascular and metabolic diseases such as heart disease, stroke and diabetes are major killers in most developed countries. These diseases consume a significant part of direct and indirect health care costs, in the billions of dollars each year. Much of the risk of these diseases can be attributed to lifestyle factors such as diet, obesity and especially physical inactivity, suggesting that we may positively influence the health of the nation by convincing people to alter their lifestyles to include regular physical activity. Physical activity also plays an important role in rehabilitation or prevention of further disease, for example, after a heart attack or stroke. The increasing recognition of the importance of physical activity for **primary** and **secondary prevention** of cardiovascular and metabolic diseases has recently provided many research and employment opportunities for exercise managers.

The terms *primary* and *secondary prevention* are now widely used to describe health promotion strategies and medical interventions aimed at preventing or slowing the progress of disease, particularly cardiovascular diseases. Primary prevention refers to strategies and interventions to avert the initial occurrence of disease (i.e., in healthy people). Secondary prevention describes strategies and interventions aimed at preventing further disease progression, and its associated morbidity, mortality and disability, in individuals with disease. Secondary prevention also focuses on enhancing quality of life for those with known disease. Many strategies are similar for both primary and secondary prevention, although there may be differences in the approach. For example, recent public health campaigns (described in chapter 3) encourage all individuals to maintain a physically active lifestyle; however, different types of physical activity programs may be needed for a healthy individual compared with someone diagnosed with heart disease.

This chapter focuses first on the role of physical activity in preventing major cardiovascular, respiratory and metabolic diseases or impairments (primary prevention) and then on extension and modification of the basic principles of exercise prescription (as described in section 2) for individuals with known disease or impairment (secondary prevention).

Cardiovascular Disease

The most common cause of death in most developed countries, cardiovascular disease comprises a range of conditions of the heart and blood vessels, such as coronary heart disease (CHD), chronic heart failure, hypertension, stroke and peripheral vascular disease. In Australia, CHD is the second, and stroke the third, most frequent cause of death (refer to chapter 2). In many developed countries, cardiovascular disease and CHD mortality peaked around 1968 and have been declining since, primarily because of advances in medical care (e.g., screening, medication, surgery, rehabilitation) and health promotion campaigns to encourage lifestyle interventions (e.g., low-fat diet, avoiding cigarette smoking). The causes of cardiovascular disease are multifactorial and are determined by both genetic and environmental factors. As described in chapter 2, major contributors to CHD include family history, age and sex, hypertension, cigarette smoking, dyslipidaemia (abnormal blood lipid profile), physical inactivity, obesity (especially abdominal obesity) and diabetes or impaired glucose tolerance (see table 2.6). Psychological stress may also be a contributing factor to CHD.

Clinical manifestations of CHD include **angina** (chest pain or discomfort due to myocardial ischaemia), acute myocardial infarction (heart attack), left ventricular dysfunction and sudden cardiac death (cardiac arrest). Fatality rates increase after about age 35 years in men and after menopause in women. CHD and some other cardiovascular conditions (e.g., stroke, peripheral vascular disease) result from degenerative changes in blood vessels (termed **atherosclerosis**). Pathogenesis involves accumulation of lipid (cholesterol) and fibrous tissue in the arterial wall, which permits infiltration of the vessel wall by inflammatory cells and a subsequent increase of arterial smooth muscle cells in the vessel's lumen. Accumulation of smooth muscle cells and associated substances reduces the artery's cross-section, limiting blood flow. Depending on the degree of occlusion of the vessel, myocardial (or other tissue) oxygen supply may be compromised. Ischaemia, caused by inadequate blood flow to the myocardium, reflects an imbalance between oxygen demand and supply and may be perceived as pain in the chest (angina) or leg (claudication). In some people, ischaemia occurs without overt symptoms (termed *silent ischaemia;* this is of particular concern because the individual may not be aware of the presence of disease). Myocardial oxygen demand increases with the work of the heart and can be mea-

sured as the rate pressure product (RPP), which is a function of systolic blood pressure and heart rate; RPP gives a non-invasive indication of the work of the heart. When heart rate is elevated (e.g., during physical stress such as exercise), oxygen supply to the heart may become inadequate. Atherosclerosis becomes clinically significant when >75% of a coronary vessel is occluded.

Physical Activity and Cardiovascular Disease

It is now well accepted that regular physical activity reduces mortality and morbidity from cardiovascular disease through many mechanisms (discussed in chapter 2). Biological mechanisms may be both direct and indirect, for example, direct by strengthening the heart and indirect by beneficially altering cardiovascular disease risk factors. Regular exercise has a direct effect on the heart by

- ▶ enhancing myocardial oxygen delivery by delaying the development of atherosclerosis,
- ▶ reducing myocardial oxygen demand and work of the heart at rest and during submaximal exercise,
- ▶ decreasing catecholamine output at rest and during submaximal exercise, and
- ▶ helping to stabilise the heart's electrical activity at rest and during exercise.

Exercise training also indirectly reduces risk of disease by improving the blood lipid profile, reducing body fat levels and especially abdominal obesity, decreasing blood pressure and improving glucose tolerance. These beneficial effects are inter-related and synergistic. For example, an exercise-induced decrease in body fat will also help reduce blood pressure and improve glucose tolerance and the blood lipid profile.

Regular exercise also exerts anti-thrombotic effects (i.e., inhibits formation of blood clots) by reducing blood viscosity (through plasma volume expansion), regulating enzymes involved in clot formation (e.g., fibrinogen), enhancing fibrinolysis (the body's natural system of preventing blood clots) and inhibiting platelet aggregation. These direct positive effects on blood clotting mechanisms help reduce the risk of myocardial infarction and stroke. In addition, obesity (especially abdominal obesity) adversely alters the blood's fibrinolytic capacity. Thus, physical activity that induces loss of body mass and fat indirectly contributes to enhanced anti-thrombotic effects as well. Regular exercise also improves exercise tolerance in cardiac patients with other conditions such as heart failure or cardiac transplant. For these patients, improvement in functional capacity does not alter the disease process itself, but it contributes to enhanced quality of life.

Medications and Medical Interventions for Cardiovascular Disease

Cardiovascular disease is treated with a variety of medications. Many of these influence exercise capacity, interpretation of exercise or fitness test results, and exercise prescription. Table 8.1 provides a summary of the general classes of medications to treat

cardiovascular disease. Common surgical procedures include coronary arterial bypass graft (CABG) and percutaneous transluminal coronary angioplasty (PTCA). CABG involves replacing a blocked coronary artery with a synthetic graft or a vein from another part of the body. In PTCA, a small balloon is inserted via a catheter into the blocked vessel and inflated to compress the material blocking the vessel; a small device called a stent may be inserted at the site of PTCA to maintain an open vessel. Secondary prevention or cardiac rehabilitation includes patient education and support to change lifestyle factors, such as diet, physical activity and stress management.

TABLE 8.1—Some Classes of Medications Prescribed for Cardiovascular, Respiratory and Metabolic Disorders

Class of medication	Disease/condition for which prescribed	Effects on exercise capacity or test results
Beta-antagonists	Hypertension, angina	↓ HR and BP at rest and exercise ↑ exercise tolerance in angina
Calcium channel blockers	Hypertension, angina	↓ or ↑ HR, ↓ BP ↑ exercise tolerance in angina
Diuretics	Hypertension	No changes
Peripheral vasodilators	Intermittent claudication	↑ exercise tolerance
Angiotensin-converting enzyme (ACE) inhibitors	Hypertension	↓ BP
Antihyperlipidaemic agents	Dyslipidaemia	Generally no changes; some may cause ECG changes
Anti-inflammatory agents		
NSAIDs	Arthritis, acute injury	No changes; may ↑ exercise tolerance in arthritis if limited by pain
Aerosol corticosteroids	Asthma	No changes or ↑ HR and BP
Bronchodilators	Asthma, COPD	↑ exercise tolerance if limited by bronchospasm
Hypoglycaemic agents		
Insulin	Type 1 diabetes	No changes
OHA	Type 2 diabetes	No changes

Abbreviations: HR = heart rate; BP = blood pressure; ECG = electrocardiogram; NSAIDs = non-steroidal anti-inflammatory drugs; COPD = chronic obstructive pulmonary disease; OHA = oral hypoglycaemic agents.

Compiled from American College of Sports Medicine, 2000, *ACSM's guidelines for exercise testing and prescription*, 6th ed. (Philadelphia: Lippincott Williams & Wilkins); American College of Sports Medicine, 1997, *ACSM's exercise management for persons with chronic diseases and disabilities*. (Champaign, IL: Human Kinetics).

Metabolic Syndrome

Certain diseases or conditions often occur together, a phenomenon known as clustering. One common example among adults in developed countries is the so-called **metabolic syndrome (syndrome X),** which consists of obesity, glucose intolerance or hyperinsulinaemia (high blood insulin levels), dyslipidaemia (blood lipid levels outside the recommended ranges) and hypertension. Each component of the syndrome itself elevates risk of cardiovascular disease, but there is a compounded effect when an individual has two or more risk factors. Although there is a genetic predisposition, it is currently acknowledged that lifestyle factors such as physical inactivity, diet, obesity and smoking are major contributing factors. In recent years, the incidence of obesity has increased, while rates of adult participation in physical activity have remained relatively low. It is believed that these two factors together result in an increase in the number of adults exhibiting metabolic syndrome and the appearance of the syndrome at progressively younger ages. Approximately 70% of the Australian population over age 25 years is estimated to have at least one component of metabolic syndrome. Regular physical activity can be important for prevention and treatment of metabolic syndrome through its independent and interactive effects on body mass and composition, blood lipids, blood pressure and glucose tolerance. Indeed, increasing physical activity, along with dietary intervention, is the treatment of choice for many individuals with metabolic syndrome.

The following section discusses each component of metabolic syndrome and the role of physical activity in its prevention and treatment. Since these components often appear together and exercise interventions are inter-related, a combined discussion of exercise capacity and prescription for metabolic syndrome is presented at the end of this section.

Obesity

Obesity is defined as an excess of adipose tissue (body fat). Obesity may be assessed by several measures, the simplest being body mass index (BMI; kg · m^{-2}). The recommended BMI range for good health is generally 20 to 25 for both males and females, although there are slightly different scales depending on the source of information. A BMI between 25 and 27 is considered overweight, between 27 and 30 is considered moderately obese, between 31 and 40 markedly obese, and above 40 morbidly obese. Obesity may also be assessed by body composition analysis. A percentage body fat greater than 20% for males or 30% for females is often used to define obesity. Body fat levels above 25% in men and 32% in women increase risk of cardiovascular disease. However, body composition analysis is not practical for methodological reasons. For example, sophisticated imaging techniques are expensive and the validity of hydrostatic weighing has been questioned because of inter-individual differences in bone density. Relatively easy measures of obesity (particularly abdominal obesity) are the **waist to hip ratio (WHR)** or simple waist circumference. The waist measurement is an important indicator of abdominal obesity, which is associated with increased risk of cardiovascular disease and type 2 diabetes. Recommended WHRs are given in table 8.2.

Obesity is a contributing factor to a number of diseases or conditions, such as hypertension, dyslipidaemia, cardiovascular disease, glucose intolerance and type 2 diabetes, osteoarthritis, certain forms of cancer (bowel, breast, reproductive system) and increased risk of surgical complications. The incidence of obesity has increased over the past 10 to 20 years in most developed countries, despite a concomitant decline in fat consumption. In Australia, approximately 50% of the adult population is now considered to be overweight or obese (about 60% of men and 47% of women). The increasing incidence of obesity among children and adolescents is particularly alarming since obesity at an early age greatly increases risk of adult obesity and associated diseases; about 20% of children and adolescents are now considered overweight or obese. Physical inactivity appears to be a major contributor to this increasing prevalence of obesity.

It is now accepted that there is a genetic predisposition toward obesity, particularly if both biological parents are obese. Research on animal models and humans have isolated more than one gene contributing to obesity. However, it is believed that development of obesity requires combined genetic and environmental factors (e.g., excess energy intake and physical inactivity).

Abdominal (central, or visceral) obesity is defined as excess fat in the abdominal region (see figure 8.1); it is a particular health concern because it is associated with increased risk of cardiovascular disease, hypertension, dyslipidaemia and glucose intolerance or type 2 diabetes. Middle-aged and older men are more likely to exhibit this pattern of obesity. Abdominal obesity occurs less frequently in women, who generally increase fat around the hips and thighs (see figure 8.1), but when present, it is associ-

TABLE 8.2—Recommended Ranges of Simple Variables Used in Health Risk Screening and Exercise Prescription

Variable	Recommended range	Usual intervention when value is out of recommended range
Body mass index	20-25	25-30: diet, physical activity >30: very low-energy diet Medication[a][b] may be used if diet + physical activity are not effective
Waist circumference	Females: <90 cm Males: <100 cm	Weight loss, diet, physical activity
Waist to hip ratio	Females: <0.85 Males: <1.0	Weight loss, diet, physical activity
Blood pressure	<120/80 mmHg	130-140/80-90: weight loss, diet, physical activity >140/90: medication[a], weight loss, diet, physical activity
Blood lipids	TC: <5.3 mmol · L^{-1} LDL-C: <3.4 HDL-C: >0.9 TC to HDL-C ratio: <4.5 Tg: <2.3	Weight loss, low-fat diet, physical activity Medication[a] if above not effective or values very high
Blood glucose	<6.1 mmol · L^{-1} fasting	Investigate cause of elevated glucose Type 1 diabetes: insulin[a], controlled diet Type 2 diabetes: weight loss, diet, physical activity; insulin[a] or OHA[a]

[a]Medication as prescribed by client's medical practitioner.

[b]Pharmacological treatment of obesity is controversial at present.

Abbreviations: TC = total cholesterol; LDL-C = low-density lipoprotein cholesterol; HDL-C = high-density lipoprotein cholesterol; Tg = triglycerides; OHA = oral hypoglycaemic agents.

ated with increased risk of disease. Even among individuals of similar BMI, abdominal obesity confers an elevated risk of cardiovascular disease. Fat is more easily mobilised from abdominal sites compared with other sites such as the hips and thighs. It is thought that fat released from abdominal sites readily enters the portal circulation, where elevated fatty acid concentration increases liver synthesis of detrimental lipoproteins. Aerobic exercise reduces fat in the trunk and abdominal regions more effectively than in the extremities and hips. These differences in fat deposition patterns and metabolic activity may help explain why physical activity is more effective for reducing abdominal obesity and why weight loss through diet and exercise may be more difficult for women than for men.

Physical Activity and Obesity

Epidemiological evidence shows an increase in the incidence of obesity and physical inactivity over recent years. By increasing daily energy expenditure, physical activity would seem a logical intervention for prevention and management of obesity. Physical activity without dietary intervention may induce slight to moderate weight loss in overweight but not obese individuals. For example, a gradual loss of ≤10 kg may be possible over several months. However, exercise by itself is usually insufficient for effective and permanent weight loss in obese individuals, who require dietary intervention combined with physical activity. It is important to note that low- to moderate-intensity exercise improves conditions

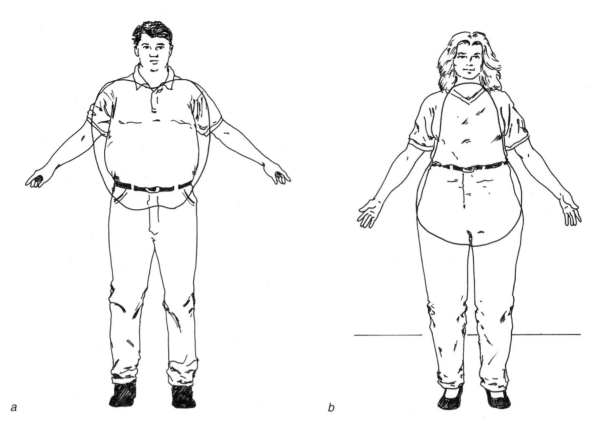

a   *b*

FIGURE 8.1   Pattern of fat distribution in the body: *(a)* android, or male pattern ("apple" shape) and *(b)* gynoid, or female pattern ("pear" shape).

of metabolic syndrome (e.g., glucose tolerance, blood pressure and abdominal obesity) with only modest changes in body mass or fitness level in overweight or moderately obese individuals. Relatively small changes in body mass or waist circumference are also associated with large changes in abdominal fat. For example, a 12-kg loss of body mass or a 7-cm decrease in waist circumference equates to a 30 to 35% reduction in visceral adipose tissue (Ross et al. 2000).

In formerly obese individuals, long-term success of weight loss programs is often poor because of the changes in basal metabolic rate (BMR) that accompany weight loss. BMR accounts for a major portion of total daily energy expenditure and is related to age, sex, body surface area and lean body mass. Weight loss through diet but without exercise causes BMR to decline by up to 15 to 20%, partially because of loss of muscle mass and an apparent increase in metabolic efficiency (that is, the body uses less energy for normal functions). This is one reason why

formerly obese individuals often regain weight after extended dieting. In contrast, including physical activity in a weight loss program maintains or may even increase muscle mass, which in turn helps to maintain or increase BMR. Exercise programs that specifically increase muscle mass (e.g., resistance training) in addition to increasing energy expenditure may be needed for permanent weight loss in obese individuals.

Dyslipidaemia

Lipids (fats) essential for body function are carried in the blood in a number of forms, primarily combined with proteins (lipoproteins) or as triglycerides. Dyslipidaemia is a general term reflecting various types of abnormal blood lipid profiles, which can be further classified by the ratios and concentrations of lipoproteins. There are both genetic and environmental contributing factors (e.g., diet, physical inactivity). Dyslipidaemia is a major risk factor for cardiovascular disease, elevating risk two- to three-fold and possibly higher depending on the concentrations of various blood lipid components. Up to half of the Australian adult population exhibits some aspect of dyslipidaemia, usually elevated blood cholesterol levels.

The most commonly encountered abnormal lipid profile is elevated levels of serum total cholesterol (TC), low-density lipoprotein cholesterol (LDL-C) and triglycerides (Tg) and reduced levels of high-density lipoprotein cholesterol (HDL-C). Abnormal blood lipids are also reflected in the levels of associated proteins, such as the apolipoproteins. Low concentrations of TC, LDL-C and Tg and high HDL-C concentrations represent a favourable blood lipid profile. Recommended levels are given in table 8.2. High levels of cholesterol carried in the LDL-C fraction contribute to atherosclerosis, whereas a high level of HDL-C is considered protective because it is involved in removal and degradation of potentially damaging cholesterol. The ratio of TC to HDL-C (TC:HDL-C) is another important measure in assessing risk of cardiovascular disease.

Physical Activity and Dyslipidaemia

Elevated TC, LDL-C and Tg and low HDL-C levels occur in association with the metabolic syndrome, in particular type 2 diabetes and abdominal obesity. TC, LDL-C and Tg concentrations tend to increase with age in men and after menopause in women. When elevated, the risk of cardiovascular disease is greatly increased. Dietary and physical activity interventions are the non-pharmacological methods of choice for normalising the blood lipid profile. Medication may be required when high TC, LDL-C or Tg levels appear resistant to such intervention or in familial (genetic) dyslipidaemia. Weight loss, especially reduction of abdominal fat, induces favourable changes such as decreased TC, LDL-C and Tg and increased HDL-C concentrations. Exercise by itself (i.e., without weight loss) does not generally influence TC or LDL-C, although it does increase HDL-C and reduce Tg levels.

Endurance exercise is now recognised as the most effective means of increasing HDL-C levels, particularly by increasing the concentration of the most protective HDL_2-C subfraction. Endurance athletes such as distance runners and cross-country skiers exhibit the highest HDL-C concentrations (often in the range of 1.5-2.5 mmol $\cdot$ L^{-1}) and correspondingly high HDL_2-C subfractions. Although such exercise is unrealistic for most non-athletes, regular moderate physical activity by the overweight and moderately obese (BMI of 25 to 30) increases HDL-C con-

centration and reduces Tg concentration and the TC:HDL-C ratio, even without weight loss. However, for the obese individual, weight loss achieved through a combination of dietary and exercise interventions is necessary to significantly alter the blood lipid profile. Fat loss appears to be the most important factor for normalising blood lipids in the obese.

The effects of exercise on HDL-C concentration depend on several factors including initial body mass and HDL-C level, training volume and duration, and extent of weight and fat loss during training. Increased HDL-C and HDL_2-C concentrations have been observed after several months of endurance training without loss of body mass (Nicklas et al. 1997; Thompson et al. 1997) in lean and overweight men (BMI <30). The increase in HDL-C level is smaller than the increase in the cardioprotective subfraction HDL_2-C (5-10% and 30-80%, respectively). Although changes in HDL-C are modest, they are sufficient to reduce the risk of heart disease. For example, it has been estimated that each 0.026 mmol $\cdot$ L^{-1} increase in HDL-C concentration reduces risk by 2 to 4%, thus an increase of 0.1 mmol$\cdot$ L^{-1} may reduce risk by as much as 15%. A minimum of 1,000 to 1,200 kcal/wk energy expenditure in exercise is deemed necessary to increase HDL-C levels (refer to chapter 7 for estimation of energy expenditure during physical activity).

Training-induced changes in HDL-C and HDL_2-C levels appear to be blunted in the obese and in those with initially low HDL-C concentrations (<0.9 mmol $\cdot$ L^{-1}) (Nicklas et al. 1997). In these individuals, exercise appears to increase HDL-C levels only when body mass is also reduced. Changes in free fatty acid and Tg metabolism may be responsible for this lack of exercise effect on HDL-C. Training-induced changes in HDL-C and HDL_2-C levels tend to be higher in leaner individuals with high initial HDL-C concentration and $\dot{V}O_2$max.

Diabetes

Diabetes is a metabolic disease resulting in abnormally high blood glucose levels (>7.0 mmol $\cdot$ L^{-1} fasting or >11.1 mmol $\cdot$ L^{-1} non-fasting). A fasting blood glucose level of <6.1 mmol $\cdot$ L^{-1} is recommended (refer to table 8.2). Values between 6.1 and 7.0 mmol $\cdot$ L^{-1} indicate impaired glucose tolerance and a higher risk of developing diabetes. There are two main forms of diabetes: insulin-dependent diabetes mellitus (IDDM, or type 1) and non-insulin-dependent diabetes mellitus (NIDDM, or type 2). Type 1 diabetes usually (but not always) begins in childhood or adolescence. It is an autoimmune disease in which the body's immune system attacks the insulin-producing beta cells of the pancreas, leaving an insulin deficit that must then be replaced exogenously by daily injection. Type 2 diabetes usually begins after age 40, although it can occur earlier; it is characterised by a relative insulin deficiency due to insulin insensitivity. That is, the body produces some insulin, but receptors on peripheral tissues (e.g., adipose, liver, skeletal muscle) are insensitive to the insulin. Since insulin is required to stimulate cellular uptake of glucose, any deficit in the amount of available insulin (type 1) or the ability of cells to respond to insulin (type 2) results in elevated blood glucose concentration. If left untreated for extended periods, elevated blood glucose levels may lead to myriad pathologies such as damage to blood vessels and peripheral nerves.

Diabetes is a major risk factor for cardiovascular conditions such as heart disease, stroke and peripheral vascular disease, and it also contributes to eye and kidney diseases. The risk of mortality is two to three times higher in diabetics than in non-diabetics. Diabetes is increasing in prevalence in Australia and many developed countries, mainly because of an increased incidence of type 2 diabetes, which accounts for about 80 to 90% of cases in this country (about 3% of the adult population). The incidence of type 2 diabetes has doubled in the past 20 years, and it is also occurring earlier, even in some teenagers. This is especially alarming since earlier onset leads to an even higher prevalence among adults, and a longer duration increases risk of cardiovascular disease or other complications. In Australia, diabetes is the eighth leading cause of death and seventh leading cause of disability-adjusted life years (DALYs; refer to chapter 2); it also contributes to CAD (second leading cause of death and most prevalent cause of DALYs). As discussed in chapter 2, diabetes is one of the six major areas of health concern (Australian Institute of Health and Welfare 2000), and annual medical costs of diabetes have been estimated at >$1 billion. Although type 1 diabetes cannot at present be prevented, type 2 diabetes has a significant lifestyle-associated component. There is a genetic predisposition to both forms of diabetes; however, in individuals genetically predisposed to type 2 diabetes, the incidence of disease may be reduced by 50% with appropriate dietary and physical activity intervention.

Risk factors for type 2 diabetes include genetic predisposition, hyperinsulinaemia (high blood insulin levels), obesity (especially abdominal obesity) and physical inactivity. Physical inactivity is an in-dependent risk factor for type 2 diabetes, that is, physical inactivity by itself increases the risk of type 2 diabetes, independently of other risk factors. Type 2 diabetes usually develops over time, such that hyperinsulinaemia precedes impaired glucose tolerance. It is thought that regular exercise may prevent the progression from hyperinsulinaemia to impaired glucose tolerance and the subsequent diagnosis of type 2 diabetes. More than 90% of people with type 2 diabetes are obese, and weight gain as an adult is especially associated with type 2 diabetes. Obesity reduces both the number and sensitivity of insulin receptors; that is, there are fewer receptors for insulin, and each one is less sensitive to a given level of insulin in the blood. Skeletal muscle appears to be a major site of insulin insensitivity. Insulin sensitivity varies by skeletal muscle fibre type; slow twitch (ST, or type I) and fast twitch a (FTa, or IIa) fibres exhibit higher insulin sensitivity than fast twitch b (FTb, or IIb) fibres.

Type 1 diabetes requires exogenous insulin injection and dietary modification to regulate blood glucose levels. The first choice of treatment for type 2 diabetes is dietary modification and regular exercise to reduce body fat levels and to increase insulin sensitivity. Insulin sensitivity and glucose tolerance may be significantly improved with only marginal (5-10%) loss of body mass. Exercise without weight loss may also enhance insulin sensitivity. When diet and exercise are not effective, oral hypoglycaemic agents (OHA) may be prescribed to increase insulin production and reduce hepatic glucose output. If these treatments prove unsuccessful, some patients with type 2 diabetes will also require insulin injection.

Physical Activity and Diabetes

Regular physical activity is advocated for all individuals with diabetes, provided that blood glucose levels are well controlled. Muscular contraction stimulates glucose uptake into skeletal muscle cells via an insulin-independent pathway (i.e., the GLUT-4 receptor), and this helps lower blood glucose levels. Physical activity also enhances insulin receptor sensitivity, increasing insulin-dependent glucose uptake into several tissues. Stimulatory effects of exercise on insulin-independent glucose uptake occur both chronically with exercise training and acutely after each session of activity; a single bout of exercise may stimulate glucose uptake for 24 to 48 h afterward. Moreover, regular exercise may also indirectly enhance insulin receptor sensitivity and glucose tolerance by reducing fat mass, increasing muscle mass and capillarity (number of capillaries around each muscle fibre), and perhaps inducing a transition in the metabolic characteristics of skeletal muscle fibre type (e.g., from FTb to FTa). Glucose tolerance may be improved by regular moderate exercise even in overweight/obese individuals with type 2 diabetes. Although physical activity is recommended for those with diabetes, blood glucose levels need to be monitored because there is a risk of **hypoglycaemia** during or after exercise.

Hypertension

An individual is considered to have hypertension when systolic blood pressure is 140 mmHg or higher, diastolic blood pressure is 90 mmHg or higher, or if taking antihypertensive medication. National surveys by the National Heart Foundation of Australia report that the incidence of hypertension is 13% of women and 17% of men over age 20. Blood pressure increases with age (systolic more than diastolic) and so too does the prevalence of hypertension; 54% of women and 37% of men aged 65 to 69 years have high blood pressure. The Heart Foundation and World Health Organization classify values as

- ▶ normal: <140/90,
- ▶ borderline hypertension: between 140/90 and 160/95,
- ▶ high blood pressure: >160/95, and
- ▶ very high blood pressure: >180/110.

Hypertension is a major risk factor for cardiovascular disease including heart disease and stroke, renal disease and peripheral vascular disease, all leading causes of death and disability in Australia (discussed in chapter 2). However, blood pressure can be modified through a combination of interventions. For borderline hypertension, lifestyle changes include weight reduction, dietary sodium restriction, moderate alcohol consumption and physical activity; for high and very high blood pressure, various types of medications can be prescribed in addition to lifestyle modification. It is estimated that even small changes in blood pressure, as little as 2 to 5 mmHg, result in large decreases in the incidence of hypertension and associated diseases across the population.

Physical Activity and Hypertension

Regular physical activity is often recommended as a non-pharmacological intervention for borderline hypertension. Epidemiological and intervention studies demonstrate an inverse association between physical activity and blood pressure. Exercise intervention has been shown to lower diastolic and systolic blood pressure by approximately 6 to 7 mmHg in both normotensive and hypertensive individuals; some studies have reported 10 mmHg decreases in blood pressure. Such alterations appear to occur independently of loss of body mass. Moreover, exercise training reduces blood pressure at a given submaximal work rate, reducing rate pressure product (heart rate × systolic blood pressure) and thus myocardial oxygen demand and stress on the heart. If maintained for years, regular exercise may also reduce the magnitude of the age-related rise in blood pressure. The exact mechanisms responsible for the decreases in resting and exercise blood pressure are not clearly known, but they may relate to a combination of factors such as reduced cardiac output, catecholamine release and sensitivity, and peripheral resistance in the blood vessels.

Exercise Capacity and Metabolic Syndrome

All components of the metabolic syndrome are major risk factors for cardiovascular disease. Consequently, pre-screening for cardiovascular disease is essential and medical examination is warranted before any maximal fitness testing or vigorous exercise program. As discussed in chapter 5, a medical examination is required for individuals over age 35 with type 2 diabetes wishing to perform moderate to intense exercise (i.e., more than moderate walking). This examination should include an exercise stress test to identify any undiagnosed cardiovascular disease or abnormal blood pressure response to exercise and to diagnose other conditions such as retinopathy or neuropathy. Because familial dyslipidaemia (i.e., genetically caused) may occur in young adults and may not necessarily be accompanied by other abnormalities, it is helpful to have access to the blood lipid profiles of all clients if possible; it is estimated that about half of those with elevated blood pressure or glucose intolerance may be unaware of their condition. Blood pressure and blood glucose levels also provide important information for screening and assessment. Table 8.3 briefly summarises recommendations for fitness testing in individuals with cardiorespiratory and metabolic diseases.

Fitness testing and anthropometric assessment may not be necessary for the inactive, obese, non-hypertensive individual. Fitness level will often be low because of inactivity and high body mass; these measures may be meaningless and may discourage the obese client. Any program prescribed should first aim to encourage adoption of regular moderate physical activity sufficient to induce some weight and particularly abdominal fat loss. Fitness testing and

TABLE 8.3—Summary of Assessment Recommendations for Individuals With Cardiorespiratory and Metabolic Disorders

Disease or condition	Exercise/fitness test recommended	Other useful tests or information	Contraindications, precautions or other considerations
Obesity	Testing may not be relevant; if needed, use submax, weight supported or upper body	Blood glucose level WHR or WC TC and lipoproteins BP	May have low functional capacity; $\dot{V}O_2max \cdot kg^{-1}$ will be low
Type 1 diabetes	Standard test if approved	Blood glucose level Time/location of last insulin injection	Avoid if poor blood glucose control Have glucose available
Type 2 diabetes	Submax, weight supported or upper body if obese Skinfolds if not obese	Blood glucose level WHR or WC TC and lipoproteins Medications	Avoid if poor blood glucose control Have OHA available or glucose if uses insulin As for obesity if also overweight or obese
Hypertension	Standard test if approved Measure BP during test Submax, weight supported or upper body if obese	WHR Skinfolds if not obese BP from maximal exercise test	Stop test if SBP >260 mmHg, DBP >115 mmHg or headache develops
Dyslipidaemia	Submax, weight supported or upper body if obese	WHR or WC TC and lipoproteins Skinfolds if not obese	As for obesity, if also overweight or obese
PAOD	Exercise tolerance (time to pain onset and maximum pain) Discontinuous protocol Low intensity, gradual increments	BP at rest and during exercise Pain during ADLs Gait analysis	High risk for CAD Extended warm-up needed
Asthma	Submax preferred unless max data needed Challenge test if needed to document EIB	Lung function (FEV$_1$) before and after	Use meds and warm up before Avoid when low PEF or URTI present
COPD	Cycle ergometry Low intensity, gradual increments $\dot{V}O_2max$, RPE, arterial O_2 Dyspnoea ratings	Dyspnoea during ADLs Use of supplemental oxygen Medications Spirometry data	Low functional capacity Avoid early in morning

Assuming the client has been pre-screened and cleared for testing by a medical practitioner, if needed, according to the ACSM guidelines (see chapter 5).

Abbreviations: submax = submaximal exercise test; WHR = waist to hip ratio; WC = waist circumference; TC = total cholesterol; BP = blood pressure; OHA = oral hypoglycaemic agents; SBP = systolic blood pressure; DBP = diastolic blood pressure; PAOD = peripheral artery occlusive disease; ADLs = activities of daily living; CAD = coronary artery disease; max = maximal exercise test; EIB = exercise-induced bronchospasm; meds = medications; PEF = peak expiratory flow; URTI = upper respiratory tract infection; COPD = chronic obstructive pulmonary disorder; RPE = rating of perceived exertion; FEV^1 = forced expiratory volume in 1s.

anthropometric measures may be useful after a regular program and some weight loss have been established. Waist circumference and WHR are easily measured, give a good indication of abdominal obesity, can be quickly altered by regular exercise and should be included in initial and follow-up assessment.

For individuals with high blood pressure and other risk factors for cardiovascular disease, medical screening and exercise stress testing are required before beginning moderate to intense physical activity. However, it is inadvisable to maximally test a hypertensive individual without a medical practitioner present (ACSM 2000). In hypertensive individuals, exercising blood pressure is measured during and after the exercise stress test to determine if abnormally high values are reached and at what stage of exercise. The test is stopped if abnormal responses are observed, such as systolic blood pressure >260 mmHg, diastolic blood pressure >115 mmHg, headache or failure of systolic blood pressure to rise with increasing work rate. Blood pressure measurement may also be useful during submaximal exercise (both testing and regular sessions) to ensure that blood pressure remains within the acceptable range. Maximal strength testing (i.e., 1 RM) is contraindicated for individuals with hypertension or diabetes because blood pressure may rise to dangerous levels and damage may occur in some blood vessels, particularly in the eyes.

Exercise Prescription for Metabolic Syndrome

When prescribing exercise for the individual with metabolic syndrome or its components, the choice of exercise mode, frequency and intensity is dictated by carefully balancing client readiness, needs (e.g., weight loss), other risk factors (e.g., hypertension) or conditions (e.g., disability), fitness level and likelihood of compliance (refer to chapters 4 and 5). Although exercise to achieve weight loss is important for overweight or obese clients, it may be more important from the perspective of program adoption and long-term compliance to emphasise that physical activity may be beneficial by itself even with only small changes in body mass or other factors. The primary focus should be on first establishing a routine of regular moderate and enjoyable physical activity and then later focusing on other issues such as weight loss.

Exercise Prescription for the Overweight and Obese

For the overweight or obese client, physical activity intervention should focus on increasing energy ex-

penditure sufficiently to induce loss of body mass and body fat (see table 8.4). Energy expenditure of >300 kcal (>1260 kJ) per session is recommended; approximately 7,700 kcal (32 mJ) energy expenditure is required to lose 1.0 kg of body fat. Excess body mass may limit agility and range of movement or may increase stress on joints, so simple modes such as stationary cycling, walking or water-based activities are recommended, at least at the onset. **Circuit resistance training** with relatively longer work and shorter rest intervals (e.g., 45-60 s work and 15 s rest) may prove effective by increasing energy expenditure and adding muscle mass, thereby favourably altering body composition and resting metabolic rate (as discussed previously).

Exercise should be performed daily if possible and at minimum three to four times per week to significantly increase energy expenditure. Activity accumulated over the entire day (e.g., multiple 10-min sessions) may be as effective for weight loss as a continuous daily session and may enhance compliance. Lower intensity (e.g., 40-60% $\dot{V}O_2$max to start) may be preferable for a number of reasons: the obese individual's low initial fitness level, less likelihood of injury and greater chance of subject compliance over the long term. Moreover, fatty acid mobilisation from adipose tissue and subsequent uptake and oxidation by skeletal muscle are enhanced by lower intensity exercise (e.g., <75% $\dot{V}O_2$max). On the other hand, high-intensity exercise has been associated with greater loss of subcutaneous fat than low-intensity exercise of similar energy expenditure. High-intensity exercise should therefore not be discouraged in interested overweight clients capable of intense exercise (e.g., former athletes), provided it does not impinge on compliance or cause injury. Obese individuals are less tolerant of the heat (because of a higher ratio of body volume to surface area), and this should also be considered in the exercise prescription. For example, it may be more appropriate for the obese client to undertake lower intensity exercise, exercise during cooler times of day, use water-based activities or exercise in a controlled gym-based environment. Figure 8.2 presents an example of a week's physical activity program for an overweight individual wishing to lose weight.

Exercise Prescription for the Client With Type 2 Diabetes

Regular moderate physical activity, on a daily basis if possible, is recommended for the individual with type 2 diabetes. Although higher intensity exercise (e.g., 70-85% $\dot{V}O_2$max) has been shown to induce dramatic improvement in insulin sensitivity and to re-

TABLE 8.4—Exercise Recommendations for Obese and Overweight Individuals

Exercise variable	Recommendation	Reason
Mode	Endurance	Expend sufficient energy to reduce fat
	Circuit resistance	High energy cost; increase LBM
	Weight bearing if possible	Increase energy cost
Intensity	Low at start if unfit (<70% HRR)	Prevent injury, enhance compliance, mobilise fat
	Higher if capable and interested	Increase energy expenditure, LBM, glucose tolerance
Frequency	Daily if possible or at least 2-4 d/wk	Expend sufficient energy to reduce fat
		Establish habit
Duration	>30 min or 300 kcal per session	Expend sufficient energy to reduce fat at acceptable rate
Time frame	Weeks to months, depending on starting level	Realistic rate of weight loss* = 0.5-2.0 kg/wk
		Apparent slow progress at first because increase in LBM may obscure fat loss

*Depends on the initial size and health status of the person.

Abbreviations: LBM = lean body mass; HRR = heart rate reserve.

Monday	30 min brisk walking
Tuesday	At fitness centre: 10 min aerobic conditioning on rower, stair climber or exercise bike, plus circuit resistance training (2 sets, 10-15 RM, 10 exercises of major muscles)
Wednesday	Rest day or 20 min easy walking
Thursday	30 min brisk walking
Friday	Repeat Tuesday's session
Saturday	1 h social tennis or 18 holes golf
Sunday	5-km bushwalk or mountain bike ride over gentle terrain with family

Assuming there are no contraindications and that the individual has medical approval for this program. This program would not be suitable as a beginning program for an unfit individual, who would require several weeks' gradual progression to this level.

In addition to the program detailed above, incidental physical activity should be increased, for example, walking or cycling instead of driving for local errands, walking to public transport, using stairs instead of the lift and regularly performing active household tasks such as gardening or home repair.

FIGURE 8.2   Example of a 7-day exercise plan for the individual wishing to lose weight.

duce body fat levels, this level of exercise is unrealistic for clients with type 2 diabetes who are obese or unfit. High-intensity exercise may be effective for some highly motivated individuals, such as former athletes or non-athletes after significant weight loss

and improvements in fitness levels. The main focus for most individuals should be low-intensity, long-duration exercise (e.g., 30-60 min at 40-60% $\dot{V}O_2$max), which enables sufficient energy and fat metabolism to induce weight loss and also causes favourable changes in blood lipids and glucose tolerance. Addition of circuit resistance training involving high repetitions and low weights (e.g., 10-20 RM) to an aerobic program may also be beneficial; this type of training induces high energy consumption ($\sim$10 kcal $\cdot$ min^{-1}) and an increase in muscle mass. In a recent study (Eriksson et al. 1998), the combination of aerobic and circuit resistance training was shown to improve insulin sensitivity to a greater extent than simple aerobic training. However, to avoid damage to blood vessels, resistance training is advised only for those patients with type 2 diabetes who do not have retinopathy (degenerative changes to the retina resulting from diabetes) or hypertension. Attention to footwear and foot hygiene is important because peripheral neuropathy (degenerative changes in sensory nerves resulting from diabetes) may reduce sensation in the feet. In addition, hypohydration may result from exercise in the diabetic, so adequate fluid intake before, during and after exercise is essential. Individuals with type 2 diabetes who take insulin or oral hypoglycaemic agents (OHA) should follow exercise guidelines for type 1 diabetes to avoid hypoglycaemia during and after exercise (see figure 8.3).

Exercise Prescription for the Client With Type 1 Diabetes

Individuals with type 1 diabetes are generally not restricted from any type or level of activity provided that blood glucose levels are well controlled; indeed, many professional and other high-performance athletes have type 1 diabetes. If control is good, exercise helps lower blood glucose levels. If control is poor, exercise increases the already high blood glucose levels even further, and intense exercise is contraindicated until the client seeks medical advice and returns to good control. Even in the exerciser with well-controlled diabetes, communication between the client and his or her physician is essential because regular exercise may alter the dosage of insulin required to maintain blood glucose levels. In some instances, a client's physician and exercise manager may have an established line of communication, for example, in a group practice including medical and other health practitioners. In other situations, it is advisable for the exercise manager to provide a detailed written exercise program for the client to take to his or her physician. Guidelines for exercise for the individual with type 1 diabetes are presented in figure 8.3.

INSULIN USAGE

▶ Maintain close communication with physician to monitor appropriate insulin dosage.

▶ Avoid exercise at peak insulin activity.

▶ Inject insulin away from muscles to be used during exercise.

DIET

▶ Consume carbohydrate 30-60 min before exercise.

▶ Always carry a ready supply of glucose in case of hypoglycaemia.

▶ Drink plenty of fluids before, during and after exercise.

EXERCISE SETTING

▶ Exercise daily if possible and at the same time of day, preferably not at night.

▶ Exercise in a group or with at least one other person who is aware of the condition.

▶ Avoid high-risk or isolated activities if there is a chance of experiencing hypoglycaemia.

FOOT CARE

▶ Check feet for cuts and bruises before and after exercise.

▶ Always wear appropriate and supportive footwear.

Compiled from American College of Sports Medicine, 2000, *ACSM's guidelines for exercise testing and prescription*, 6th ed. (Philadelphia: Lippincott Williams & Wilkins); B.N. Campaigne, 1998, Exercise and diabetes. In American College of Sports Medicine. *ACSM's resource manual for guidelines for exercise testing and prescription*, 3rd ed. (Baltimore: Williams & Wilkins), 267-274.

FIGURE 8.3 Recommendations for exercise for individuals with type 1 diabetes.

Consistency is essential for exercise prescription for the client with type 1 diabetes. Exercise should be performed daily if possible, and the time of day, exercise intensity and duration, and environmental conditions should also be as consistent as possible to ensure that insulin requirements remain relatively constant. This may be difficult for athletes who must vary exercise according to the demands of the sport; diabetic athletes may need to adjust insulin dosage and diet accordingly. The diabetic exerciser should avoid exercising during peak insulin activity because the combined effects of exercise and insulin in stimulating glucose uptake from the blood may cause hypoglycaemia. Insulin should not be injected into the working muscles—this increases washout of insulin into the blood and may also cause hypoglycaemia.

The diabetic should consume a carbohydrate-rich snack 30-60 min before exercise and monitor blood glucose levels before and after exercise. If the resting blood glucose level is poorly controlled, that is, less than 4.5 mmol $\cdot$ L^{-1} (indicating hypoglycaemia) or greater than 14 mmol $\cdot$ L^{-1} (indicating hyperglycaemia), exercise should not be undertaken. Hypoglycaemia during or after exercise is a potential concern for any diabetic who injects insulin or uses oral hypoglycaemic agents, regardless of the type of diabetes. Both exercise and insulin stimulate glucose uptake from the blood, albeit by different pathways; excess uptake of glucose during or after exercise may thus lead to critically low blood glucose. Because hypoglycaemia may occur up to several hours after exercise, exercise should be avoided in the hours before retiring at night to prevent hypoglycaemia during sleep. The dosage, timing and site of insulin injection may need modification based on exercise requirements. All insulin-injecting diabetics should carry a ready supply of fast-acting glucose when exercising and should avoid exercising alone or in isolated areas. To avoid hypoglycaemia during prolonged exercise, exercise duration longer than 60 min requires glucose monitoring and a carbohydrate snack every 30 min.

Diabetes may cause peripheral neuropathy, leading to loss of nerve sensation especially in the feet. Adequate supportive footwear and socks should be worn, and the feet should be frequently checked for cuts or bruises. Because high blood glucose levels may cause excessive dehydration, drinking plenty of fluids before, during and after exercise is also essential. Diabetics with retinopathy (damage to blood vessels in the retina) should avoid jarring or bouncing exercises (e.g., jogging/running, high-impact aerobics, plyometrics) since these may further damage delicate blood vessels. The diabetic is advised to avoid activities such as scuba diving, hang-gliding and sky diving because of obvious risks of becoming hypoglycaemic in such situations. In addition, activities in isolated environments (e.g., mountain climbing) are also risky because hypoglycaemia may become life-threatening without ready access to medical care.

Exercise Prescription for Dyslipidaemia

The minimal and optimal modes and amounts of physical activity required to significantly improve the blood lipid profile are not clearly known at present. Endurance training such as distance running produces a favourable blood lipid profile (i.e., low levels of TC, Tg and TC:HDL-C and high levels of HDL-C). Epidemiological studies on runners have shown that HDL-C concentration is directly related to average weekly running distance up to 80 km/wk; an apparent threshold of about 16 km/wk is required to show elevations above values of non-runners (Williams 1996). Intervention studies (Crouse et al. 1997; Nicklas et al. 1997; Thompson et al. 1997) show that the most effective program to induce increases in HDL-C without weight loss in non-obese individuals should involve the following:

▶ Duration of 30 to 60 min per session

▶ Frequency of three to four times weekly

▶ Intensity of 50 to 80% $\dot{V}O_2$max or HRR

▶ Minimal energy expenditure of 900 to 1,050 kcal/wk

▶ Minimum period of 6 months

▶ 15 to 25% increments in $\dot{V}O_2$max by 6 months

Although this level of exercise fits within the ACSM recommendations, it is higher than the minimum amount recommended by public health campaigns such as the 1996 U.S. Surgeon General's Report or the Active Australia policy (discussed in chapter 2).

Exercise intensity is less important than duration or total energy expenditure for altering the blood lipid profile; for example, when energy expenditure was held constant at 350 kcal per session, exercise at 50% and 80% $\dot{V}O_2$max produced similar increases in HDL-C levels (Nicklas et al. 1997). Many exercise modes alter HDL-C levels, including walking, jogging, rowing, skiing and cycle ergometry; the effects of swim training have not been clearly established. Fat loss and exercise have additive effects on HDL-C levels, and a combination of diet and exercise are most effective for reducing body mass and WHR in overweight and especially obese individuals.

Case Study 8.1

Andrew is 47 years old, works as a branch manager at a suburban bank located in a major shopping complex, and undertakes no physical activity during his leisure time. A recent fasting blood profile yielded the following results: total cholesterol = 7.1, LDL cholesterol = 4.8, HDL cholesterol = 0.84, triglycerides = 2.4 and glucose = 6.6 (all in $mmol \cdot L^{-1}$). Andrew has been referred by his GP, who is concerned about his sedentary lifestyle. His doctor prefers first trying lifestyle modification before considering medication.

Andrew's height is 183 cm, body mass is 90 kg, waist measurement is 100 cm and waist to hip ratio is 1.02. Andrew was physically active as a young man, having played cricket and rugby at school and university. However, over the years he has become progressively less active because of work and family commitments. His children are now fairly independent teenagers.

Write a 6-month progressive activity program for Andrew that will help address the specific health concerns raised by his doctor.

Key Issues

1. What specifically is Andrew's doctor concerned about? To what extent can physical activity alone help address these concerns? What other interventions might be needed? Why?

2. What are the main goals for Andrew in the first 6 months of his activity program?

3. At what stage of change (refer to chapter 4) is Andrew now? How will you adjust his exercise program as he moves through the various stages?

4. What factors will influence Andrew's adherence to your exercise program? How will you accommodate these in your exercise prescription?

5. Is resistance training recommended for Andrew? Why or why not?

Exercise Prescription for Hypertension

In general, exercise prescription for hypertensive individuals should include moderate-intensity exercise using the entire body or large body segments. The mode of exercise is not as important as the intensity and volume (duration, frequency). Walking, jogging, aerobics, cycling and swimming effectively lower both systolic and diastolic blood pressure in hypertensive and normotensive individuals. A recent meta-analysis of studies on blood pressure and exercise concluded that exercise three times per week between 60 and 70% $\dot{V}O_2$max is sufficient to alter blood pressure (there are too few studies of lower intensity exercise to draw any conclusions) (Halbert et al. 1997). Exercise above 70% $\dot{V}O_2$max or more than three times per week appears to have little additional effect on lowering blood pressure. Exercise studies generally show decreases of about 5 to 7 mmHg for both systolic and diastolic blood pressures, although declines of up to 10 mmHg have been reported. While these changes seem rather small, they are sufficient to bring about large changes in risk of disease.

There are too few studies to determine whether circuit resistance training by itself effectively alters blood pressure. At present, resistance training is recommended only as a complement to endurance training and only when performed as high-repetition, low-resistance activity (e.g., circuit training using sets of 8-12 RM, as recommended by the USSG and ACSM; refer to chapters 2 and 7). Circuit resistance training may be most beneficial by reducing body weight and fat levels and may thus indirectly contribute to lowering blood pressure. Because blood pressure may rise to dangerously high levels in hypertensive individuals, intense resistance training or maximal lifting is not recommended. The client should be instructed to breathe regularly during resistance training (usually exhalation during each lift or push and inhalation during recovery between each lift). Holding the breath should be avoided.

An individual with markedly elevated blood pressure (i.e., >160/100 mmHg at rest or large increases at low exercise levels) should begin an exercise program only after evaluation by a physician and while on medication. For hypertensives on medication, regular exercise may further lower blood pressure, which may require alteration of dosage; communication between patient and physician about exercise is thus very important. As previously described for the diabetic client, it is advisable to give the hypertensive client a written detailed exercise program that can be shown to the physician managing the client's hypertension.

Exercise Cardiac Rehabilitation

Physical activity has become an integral part of secondary prevention after a cardiac event (e.g., myocardial infarction, cardiac failure, surgical procedures). Cardiac rehabilitation refers to a series of programs that help patients return to an active and satisfying life after some type of cardiac episode. Cardiac rehabilitation comprises a multifaceted intervention to counsel, educate, encourage and support the patient in making lifestyle and behaviour changes. According to the National Heart Foundation of Australia (NHFA), the broad aims of cardiac rehabilitation are to maximise physical, psychological and social functioning, enabling the patient to live productively and with confidence, and to assist and encourage behaviours that may minimise the risk of further cardiac events and conditions (NHFA 1998). Programs may include interventions to facilitate weight loss, smoking cessation, management of blood pressure, lipids, medication and physical activity to prevent further disease progression and recurrence of cardiac events.

Exercise cardiac rehabilitation plays a part in comprehensive programs involving progressive physical activity. Candidates for exercise cardiac rehabilitation include patients

- at risk of cardiac or other vascular diseases;
- with stable angina pectoralis or myocardial ischaemia;
- recovering from an acute cardiac event, such as myocardial infarction, coronary arterial bypass grafts (CABG) or percutaneous transluminal coronary angioplasty (PTCA);
- with peripheral vascular disease;
- who are heart transplant recipients or have a pacemaker or valve replacement;
- with certain forms of non-ischaemic heart disease; and
- with complex conditions requiring multiple medications.

While exercise by itself probably does not halt the progression of cardiovascular disease, there is good evidence that a multifactorial intervention program including education, counselling, dieting, smoking cessation, medication and physical activity will. Documented positive outcomes of such multifactorial programs include the following:

- Increased objective measures of exercise tolerance without complications
- Enhanced compliance in physical activity
- Decreased angina occurrence and increased threshold in CAD patients
- Favourable changes in blood lipid profile
- Decreased blood pressure
- Enhanced psychological well-being
- Faster return to work after a cardiac event
- Decreased mortality from cardiovascular disease

There are many potential benefits of a supervised exercise program as part of secondary prevention during and after hospitalisation. These include counteracting deconditioning due to bed rest, providing supervision to monitor the patient, identifying abnormal responses to physical activity in a controlled setting, enhancing safety during exercise and facilitating return to normal daily and occupational activities. In the United States, the net savings of exercise cardiac rehabilitation (after adjusting for cost of the program) have been estimated at >$250 per patient in the first 2 years. That sum becomes considerable if multiplied by the number of cardiac patients throughout the country who may benefit. Although most data on the effectiveness of exercise cardiac rehabilitation relate to middle-aged men, there is good evidence that female and elderly cardiac patients show similar responses. The use of exercise programs as part of secondary prevention is one of the fastest growing opportunities for employment of exercise management graduates in Australia.

Until the late 1990s, programs were categorised into three stages in Australia and three to four stages overseas: stage 1 while the patient is in hospital, stage 2 up to 12 weeks after discharge from hospital and stages 3 and 4 starting 12 weeks after the initial event and lasting for several months or longer. In the past few years, there has been a move toward a more simplified and flexible approach. The length of programs and the duration of patient monitoring is more varied, based on many factors such as the patient's needs and level of risk, exercise history and occupational activity. This approach also aims to make programs more accessible and individualised, given that many Australians live away from major urban centres, thus limiting their access to clinic-based programs. Recent efforts focus on providing home- or community-based programs that can be safely accessed by all.

In Australia, programs are now classified into three phases:

▶ In-patient (phase 1): involves early mobilisation while the patient is still in hospital

▶ Out-patient (phase 2): lasts for 4 to 12 weeks after discharge from hospital, during which time the patient exercises in a supervised program while variables such as ECG, blood pressure and other responses to exercise may be monitored

▶ Maintenance (phase 3): open-ended (hopefully for life) and the level of structure and supervision depends on the patient's condition (NHFA 1998).

Exercise Prescription for Cardiac Patients

When prescribing exercise for the cardiac patient, the need for exercise volume and intensity sufficient to generate changes in functional capacity must be balanced with the patient's disease state, fitness level before the event, enjoyment, goals, motivation and likelihood of long-term compliance. Table 8.5 summarises general guidelines for exercise prescription for cardiac patients. In-patient exercise rehabilitation (phase 1, or mobilisation phase) aims to counteract the deleterious effects of bed rest, to promote self-confidence and to progressively increase physical capacity so that the patient may be able to perform basic self-care after release from hospital. This phase begins when the patient is clinically stable and can undertake limited activity. Activities include basic mobilisation such as sitting, walking short distances and performing **activities of daily living (ADLs)** (e.g., rising from sitting to standing, walking, dressing, showering), in addition to specific arm and leg exercises. Progress through this phase varies depending on age, extent of disease and type of cardiac event. At the end of this phase by the time of discharge from hospital, patients should be able to slowly walk for 5 to 10 min, three to four times per day, and climb one to two flights of stairs under supervision. The phase 1 patient generally performs low-intensity exercise according to comfort level. A

TABLE 8.5—General Recommendations for Exercise Cardiac Rehabilitation

Phase	Duration	Intensity	Frequency
In-patient (phase 1) (by time of discharge from hospital)	5-10 min walking One flight stairs Bathing, dressing	Resting HR + 5-20 beats · min^{-1} SBP + 10-40 mmHg	Three to four times/day
Out-patient (phase 2)			
Aerobic	10-45 min	40-70% HRR 11-13 RPE	3-5 d/wk, daily if possible
Resistance[a]	1 set, 8-10 exercises, 10-15 reps	40-70% HRR 11-13 RPE	2 d/wk
Maintenance (phase 3)			
Aerobic	30-45 min	40-80% HRR 11-14 RPE	At least 3 d/wk, daily if possible
Resistance[a]	2-3 sets, 8-10 exercises, 10-15 reps	40-80% HRR 11-14 RPE	2-3 d/wk

[a]Resistance exercise only in low-risk, clinically stable patients, as approved by medical practitioner.

Abbreviations: SBP = systolic blood pressure; HRR = heart rate reserve; RPE = rating of perceived exertion.

Compiled from National Heart Foundation of Australia, 1998, *Recommendations for cardiac rehabilitation*; American College of Sports Medicine, 2000, *ACSM's guidelines for exercise testing and prescription*, 6th ed. (Philadelphia: Lippincott Williams & Wilkins).

general guide is that exercise intensity should elicit responses of heart rate equivalent to resting heart rate plus 5 to 20 beats · min^{-1} and blood pressure equivalent to resting systolic blood pressure plus 10 to 40 mmHg.

Surgical patients (e.g., after coronary arterial bypass) have special needs for mobilisation (movement) of the upper body and for wound care (e.g., chest and leg from which the vein graft was taken). Bypass patients usually undergo extensive physiotherapy to enhance range of motion and mobilisation of the chest and upper body before discharge from hospital. Upper body aerobic and resistance exercise is generally prohibited for the first 4 to 8 weeks after bypass surgery to avoid pain and to allow the midsternal incision to heal.

After discharge from hospital, patients are referred to an out-patient exercise rehabilitation program (phase 2), which may be based in a hospital or clinic, community health centre, general practice or the patient's home (or some combination). This phase usually begins 2 to 3 weeks after discharge from hospital and may last 4 to 12 weeks depending on patient progress. For patients who have successfully completed an in-patient program, exercise is usually prescribed in the range of 40 to 70% $\dot{V}O_2$max or HRR or 11 to 13 RPE, depending on functional capacity and time since the cardiac event. The general recommendation is for the phase 2 patient to eventually be able to perform light to moderate physical activity for 30 to 45 min, three to four times per week, and to also increase incidental physical activity (e.g., using the stairs).

Risk stratification of patients early in their recovery permits low-risk patients to be identified for home- or community-based programs. Low-risk patients are those with clinically stable disease as indicated by no left ventricular dysfunction, angina, arrhythmias or complications and a functional capacity of at least 6 METs 3 weeks after the cardiac event. Higher risk patients have low functional capacity (<6 METs), angina or evidence of ischaemia, arrhythmias, left ventricular dysfunction or other complications. High-risk patients are recommended to continue exercise in a clinically-supervised setting where variables such as heart rate, RPE, ECG, blood pressure and angina or other symptoms may be monitored. The National Heart Foundation of Australia recommends that group programs be supervised by a health professional, such as a nurse, physiotherapist, occupational therapist or exercise scientist with experience in exercise cardiac rehabilitation (NHFA 1998). Weekly assessment by a member of the cardiac rehabilitation team is also recommended for home- or community-based programs,

which have been shown to be as safe and effective for low-risk patients as clinic- or hospital-based programs.

To increase muscular strength and endurance, upper body and moderate resistance training may also be recommended in addition to, but not instead of, cardiovascular conditioning. Upper body and resistance exercise may be beneficial, especially when occupation, leisure or ADLs require a certain level of strength (e.g., trades, gardening, housework). Such training has been shown to be safe for the clinically stable low-risk patient as long as certain guidelines are followed; resistance training is inappropriate for the high-risk or clinically unstable patient. For low-risk patients, upper body exercise should be performed at a heart rate about 10 to 15 beats · min^{-1} less, or power output 50% less, than for lower or whole body exercise. Previous guidelines suggested that cardiac patients should not perform resistance training for several months after a cardiac event. However, more recent practice suggests that clinically stable patients can begin resistance training earlier (2-6 weeks post-event), provided that a continuum of modalities is used (ACSM 2000). Patients start with elastic bands, light hand-held weights (0.5-2.0 kg), wall pulleys and calisthenics using the body mass as resistance, and they gradually progress to machine weights in the maintenance phase. Refer to table 8.5 for the general recommendations for starting and maintaining a resistance training program.

At the end of the out-patient phase (phase 2), it is hoped that the patient will continue regular physical activity, along with other behaviour changes, to maintain a healthy lifestyle and reduce the risk of recurrence of cardiac events. Thus, the maintenance phase (phase 3) is considered to be open-ended (and hopefully lifelong). Not all patients require structured programs and some may continue a home-based program in consultation with their physician. Other patients may find the support of a structured community- or clinic-based program beneficial for continued compliance. The guidelines for physical activity are, at this point, similar to those for the general public, as long as the patient has been cleared for exercise and there is regular follow-up with the medical practitioner. Whole body or large muscle group activities such as walking, jogging, aerobics, swimming and other aquatic activities, cycling and light circuit training (for the low-risk patient) are recommended. Standard recommendations also apply such as accumulating 30 min of daily activity at least 5, and preferably all, days per week. The mode of aerobic exercise is not as important as the choice of appropriate intensity, frequency and duration of training. Controlled experimental trials show that risk of mortality from a future cardiac event may be decreased by 25% with moderate exercise in the range of 300 to 400 kcal per session (approximately 30-45 min at 60-75% $\dot{V}O_2$max), three to four times per week.

Post-myocardial infarction and CABG patients without complications usually achieve a functional capacity of 8 to 9 METs by 6 months after the event, so moderate exercise in the range of 4 to 7 METs (e.g., walking, cycling, swimming, golf, aerobics; refer to chapters 2 and 7) would be appropriate.

Case Study 8.2

Theresa is 68 and recovering from triple coronary arterial bypass surgery 8 weeks ago. She has had no previous hospitalisations or medical complications arising from her heart condition. She attended the hospital's in-patient cardiac rehabilitation program and has been walking 5 min twice per day since being discharged 7 weeks ago. She was only somewhat active before surgery through light gardening and occasional walking. Theresa's medications include aspirin and Metoprolol (a beta-blocker), and her resting blood pressure and heart rate are normal. Her cardiologist has referred her to you for an out-patient exercise program. Write a progressive 12-week program for Theresa.

Key Issues

1. What factors influence exercise adherence in female cardiac patients? How are these incorporated into an exercise program?

2. What are the main goals of Theresa's exercise program for the next 12 weeks?

3. What particular types of exercise are recommended at this stage in Theresa's recovery? Why?

4. Is it necessary to monitor Theresa during exercise? What criteria are used to make this decision?

5. What influence, if any, will her medication have on her exercise capacity or other exercise-related factors?

6. How much progress do you expect over the next 12 weeks?

Case Study 8.3

Mike is 57 years old and has been referred to your out-patient exercise cardiac rehabilitation program 12 weeks after PTCA and a stent inserted in the circumflex artery. His diagnosis and the subsequent procedure followed a routine stress test. Before the intervention, Mike cycled five times per week for 35 min during his lunch hour. His medications include aspirin and Pravastatin. He returned to work 5 weeks ago and would like to resume cycling as soon as recommended.

Write an exercise program that gradually returns Mike to his previous fitness level and exercise habits.

Key Issues

1. What modes of exercise will you start Mike with? In what settings (e.g., road cycling, gym-based, supervised clinical program)? Why?

2. Does Mike need to be monitored during exercise? Why or why not?

3. What precautions will be needed as Mike gradually increases his exercise volume (intensity and duration)? Why? What are the potential health risks and likelihood of them occurring?

4. Will Mike be able to regain his previous fitness level and exercise habit? Why or why not? If yes, how long do you expect it will take? Why? Explain this in terms that Mike can understand.

Peripheral Artery Occlusive Disease (PAOD)

Peripheral artery occlusive disease (PAOD) is a general term to describe conditions that affect the peripheral circulation. PAOD commonly involves atherosclerosis or arterial stenosis in the legs, both of which cause narrowing of the lumen in the arteries and thus reduced blood flow. A simple clinical measure of PAOD is the ratio of systolic blood pressure in the ankle compared with brachial systolic blood pressure, called the ankle-brachial index (ABI). The incidence of PAOD increases with age, and about 20% of older individuals exhibit its symptoms. Risk factors for PAOD are similar to those for cardiovascular disease, in particular hypertension, diabetes, cigarette smoking and dyslipidaemia, since the mechanisms of arterial damage are similar regardless of location.

PAOD causes transitory ischaemic pain (called intermittent claudication) in the affected area. Pain occurs during exertion, increases with exercise intensity or duration and generally subsides at cessation of exercise (hence the term *intermittent*). Ischaemia results from an imbalance between demand for oxygen by the working muscles and supply through the narrowed arteries. The pain may be described as a burning, cramping or aching feeling, usually in the calf but sometimes in the leg or buttocks as well. Treatment for PAOD may include exercise (to improve oxygen extraction by skeletal muscle), medication (to decrease blood viscosity and enhance blood flow) and possibly surgery (e.g., bypass, angioplasty) when pain is intense and exercise and medication are ineffective.

Because individuals with PAOD tend to avoid physical activity because of the pain, functional capacity and activities of daily living (ADLs) are compromised. These in turn may lead to a loss of ability to work or live independently. The major goals of exercise rehabilitation for the PAOD patient are to relieve symptoms during exertion, restore functional capacity and the ability to perform ADLs, and decrease risk factors for cardiovascular disease. Some of the documented benefits of exercise include

- increased exercise capacity (e.g., walking distance) by two- to threefold,
- increased exercise oxygen consumption,
- decreased pain during walking or ability to walk further before pain begins,

- increased habitual physical activity,
- enhanced perception of well-being and functional capacity,
- decreased blood viscosity (enhances blood flow), and
- increased mechanical efficiency during walking (more work at same metabolic cost).

It is not clear by which mechanisms exercise training enhances functional capacity. It likely involves a combination of increases in skeletal muscle oxidative capacity, pain threshold and mechanical efficiency.

Exercise Capacity and PAOD

Because of the associated risk of cardiovascular disease, patients with PAOD need medical examination and clearance before undertaking exercise testing or programs. Assessment usually includes an exercise test to determine functional capacity and onset of ischaemic pain, a medical exam to assess the severity of disease, and questionnaires to identify the extent that PAOD limits functional capacity and ADLs. Exercise testing attempts to determine pain-free walking distance (threshold at which pain occurs) and total walking distance (before pain limits exercise capacity). Gait analysis (refer to chapter 9) may be of benefit because mechanical efficiency is often affected by pain.

The standard exercise treadmill test must be modified to accommodate the low functional capacity and presence of pain. A multi-stage discontinuous treadmill protocol, starting at a slow speed with gradual increments and including rest between work intervals, is better tolerated than standard tests. Alternatively, a useful field test is the 12-min walk test (i.e., the distance covered in 12 min). Assessing the patient's perception of pain using a standard 0 to 4 scale (no pain to extreme pain) is useful for determining the test end-point and for subsequent exercise prescription. Depending on the severity of pain, an accurate measure of $\dot{V}O_2$max may be impossible to obtain if pain rather than metabolic fatigue limits exercise capacity. However, $\dot{V}O_2$peak (maximum oxygen consumption achieved during symptom-limited test) may be useful for exercise prescription and for assessing progress.

Exercise Prescription for PAOD

Exercise should be performed at least three times per week and daily if possible. Supervised programs, such as an out-patient exercise rehabilitation program, may result in better long-term compliance. Weight-bearing exercise (e.g., walking) is preferable because it produces favourable changes in leg muscle oxidative metabolism and is more specific to ADLs. However, weight-supported exercise (e.g., cycling) can be used if severe pain limits walking ability or to increase exercise duration or intensity sufficiently to induce training adaptations. Because pain appears during exertion and subsides with rest, interval exercise is better tolerated than continuous exercise.

The exercise session should consist of at least 5 min of aerobic and musculoskeletal warm-up and cool-down before and after exercise (refer to chapter 7). The warm-up, which may need to be longer if exercising in cold weather, is especially important because it facilitates dilation of peripheral vessels. Exercise intensity and volume should accommodate the initial low functional capacity of the client. To start, beneficial effects may be realised from interval walking, starting with 10 to 15 min total walking and gradually increasing to 35 min total walking time per session. Intensity should start at about 50% of maximum capacity, as measured in the exercise test, and progress to 80% over several months. Ratings of perceived exertion and perception of pain (0-4 scale) are more effective for gauging exercise intensity than percentage of maximum heart rate. The patient should walk to a rating of 2 to 3 (moderate to intense pain) on the 0 to 4 scale, rest until pain subsides, then begin walking again; this should be repeated until the total walking target time is reached. A total session time of 1 h may be necessary to accommodate the warm-up, walk/rest intervals and cool-down. Progress may be slow, and 4 to 6 months may be required to see significant changes. Gradually, total and pain-free walking distance will increase, requiring fewer rest intervals. There is little evidence that resistance training helps PAOD, but it should not be discouraged as a supplemental program if the client is interested, there are no contraindications, the resistance training does not induce extreme pain and the walking program is not compromised.

Pulmonary Disorders

Chronic obstructive pulmonary disorder (COPD) is a general term to describe a group of conditions characterised by airway obstruction; asthma, emphysema and bronchitis are the most common forms. COPD is a major cause of morbidity, disability and the need for medical treatment in Australia. As noted in chapter 2, COPD is the fourth leading cause of death and third leading cause of DALYs in Australia.

The severity of COPD varies widely depending on the type and cause, age of patient and duration of disease, and it is difficult to group all COPDs together into a single category for purposes of exercise prescription. Chronic airflow obstruction is defined functionally by changes in spirometric measures, such as forced expiratory volume in 1 s (FEV_1) and vital capacity. Airflow can be obstructed by structural changes in the lungs and airways such as thickened bronchial walls and secretions (bronchitis), loss of elasticity in the alveoli (emphysema), or airway narrowing due to inflammation or bronchoconstriction (asthma). In addition, structural and functional changes in the lungs may result in underperfusion or underventilation of parts of the lungs, resulting in poor oxygenation of blood and possibly fluid retention.

Regular physical activity plays an important role in management of pulmonary disorders such as COPD. A regular program may enhance exercise capacity, lung function during exercise, and quality of life while increasing the threshold of physical activity at which **dyspnoea** (difficult or laboured breathing) occurs. Pulmonary disorders can sometimes be psychologically debilitating because impaired physical capacity and symptoms such as shortness of breath may lead to anxiety and social isolation; group-based physical activity programs may help address psychological as well as physical effects of the disorder. Depending on the severity of disease and the patient's functional capacity and age, a medically supervised program may be warranted, including multifaceted care from respiratory, physical and occupational therapists and medical specialists.

Emphysema and Chronic Bronchitis

Diseases such as emphysema and chronic bronchitis develop slowly over a period of years, often in long-time cigarette smokers. Chronic bronchitis is characterised by chronic cough and excessive production of sputum. The airway wall thickens as a result of chronic inflammation and increased production of mucus, narrowing the large bronchi and increasing resistance to air flow, eventually leading to arterial hypoxemia (low blood oxygen content). Emphysema, which affects the small airways, is caused by an imbalance of proteolytic enzymes in the lungs that eventually leads to destruction of alveoli. Expiratory flow becomes limited because of loss of elastic recoil, and ventilation may not be uniformly distributed throughout the lungs. In moderate emphysema, arterial oxygen content may be normal, but more advanced disease may cause blood oxygen levels to decline. Both emphysema and chronic bronchitis can lead to right heart failure through increased pulmonary vascular resistance.

Exercise Capacity and Emphysema and Chronic Bronchitis

Ventilation is not considered a limiting factor to exercise capacity in healthy individuals. For the pulmonary patient, exercise capacity may be limited by factors related to ventilation such as reduced vital capacity and arterial oxygen saturation. Impairment of expiratory flow increases dead space and decreases tidal volume, causing an increase in respiratory rate and fatigue of respiratory muscles. Gas exchange and oxygenation of blood are restricted, ultimately causing symptoms of dyspnoea, which limits exercise tolerance. Depending on the severity of disease, exercise tolerance may be limited by the discomfort of dyspnoea rather than metabolic factors as in healthy individuals. Clinical exercise testing by a pulmonary specialist provides valuable diagnostic data for determining the type of illness, causes of low functional capacity and other factors (e.g., presence of heart disease). Exercise testing is best performed on a cycle ergometer to provide reliable measures of work capacity and so that work rate can be gradually increased. The test usually consists of 3-min stages starting at very low power output and progressing gradually (e.g., 10-20 W · min^{-1}). Oxygen consumption, arterial oxygen saturation, blood pressure, RPE, dyspnoea, ECG, expired CO_2 content and possibly blood lactate levels are assessed.

Exercise Prescription for Emphysema and Chronic Bronchitis

For COPD, the general principles of exercise prescription may be used, with some modifications to ensure individualisation of the program. Whole body exercise or activities using large muscle groups (e.g., walking, cycling, rowing, water-based) are recommended. Exercise should be performed for up to 30 min at least three times per week and more frequently if possible. Since many COPD patients have low exercise tolerance, interval training or several short bouts (10 min) of activity repeated through-

out the day may help in the early stages. Although there is no clear recommended range, exercise should begin at low intensity (e.g., 40-50% $\dot{V}O_2$max or 11-13 RPE) for inactive individuals, gradually increasing to a higher yet still tolerable range. Use of target heart rates should be based on actual measured maximum heart rates rather than predicted values because the relationship between heart rate, work rate and oxygen consumption is not the same for pulmonary disease as in healthy populations. Patients may prefer relying on perception of effort (RPE scale) or breathing discomfort (dyspnoea rating) rather than HR to determine exercise intensity. Exercise up to 2 (on a 0-4 scale), indicating moderate dyspnoea, is recommended.

Exercise is best avoided in the early morning when symptoms are usually at their worst. "Pursed lip" breathing is recommended to increase tidal volume while decreasing respiratory frequency, thus improving oxygenation and reducing symptoms of dyspnoea. The patient is instructed to use controlled breathing by inhaling through the nose and exhaling steadily through pursed lips (i.e., lips firmly together except at the centre); exhalation should take twice as long as inhalation. Supplemental oxygen may be required for pulmonary patients exhibiting reduced oxygen saturation (≤88%) during exercise; this would generally be used only in a clinical rehabilitation program. Moderate muscular strength and flexibility training, especially for the upper body or respiratory muscles, is also recommended two to three times per week. Strength training should incorporate high-repetition, low-resistance movements of the arm, shoulder and trunk muscles using light hand-held weights, elastic bands, weight machines or the body as resistance. Muscular strength and endurance exercises should focus on enhancing the ability to perform ADLs without causing breathlessness. Respiratory muscle training based on lung function data may enhance respiratory muscle strength and endurance and therefore improve breathing efficiency.

Asthma

Asthma is a chronic inflammatory disorder of the large airways in the lungs. The airways of an asthmatic become inflamed when exposed to certain airborne irritants such as allergens, dust or cold dry air; constriction of smooth muscle cells lining the airways further restricts air flow to and from the lungs. Asthma is the most common chronic respiratory disorder in children and young adults and the most common reason for hospitalisation among young people. For reasons unknown, the incidence of asthma has increased throughout the world over the past 10 years. Australia and New Zealand exhibit the highest rates of asthma, estimated to occur in 11% of the overall population and up to 20% of children. Approximately 2 million Australians exhibit some aspect of asthma, and the costs are estimated at about $585 to $725 million each year. There is a genetic predisposition to asthma; it has recently been proposed that genetic predisposition combined with exposure to various environmental and infectious agents in infancy may account for the increasing prevalence.

Exercise-induced asthma (EIA), more recently termed **exercise-induced bronchospasm (EIB),** is an acute airway narrowing during or after strenuous exercise. EIB occurs in 40 to 80% of all asthmatics and in 40% of those with allergic rhinitis (hay fever). It may be the only manifestation of the disorder in individuals with mild asthma. EIB is defined as a decline of 15% or more in the FEV_1 (forced expiratory volume in 1 s, a standard pulmonary function measure) after exercise. As exercise intensity increases above the ventilatory (anaerobic) threshold, minute ventilation increases disproportionately to work rate, requiring heavy mouth breathing. As ventilation increases in susceptible individuals, water and heat are lost from the lower airways, causing release of inflammatory mediators and resulting in bronchoconstriction. Symptoms of EIB usually begin after 3 to 8 min of intense exercise and include chest tightness, coughing, wheezing and dyspnoea. Symptoms are at their worst 8 to 15 min post-exercise and are normally resolved 30 to 60 min post-exercise. EIB usually occurs only during or after intense exercise—above the ventilatory threshold, or about 60 to 75% $\dot{V}O_2$max in untrained and 70 to 90% in endurance-trained individuals. EIB is unlikely to occur during light to moderate activity.

Exercise Capacity and Asthma

If asthma is well controlled, the asthmatic may exhibit no impairment of exercise capacity; indeed, many high-performance athletes in a number of sports have asthma. The availability of recently developed drugs (e.g., preventers, bronchodilators) allows most asthmatics to participate in virtually any level of exercise, provided certain precautions are met (discussed in the following section). Because of the high prevalence in Australia, all pre-program screening (refer to chapter 5) should include some method of identifying symptoms, severity of EIB when it

occurs and the overall level of control. The asthmatic is strongly encouraged to develop a management plan, in consultation with a physician, that should include details on medication and physical activity. Regular monitoring of peak expiratory flow (PEF) using a peak flow meter is also recommended. Submaximal rather than maximal fitness testing is preferred for non-athletes, since it is less likely to induce EIB. Maximal fitness testing may be appropriate for the competitive athlete whose asthma is well controlled and whose PEF is stable, provided that appropriate preventer and reliever medications are used. Children with asthma may exhibit lower aerobic and anaerobic fitness levels than their non-asthmatic peers.

Exercise Prescription for Asthma

Regular physical activity is strongly encouraged for the asthmatic. Physical conditioning reduces the risk of diseases related to inactivity (e.g., cardiovascular and metabolic diseases) and also raises the threshold at which EIB occurs. For children, physical activity is strongly advocated because of its important role in developing physical skills and social interactions. Most episodes of EIB can be prevented using appropriate medication and exercise prescription. Non-pharmacological means to prevent EIB include maintaining physical fitness, performing a proper warm-up and cool-down, and choosing the least asthmagenic environment (e.g., avoiding pollutants or irritants) and types of exercise. Specific guidelines are given in figure 8.4.

Maintaining physical fitness through regular aerobic training increases the ventilatory threshold, raising the threshold at which EIB occurs and thus reducing the likelihood of an attack during moderate exercise. Many asthmatics exhibit a refractory period after vigorous exercise during which bronchoconstriction seems to be inhibited for 1 to 2 h. For these people, a controlled 10-min warm-up consisting of light distance exercise followed by five to seven 30-s sprints may protect against EIB for up to 2 h. After warm-up, a slow rather than sudden increase in exercise intensity is preferred to allow minute ventilation to increase gradually. Exercising in a controlled environment free from irritants (e.g., indoors on cold or dry days, away from pollutants and dust) or with high humidity (e.g., water-based activities) is also advised.

Exercise prescription for asthmatics should include the same general recommendations for developing cardiovascular fitness and muscular strength as for healthy non-athletes, along with encouraging

▶ Use bronchodilator and other preventer medications before exercise and have them available during exercise.

▶ Avoid exercise when PEF is reduced or during URTI.

▶ Choose less asthmagenic activities and environments (e.g., interval and low-intensity exercise, water-based activities, avoid cold air).

▶ Warm-up should include 10 min submaximal exercise plus five to seven sprints before activity.

▶ Gradually increase exercise intensity at onset of session.

▶ Exercise below EIB threshold.

▶ Breathe through nose as much as possible (this warms and humidifies air).

▶ Maintain a regular program and consistent fitness level.

Abbreviations: PEF = peak expiratory flow; URTI = upper respiratory tract infection; EIB = exercise-induced bronchospasm.

Compiled from R.C. Tan and S.L. Spector, 1998, "Exercise-induced asthma," *Sports Medicine* 25: 1-6; R.F. Lemanske and W.W. Busse, 1997, "Asthma," *JAMA* 278: 1855-1873; G.E. D'Alonzo and D.E. Ciccolella, 1999, Asthma, In *Lifestyle medicine*, edited by J.M. Rippe (Malden, MA: Blackwell Scientific), 460-476.

FIGURE 8.4   Exercise recommendations for individuals with asthma.

long-term compliance (refer to chapters 4 and 7). EIB is more likely to result from prolonged high-intensity exercise (e.g., distance running) and less likely to occur during lower intensity continuous or interval exercise. Thus, physical activity might include circuit resistance training, longer interval training (e.g., 2-5 min), cycling, aerobics, walking or many team sports (e.g., soccer, hockey). Swimming or other water-based activities (e.g., water running, aquaerobics) are also recommended because the humidified environment is thought to reduce the risk of EIB. The high-performance athlete obviously needs to train according to the demands of the sport, and there are no restrictions on such training provided there is good control and appropriate medication is used. Activities such as scuba diving and high-altitude mountain climbing are generally contraindicated because of the prolonged exposure to cold, dry air—which may precipitate an acute attack—and lack of ready access to medication and emergency facilities.

Medications to Treat Asthma

There are two general classes of asthma medications—preventers (e.g., inhaled corticosteroids, mast cell stabilisers) and relievers (e.g., bronchodilators). Recently developed drugs (e.g., antileukotrienes), although not commonly used at present in Australia, show good potential for preventing EIB. Preventers such as inhaled corticosteroids prevent local inflammation but exert little acute effect and require long-term use. Other preventers such as mast cell stabilisers have been shown to prevent EIB if used 10 to 20 min before exercise. Bronchodilators such as beta-agonists are the preferred treatment for those with mild to moderate asthma; these should be used before exercise and on appearance of EIB symptoms and, as such, should be readily available throughout exercise. If symptoms appear, the asthmatic should stop exercise and use the bronchodilator; if symptoms persist for 15 to 20 min despite repeated use of the bronchodilator, immediate medical treatment should be sought. Some of these medications are banned for use in competitive sport because they are ergogenic, so the competitive athlete along with his or her physician must carefully choose the appropriate medication and form (e.g., oral, nasal, inhaled).

Cystic Fibrosis

Cystic fibrosis (CF) is the most commonly occurring inherited disease causing early death in Caucasians; the current life expectancy is about 30 years. CF is caused by a genetic defect that alters cellular transport of chloride ions, affecting hydration of cells and resulting in excessively salty sweat and thick mucus. The lungs and pancreas are the major organs affected by CF. Accumulation of thick mucus in the lungs causes frequent infection, which may lead to scarring, and in the pancreas may prevent normal action of digestive enzymes, leading to undernutrition. For a number of reasons, regular exercise is now recommended for the CF patient. Aerobic fitness and exercise tolerance are prognostic of disease severity; that is, regular exercise and good physical fitness levels predict long-term survival. Regular exercise increases lung function and may prevent loss of body mass in the CF patient. Exercise in combination with chest physiotherapy enhances sputum production and clearance from the lungs better than either alone, reducing the risk of recurrent infection. Physical activity is also a normal part of school life and social development for children.

Exercise Capacity and CF

Given the average life expectancy, many CF patients are young, so exercise testing and prescription must take into account not only the disease but also special needs of younger individuals (refer to chapter 9). In the child with CF, exercise capacity appears to be directly related to pulmonary function as measured by FEV_1 and may be limited more by ventilatory factors (e.g., dyspnoea) than cardiovascular or metabolic factors. During exercise, minute ventilation increases disproportionately in relation to workload, more so than in the healthy individual; thus, CF patients may experience respiratory muscle fatigue. Exercise capacity may be normal in the CF patient but may deteriorate with disease progression. Minute ventilation and respiratory rate at each workload are higher compared with normal values. In severe disease, arterial oxygen saturation may decline. If ventilatory factors limit exercise capacity, maximum heart rate achieved will be significantly lower than age-predicted values; lower exercise capacity may also result from deconditioning secondary

Case Study 8.4

Mary is 42 years old, slightly overweight at 170 cm and 75 kg, and works in a day care centre provided for children of employees of a large company. She has experienced moderate and sometimes severe asthma since childhood and is now managed on daily inhaled corticosteroids and bronchodilators. She has not exercised since school (i.e., in 25 years) because of her fear of triggering an attack.

Several of Mary's friends attend the company fitness centre in which you are employed, and they have been encouraging Mary to attend with them. She has recently been commenting to them that her work with the young children is becoming physically more demanding, and she is concerned about her lack of fitness and strength.

The fitness centre offers aerobics classes at various levels, a small gym incorporating weight machines, light hand-held weights and other exercise equipment such as stair climbers and treadmills. She feels she has limited time to exercise at work (perhaps one to two times per week) and is self-conscious about exercising with the younger, slimmer and fitter employees. Her family commitments (three children, ages 6, 8 and 10) also limit her leisure time. She has no particular preferences in terms of types of exercise but would like at least some of her program to include activities with her children.

Write a 6-month progressive exercise program that accommodates her specific health concerns and preferences.

Key Issues

1. What are Mary's goals for exercise over the next 6 months?

2. What health issues need to be considered in writing an exercise prescription?

3. What factors are likely to influence Mary's adherence to exercise? How will these be incorporated into the exercise prescription?

4. What types of activities would be most suitable to meet Mary's goals and needs?

to the disease. Cardiovascular variables such as heart rate are generally normal during submaximal exercise. Clinical exercise testing is recommended before starting an exercise program for patients with severe CF (<50% predicted FEV_1).

Exercise Prescription for CF

Because there is large variability in disease severity, responses to exercise and interests of the CF patient, exercise prescription should be individualised. Many CF patients are children or adolescents, so special needs of these groups must also be considered (see chapter 9). Provided that the prescription is based on accurate assessment and that certain guidelines are followed, there are no a prior restrictions on exercise—some adult CF patients have even run marathons.

Long-term compliance is important, and the client's enjoyment of the activity should be paramount. Interval exercise or sports requiring interval work (e.g., soccer, hockey) may be well tolerated since they permit the client to rest and cough to clear mucus if needed (exercise induces cough in the CF patient). Coaches and teachers who supervise physical activity of a child with CF should be educated as to specific guidelines for exercise. Children may choose a variety of activities such as swimming, cycling, aerobics, jogging or a particular sport. Exercise should be performed at least three times per week and perhaps daily if not excessively intense, and it is most effective if performed after chest physiotherapy and use of bronchodilator medication. Patients should start with 10 min and gradually increase to a total of 20 to 30 min per day, unless more is required for a particular sport. Intensity should be based on the initial fitness level and needs of activity (i.e., sport training); an inactive individual with low initial fitness will need to start at a low level. Intensity within the range of 60 to 80% actual maximum heart rate as measured in a clinical exercise test or 55 to 90% HRR is recommended once fitness has improved and there is no evidence of excessive dyspnoea (shortness of breath) or arterial desaturation (reduction in oxygen content of blood). As the program progresses, it is preferable to increase duration rather than intensity. Oxygen supplementation (in the clinical setting) or lower intensity, shorter duration exercise may be needed for those who exhibit arterial desaturation below 93% during clinical exercise testing. A general rule for arterial desaturation is that exercise intensity should be set at a heart rate 10 beats · min^{-1} lower than the point

at which desaturation or dyspnoea occurred in the exercise test.

There are no restrictions on resistance training to improve muscular strength and endurance and increase lean body mass provided that programs are scientifically based and, for children, the guidelines for strength training in children are followed (discussed in chapter 9). However, resistance training is recommended as a complement to rather than instead of aerobic training because improved respiratory function seems to occur only with aerobic exercise.

Proper hydration is important for the CF patient. Although tolerance to exercise in the heat is normal (i.e., core temperature rises to similar levels as in healthy subjects), in the CF patient sweat contains more sodium and chloride, and thus blood levels of these electrolytes may decline after exercise. CF patients have been shown to underestimate fluid needs and not adequately voluntarily replace fluids during and after exercise. The CF patient should drink water or a sports beverage every 20 to 30 min during activity, and fluid intake should be closely monitored in children with CF.

Summary

Physical inactivity is now considered a major risk factor for cardiovascular disease, presenting about the same risk as hypertension, cigarette smoking and high blood cholesterol level. Regular moderate physical activity is important for primary prevention of cardiovascular and metabolic conditions such as coronary heart disease, hypertension, obesity and impaired glucose tolerance or type 2 diabetes. Regular physical activity exerts both direct and indirect effects on the risk of disease. Moreover, moderate physical activity is an effective component of multifaceted secondary prevention (rehabilitation) for patients with cardiovascular, respiratory and metabolic diseases. For people at risk of or with known disease, physical activity has many benefits in terms of altering risk factors or possibly disease progression and enhancing functional capacity, ability to perform activities of daily living and quality of life. Effective physical activity prescription for patients with any disease or impairment builds on the basic principles of exercise prescription together with knowledge from scientific studies of adaptations to exercise for those with disease.

Selected Glossary Terms

activities of daily living (ADLs)—Physical tasks required of independent living, such as dressing and feeding oneself, walking, transferring into and out of bed or a chair, housework and stair climbing.

angina—Discomfort or pain in the chest, often radiating to the shoulders, arms, neck or jaw, resulting from myocardial ischaemia.

atherosclerosis—A pathological process resulting in potentially obstructive lesions in the major arteries, in particular the aorta, and coronary, carotid, iliac and femoral arteries.

chronic obstructive pulmonary disorder (COPD)—A group of conditions characterised by airway obstruction; the most common forms are asthma, emphysema and chronic bronchitis.

circuit resistance training—Resistance training in which the subject moves quickly between exercise stations, with little rest (<1 min) between different exercises; a good way to combine muscular and aerobic conditioning.

cystic fibrosis (CF)—A genetic disease affecting primarily the lungs in which altered cellular transport of chloride ions affects hydration of cells, resulting in excessively salty sweat and thick mucus. Accumulation of thick mucus in the lungs causes frequent infection, which may lead to scarring and permanent damage.

dyspnoea—Shortness of breath or difficult or laboured breathing, especially during physical activity, associated with pulmonary and some types of cardiovascular disorders.

exercise-induced asthma (EIA) or bronchospasm (EIB)—Acute narrowing of the airways during or after strenuous exercise, defined as a decline of 15% or more in FEV_1 after exercise; occurs in 40 to 80% of asthmatics.

hypoglycaemia—Low blood glucose level below 3.5 mmol · L^{-1}, which in the diabetic may result from the combined effect of insulin injection and exercise, both of which enhance glucose uptake by the tissues.

metabolic syndrome (syndrome X)—A clustering of risk factors for cardiovascular disease, including impaired glucose tolerance, obesity, hypertension and dyslipidaemia.

primary prevention—Interventions aimed at preventing the development of disease in healthy people or those without known disease.

secondary prevention—Interventions aimed at preventing further disease progression, or restoring functional capacity, in those with documented disease.

waist to hip ratio (WHR)—The ratio of circumferences of the waist to hip; gives a simple, non-invasive indication of the degree of abdominal fat deposition.

Student Activities and Study Questions

1. By what physiological mechanisms does exercise enhance glucose tolerance? What are the implications for exercise prescription for diabetics?

2. What is the relationship between exercise intensity and blood pressure *during* exercise (i.e., not the chronic effects of exercise training on resting blood pressure)? What are the implications for exercise prescription for hypertensive individuals?

3. By what physiological mechanisms does regular exercise improve exercise tolerance in PAOD?

4. Locate and visit a local exercise cardiac rehabilitation program. What types of patients access this program? Ask the program manager if you can meet and briefly discuss with a patient his or her perceptions of the benefits of exercise. What does this patient like about the program? What benefits does he or she feel result from the program?

5. Visit a local fitness centre or community physical activity program during a time of peak client use. Observe (discretely) how many clients are overweight/obese. Is your observation consistent with the percentage of the general population that is overweight/obese? (Probably not.) Why do you think this is so? What simple things can be done to increase participation by overweight people?

CHAPTER 9

Exercise Prescription Throughout the Lifespan

As discussed in section 1, recent public health campaigns arising from the U.S. Surgeon General's Report, such as Active Australia, recommend a physically active lifestyle for nearly all individuals beginning in childhood and extending into old age (unless, of course, a particular disease or condition makes activity impossible). The field of exercise management is concerned with encouraging everyone to become and remain physically active. Although the general recommendations for physical activity, as described in chapters 2 and 7, are broadly applicable to everyone, it is necessary to specifically adapt these recommendations to suit changing needs throughout the lifespan.

Exercise goals and motivations vary dramatically between children, adults and the elderly. The focus of physical activity also changes across the lifespan. Children require exposure to physical activity as part of normal physical and social development, but their smaller body size, limited exercise capacity and attention span (compared with adults), and attraction to fun activities must be considered in exercise programming. In the elderly, reduced physical work capacity may limit participation in intense activities, but there is more time for exercise and, for some, a keen interest in using physical activity as a means of enhancing health and quality of life. Pregnancy is an example of a condition requiring temporary modification of the normal activity program to accommodate the changing shape of the mother and growth of the baby. Although cancer is difficult to place within any particular context of exercise management, it is included in this chapter because of its prevalence in the community (most common cause of death; refer to chapter 2) and because its incidence increases as the population ages.

Physical Activity in Children

Physical activity plays an integral part of social and physical development in children, and most children are naturally active. Although young children are generally very active, participation declines after about age 12 to 13 years, especially in girls. Moreover, there is some thought, although not much evidence, that participation in physical activity has been declining in recent years among children and adolescents. This is probably due to several factors such as concerns for safety (e.g., children driven to school rather than walking), the popularity of sedentary leisure pursuits (e.g., television, video games and computers), an overall trend toward inactivity across the entire population (e.g., influence of family and other role models) and decreased resources for physical activity in schools. Because patterns of activity and many disease risk factors are established early in life (e.g., obesity, bone density), encouraging children to achieve an active lifestyle is critically important to long-term individual and community health. In addition, Australia has a long tradition of excellence across a wide range of sports; continued performance at this level requires broad-based opportunities for children to acquire physical and sports skills needed for both recreational and elite sport.

Exercise Capacity in Healthy Children

Compared with adults, both aerobic and anaerobic exercise capacities are lower in children and adolescents. Most components of physical fitness increase during normal growth and development, attaining adult levels after puberty and generally by age 20. It is now well accepted that, in addition to normal increases in physical capacity during growth and development, children exhibit training adaptations qualitatively and often quantitatively similar to healthy adults. In general, until about age 11 to 12, girls and boys perform similarly across most tests of physical fitness and motor skills such as running, jumping, catching and striking. There are some sex differences in performance of basic movement patterns, such as better performance of overhand throwing and kicking in boys and better performance of hopping, skipping and balance in girls. It is plausible that many of these sex differences arise for social (e.g., opportunity) rather than biological reasons.

Aerobic Exercise Capacity and Training Effects in Children

Resting and maximum heart rates are high in children, about 80 to 100 beats $\cdot$ min^{-1} at rest and often above 200 during intense exercise (recall that maximum heart rate may be predicted by 220 minus age). The relatively high (compared with adults) resting and exercise heart rates result from low stroke volume (volume of blood pumped by the heart with each beat) because of the small heart size. Resting heart rate declines to about 65 to 75 beats $\cdot$ min^{-1} in the teenage years as a result of increased heart size, stroke volume and haemoglobin levels. $\dot{V}O_2$max expressed as L $\cdot$ min^{-1} increases in proportion to body mass, while $\dot{V}O_2$max scaled to body mass (ml $\cdot$ kg^{-1} $\cdot$ min^{-1}) reaches adult values relatively early in adolescence. In contrast, although $\dot{V}O_2$max values relative to body size are similar, endurance exercise capacity is much lower in children compared with adults; this is attributable largely to lower mechanical efficiency. Both performance and mechanical efficiency im-

prove throughout childhood and adolescence. Thus, despite the seemingly high $\dot{V}O_2$max values, children have a lower capacity for sustained continuous exercise. In addition, most children have limited motivation for prolonged continuous exercise or exercise to exhaustion.

$\dot{V}O_2$max and endurance exercise capacity can be improved in children and adolescents through appropriate exercise training; however, children generally show less relative improvement (as a percentage of starting level) in $\dot{V}O_2$max compared with adults. While $\dot{V}O_2$max in adults may increase 20 to 40% after endurance training, it increases by only 5 to 20% in children. The reasons for this smaller increase are unknown but may relate to biological differences such as lower haemoglobin levels and thus lower oxygen carrying capacity of the blood in children. Improvements in endurance exercise performance (as measured by time to run a given distance) may be larger than the increase in $\dot{V}O_2$max, suggesting that factors such as economy of movement are improved with training. Endurance training induces adaptations in cardiovascular factors, such as lower resting and submaximal heart rate, in children as in adults.

Anaerobic Power, Anaerobic Capacity and Training Effects in Children

Compared with adults, children exhibit lower **anaerobic power** and **capacity,** as measured by the 10- to 30-s cycle ergometer test. This is true even when power and capacity are normalised for body mass. Children exhibit a smaller ratio of skeletal muscle mass to total body mass (i.e., less active muscle generating force), lower capacity for **anaerobic glycolysis** (because of lower activity of glycolytic enzymes), and lower mechanical efficiency. In addition, lack of motivation to perform an exercise test to maximum because it can be very uncomfortable (for example, causing nausea and vomiting), also means that any test of anaerobic capacity may underestimate the true capacity in children. During development, especially from ages 9 to 15, total work, anaerobic power and capacity and peak blood lactic acid levels all increase. These changes are due to enhanced skeletal muscle glycolytic enzyme activity, muscle mass (especially in boys), neural development and neuromuscular coordination (mechanical efficiency). Children recover from brief high-intensity exercise faster than adults do, possibly because of the lower glycolytic capacity and thus lower lactate levels.

Although not studied extensively in children, appropriate high-intensity exercise training leads to improvements in anaerobic capacity. In children, high-intensity training improves anaerobic power, anaerobic capacity and maximal blood lactate levels. This occurs despite little change in muscle mass, suggesting that biochemical (within skeletal muscle) and neural (e.g., coordination, motor unit recruitment) adaptations are responsible.

Muscular Strength and Endurance and Training Effects in Children

Since muscular strength is a function of muscle size, or cross-sectional area, strength is lower in children than in adults. Strength increases with growth and development throughout childhood and adolescence. Peak muscular strength is achieved in untrained individuals by about age 20 in males and 14 to 16 in females. Before puberty, strength is less related to muscle size, but this relationship becomes more evident after puberty. Increases in muscle strength during development result from combined effects of growth and neural maturation; **muscle hypertrophy** plays a more important role in postpubertal boys because of increased testosterone levels. In children, appropriate resistance training may increase muscular strength and endurance. Strength may increase over the short term (8-12 weeks) by 20 to 30% beyond natural increases due to maturation; more important, such changes can occur without risk of injury (discussed later in the chapter).

Fitness and Exercise Testing in Children

Submaximal or performance-related fitness tests are often used to assess physical fitness in children. Maximal testing is generally not needed for healthy children unless it is part of a sport development program. Clinical exercise testing is useful for diagnosis of some childhood diseases, in particular diseases of the cardiovascular and respiratory systems (e.g., heart disease, asthma, cystic fibrosis). Tests requiring a child to exercise to maximum capacity may be limited by the child's understanding of the task, relatively short attention span and low motivation to exercise to exhaustion. Field-based fitness tests are often used in schools because they are easily administered to large groups. Field testing usually includes a battery of four to six tests including tests of

- aerobic capacity (e.g., 12-min walk/run),
- muscular strength and endurance (e.g., sit-ups, pull-ups, grip strength),
- power and coordination (e.g., ball throw, vertical jump test),
- speed and power (e.g., 30- to 50-m sprints),
- agility and speed (e.g., shuttle run),
- muscle flexibility (e.g., sit-and-reach test), and
- body composition (e.g., skinfolds, girths).

Interpretation of data requires that appropriate norms exist for the age and population of children tested.

In a child with disease, clinical exercise testing may be useful to diagnose disease, to assess disease or treatment progress, and as a basis for individual exercise prescription. Contraindications for exercise testing, as discussed in chapter 5, are similar to those for adults. When testing children, standard exercise test protocols (refer to chapter 6) and equipment may need to be modified. For example, tests of aerobic capacity need to start at a low intensity and progress gradually (e.g., 12-25 W to start, with 12- to 25-W increments when testing on a bicycle ergometer). Treadmill walking may be preferable to cycle ergometry because there is less peripheral fatigue to limit performance and the pace is externally set (by the treadmill speed). If using a cycle ergometer, a smaller frame may be needed for children less than 125 cm in height. Children, whether healthy or with disease, have a limited attention span, so the test should be designed to reach its end-point within a relatively short time frame. It is questionable as to whether young children will understand and give consistent responses to the RPE scale (refer to chapter 6).

Exercise Prescription for Healthy Children

Most children are naturally active, although their limited attention spans and endurance exercise capacities favour activity in short bursts (e.g., the games of "tiggy" or "red rover"). As for adults, the optimal exercise prescription is individualised to the child's needs, interests, physical capacity, health impairment, if any, and level of maturity. In reality, however, few children have access to such individualised service. As a general rule, recommendations from the U.S. Surgeon General's Report and Active Australia (refer to chapter 2) also apply to children over the age of 6; that is, at least 30 min of moderate activity should be undertaken on most if not all days. For younger children, daily physical activity through enjoyable and creative play, preferably outdoors, is encouraged. Since natural activity levels generally decline around ages 11 to 13, especially in girls, older children may need more

PRE-ADOLESCENTS

▶ As for adults, children should participate in at least 30 min of activity on most if not all days; activity can be accumulated through several shorter bouts of ≥10 min each.

▶ All children should undertake vigorous activity at least three times per week; this does not have to be in organised or competitive sport.

▶ Physical activity should be enjoyable, chosen by the child and self-paced to ensure long-term compliance and the likelihood of acquiring a lifelong habit.

▶ Whenever possible, outdoor activities involving natural recreation (e.g., bushwalking, mountain bike riding, cycling) should be encouraged.

▶ Organised sport should take a long-term view of focusing on skill and social development (e.g., teamwork) rather than short-term outcomes such as winning.

▶ Active and positive adult role models are essential for encouraging children's continued participation.

ADOLESCENTS

▶ As for adults, at least 30 min of moderate physical activity should be performed daily or on most days; activity can be accumulated in shorter bouts.

▶ A variety of activities involving recreation, sport, work, transport and planned exercise is encouraged.

▶ Physical activity should occur within a variety of settings, such as school, family, sport and community.

▶ To ensure compliance, physical activity should be enjoyable and chosen by the individual.

▶ To optimise bone deposition, physical activity should include both endurance weight-bearing exercise and muscular conditioning activities.

▶ In addition to daily moderate physical activity, adolescents should undertake ≥20 min of vigorous activity at least three times per week; this does not have to be in organised or competitive sport.

Compiled from G. Rogers and L. Hampel, 2000, *Active Australia Children and Youth*. (Hindmarsh, SA: Australian Council for Health, Physical Education and Recreation), 9-19.

FIGURE 9.1　General recommendations for exercise prescription for children and adolescents.

structured and focused opportunities for participation. For older children, 20 to 30 min of vigorous exercise at least 3 days per week is advised in addition to moderate activity on most days. General guidelines for children and adolescents are presented in figure 9.1.

Exercise mode should be varied to accommodate interests of children and the need for skill acquisition across a range of activities. Load-bearing activities using large muscle groups (e.g., running, ball and team games) stimulate bone deposition, especially during adolescence, a critical time to maximise bone density to prevent osteoporosis later in life (refer to chapter 10). To foster lifetime commitment to a physically active lifestyle, the focus should be on enjoyment, participation by all children, skill acquisition and social development.

Continuous endurance exercise such as long distance running is generally not advised for young children because of their lower mechanical efficiency, limited endurance exercise capacity, short attention span and potential for heat illness (discussed in the next section). Given their limited anaerobic exercise capacity and rapid recovery after exercise, children are naturally attracted to interval exercise as performed in many sports (e.g., swimming, soccer, football, hockey, netball) or recreational pursuits (e.g., cycling, in-line skating, skateboarding). Except for athletes in training or in the clinical setting, it is not necessary to monitor exercise intensity in the healthy child, and the child's self-perception of intensity is usually sufficient. As a rule, children will rest when needed and are not interested in self-assessment of heart rate or RPE.

Muscular strength and endurance are important for normal development, bone health and performance in some sports (e.g., swimming). There is no reason why healthy children cannot participate in resistance training provided that programs are supervised by adults and modified to suit the needs of children. The American College of Sports Medicine and Sports Medicine Australia have issued recommendations for participation in resistance training by children; a summary of these guidelines is provided in figure 9.2. The focus of resistance training in children should be on developing muscular endurance and, to a limited extent, strength, while emphasising proper form and technique. The major concern is that improper technique or maximal lifts can damage growing bones, in particular the epiphyses (growth plates), and tendons and ligaments that are not yet fully mature. It is important that children and adolescents be discouraged from "proving" their strength through formal or informal competition in the gym. During childhood and early adolescence, there is limited capacity for muscle hypertrophy, primarily because of low testosterone levels, although muscular strength, endurance and "definition" may be enhanced to a limited extent.

MODE/TECHNIQUE

▶ Use pin weights or other machines whenever possible.

▶ Use sport-specific exercises whenever possible.

▶ Resistance training using body weight as resistance is best for younger children.

▶ Use large muscle groups and multi-joint exercises over the full range of motion.

▶ For free weights, focus on proper technique with minimal weight (e.g., bar only).

▶ Plyometrics are generally not recommended until age 16.

▶ Use resistance training as an adjunct to other forms of training.

INTENSITY/FREQUENCY/VOLUME

▶ Use higher repetition, lower resistance training (e.g., 8-12 reps) to avoid injury.

▶ Low volume (e.g., ≤ 2 sets) is recommended to avoid injury and overtraining.

▶ Incorporate rest intervals of 1 to 2 min between sets.

▶ Train no more than 2 days per week with rest days between sessions.

▶ Avoid resistance training when fatigued (e.g., do not perform at end of endurance session).

PRECAUTIONS

▶ Adult supervision is strongly recommended.

▶ Identify and correct muscle imbalances and problems with technique or range of motion.

▶ No maximal lifts until ≥16 years (Tanner Stage 5 or physically fully mature)

▶ Avoid competition between children.

▶ Avoid powerlifting and bodybuilding.

▶ Include proper warm-up and cool-down plus stretching to maintain or improve flexibility.

▶ Use proper breathing technique.

▶ Control speed in lift and recovery.

Compiled from American College of Sports Medicine, 2000, *ACSM's guidelines for exercise testing and prescription*, 6th ed. (Philadelphia: Lippincott, Williams & Wilkins); Sports Medicine Australia, 1997, *Safety guidelines for children*. Canberra.

FIGURE 9.2   Summary of guidelines for resistance training for children and adolescents.

Case Study 9.1

You are an exercise scientist contracted by a large state high school to provide advice to students and staff wishing to become physically active. The school's enrollment is 800 students, about 30% of whom are first- or second-generation immigrants from South and Southeast Asia and the Middle East. The school's administration and students strongly support your appointment, and the school has set aside a large covered outdoor area for physical activity programs. Although your salary is paid by a community grant, there is little funding for equipment, and the school wants the programs to be free of charge for staff and students.

Naila is a 15-year-old girl in year 10. She approaches you on behalf of a group of 20 Muslim girls who wish to exercise to "lose weight and tone up". Some of their parents have traditional views and are uncertain about their participation in an exercise program. The girls feel their parents may allow them to participate if the program incorporates the parents' concerns, specifically that the girls dress modestly, their program is restricted to girls only (and of course, the instructor is female), there is some level of privacy for the girls when they exercise and extremes of body shape are discouraged (i.e., neither too thin nor too muscular).

Develop a 6-week activity program for these girls that incorporates their goals and their parents' concerns.

Key Issues

1. How will you determine if the girls really need to lose weight? How important is weight loss in this program?

2. How will you provide an enjoyable and varied program that will maintain the girls' interest and help them achieve their goals?

3. What types of programs can be offered to these girls, given the financial constraints? Are there ways to enhance the programs with minimal budget?

4. What cultural factors will you need to address when developing this program?

Thermoregulation During Exercise in Children

Compared with adults, children are less tolerant of intense exercise in the heat. In children, lower mechanical efficiency and higher metabolic rate cause the body to generate more heat at a given work rate than in an adult. Children also have a lower rate of sweating, begin to sweat at a higher core temperature and rely more on circulatory adjustments and less on evaporative cooling (sweating) to lose heat. Moreover, the higher surface to body mass ratio in children favours heat gain if environmental temperature exceeds core temperature. These factors combined with a lesser ability to acclimatise to exercising in the heat and a less responsive thirst mechanism leave children more susceptible to heat illness as a result of intense prolonged exercise.

During exercise, core temperature increases in relation to exercise intensity, so moderate exercise is less likely to cause an excessive rise in core temperature. Interval exercise and games that permit substitutions provide opportunities for children to rest and drink fluids. If children must exercise in hot environments, they should be encouraged to wear appropriate clothing (light, loose-fitting) and to drink frequently. Sport or flavoured drinks are generally more palatable than plain water, may be absorbed faster and may thus encourage children to drink more during and after exercise. Whenever possible, matches should be scheduled during the cooler times of day.

Child Athletes

Children participate in a wide range of sports in Australia, probably because of the long tradition of excellence in sport and the well-established networks of local and national sporting organisations. Training children for sport, however, requires models that are specific to their unique requirements, based on the physiological, anatomical and psychological needs of young people; that is, children cannot be viewed simply as scaled-down adults. Moreover, children and adolescents differ in their exercise capacity, motivation and attention span, and working with young athletes requires modification of general principles of exercise training.

Young children are advised to participate in a wide variety of sports and to delay specialising until adolescence, after about age 12 to 13 in girls and 14 to 15 in boys. Common sense dictates that children should learn a variety of movement and sports skills to enhance their motor development and enjoyment. It can also be argued that only through exposure to different sports can an individual child (and coaches and parents) recognise talent. Experience and empirical data also show that elite young adult athletes are those who participated in a variety of sports as children. Talented young athletes who experience early "burn-out", overtraining or overuse injuries are usually those who specialised or began intensive training programs too early. Sport for pre-pubertal children should emphasise skill acquisition, social development, fitness, enjoyment and participation.

It has already been established that exercise training does improve performance, and child athletes obviously need to train to improve speed, strength and endurance. Training child athletes involves a careful balance between the amount of exercise required to elicit adaptations and the need to avoid injury and other potentially harmful outcomes such as burn-out, overtraining and growth retardation.

For pre-pubertal children, specific speed training beyond simple relays and practice games is generally unnecessary. Training using repeated sprints should not normally be performed until late childhood. As mentioned previously, anaerobic glycolytic capacity is lower in children/adolescents compared with adults. For example, for many young children, the physiological and psychological demands of repeated sprint training are likely to discourage the child athlete, unless they can be performed in a fun context (e.g., relays, simulated games) with appropriate rest intervals. Sprinting requires a larger aerobic component for children than adults; thus, endurance training will benefit the child involved in sprint/speed activities. Sprint/speed training should be specific to the needs of the sport; some points to consider when designing a sprint/speed program for older child athletes include the following:

▶ Is maximum speed required (e.g., sprint runner, swimmer)?

▶ Is the ability to sprint repeatedly required (e.g., football, hockey, soccer)?

▶ What movement patterns are required in addition to speed (e.g., straight speed such as running or swimming vs. agility such as soccer, tennis or netball)?

Several factors important for speed performance may be improved through training. Acceleration may be enhanced by working on rapid changes in pace, especially from a relevant position such as the starting position in sprinting or football. Sprinting on cue helps to develop reaction time. Balance and the ability to regain balance are important to sports such as football, hockey and tennis and may be developed through agility drills such as shuttle runs on the playing field. If maximum speed over the straight is needed, as in sprint running or swimming, athletes often work at race pace but over a shorter distance. Many sports require repeated sprints and the ability to cope with fatigue; this may be trained through multiple sprints with relatively short rest periods to improve lactate tolerance. Plyometric training is usually not recommended until after age 16 because the high-impact forces increase risk of injury to the epiphyses, immature muscles and connective tissue (discussed in chapter 11).

Endurance exercise performance may also be improved with appropriate training. Generally, a high relative intensity of exercise (i.e., >70% APMHR) is needed to show improvements in $\dot{V}O_2$max and endurance exercise capacity. For the post-pubertal child, endurance training is recommended for 20 to 40 min per session, three to five times per week. Exercise intensity should vary from 60 to 90% APMHR over the season; for example, lower intensity exercise (60-70% APMHR) early in the season, working up to more intense exercise (80-90%) later in the season. A general rule is that children under age 10 should perform at least 90% of their endurance work at an intensity of 80% APMHR or less. The amount of high-intensity work will gradually increase with age, such that a 16-year-old may perform 20 to 30% of endurance work at an intensity >80% APMHR. Because of their relatively low capacity for anaerobic glycolysis and their shorter attention span, children often find interval exercise more attractive and tolerable than continuous exercise; children also recover better than adults from repeated interval work. Even endurance work can be accomplished with interval training (e.g., using work intervals of 3-5 min).

Sports Injuries in Children and Adolescents

Although generally associated with excessive exercise in adults, overuse injuries may also occur in children. It has been estimated that up to one half of all overuse injuries in children may be prevented. Common overuse injuries in young athletes include acute injuries such as muscle strains and ligament sprains and chronic injuries such as tendonitis, stress fractures, medial tibial stress syndrome (MTSS, or shin splints) and patello-femoral disorders.

Damage to the epiphyses (growth plates) may result from acute macrotrauma, such as a direct blow to the bone, or from repetitive microtrauma, such as multiple footstrikes in distance running or use of the wrist in gymnastics. Epiphyseal damage is most likely to be associated with poor technique, inappropriate exercise or overtraining, and there is little evidence to suggest that this is a frequent injury in children who are training appropriately.

Stress fractures, minute fractures within a bone, result from excessive and repetitive loading of a bone. Lumbar spine stress fractures may occur in sports such as gymnastics or cricket (fast bowling) in which there is repetitive arching or twisting of the spine. Activities requiring prolonged running or jumping on hard surfaces (e.g., distance running,

basketball) may lead to stress fractures of the tibia. MTSS, commonly known as shin splints, is an inflammation of the muscular attachments to the tibia; it occurs in similar situations to tibial stress fractures. Poor muscle flexibility in the ankle and lower leg and incorrect footstrike contribute to the risk of stress fracture of the tibia and MTSS. Patellofemoral disorders are characterised by pain in the anterior or medial aspects of the kneecap, especially on bending the knee, running or jumping. The pain is caused by inflammation of the cartilage under the patella, resulting from movement of the patella during activity.

Overuse injuries tend to occur more frequently during the child's "growth spurt" around the time of puberty. Risk factors for overuse injuries include

▶ sudden change in intensity, frequency, duration or mode of exercise;

▶ sudden change in technique;

Case Study 9.2

You are an exercise physiologist working with a group of physiotherapists specialising in sports injuries. Your practice is located within a large commercial fitness centre that includes a well-equipped gym (free weights and weight machines), electronic exercise equipment (bikes, rowers, stair climbers, treadmills), heated 25-m pool of uniform 1.2-m depth and other apparatus such as boxacise equipment and Swiss Balls. The fitness centre is located near a skateboard park, paved bike path and grass athletics track.

Scott is a 12-year-old boy who participates in track and field in summer and soccer in winter. He is being treated by one of the physiotherapists for severe medial tibial stress syndrome (shin splints), which the therapist believes resulted from training for sprints and jumps. He is 170 cm tall, weighs 60 kg and has grown 8 cm in the past 2 months. Scott has completed 8 weeks of therapy to improve flexibility of his lower limbs. Although the pain has subsided considerably, it is still present in impact activities such as jumping. The therapist has given him a stretching program to further develop muscle flexibility.

You are asked to provide a program to help Scott regain his fitness as the soccer season approaches. He is bright, articulate and full of energy, but he does not like to train ("too boring"). He enjoys in-line skating, bike riding and swimming and expresses an interest in resistance training. Scott also develops mild exercise-induced asthma (bronchoconstriction) but only during continuous high-intensity activity such as distance running. Write an 8-week progressive training program leading up to the start of the soccer season.

Key Issues

1. What are Scott's major concerns and goals over the next 2 months? How should the program be written to accommodate his injury, demands of soccer and mild asthma?

2. Should Scott start resistance training? What are the possible benefits? What precautions should be taken? What type of resistance training is best for his sports?

3. How will you get Scott to be active and improve his fitness without "training"?

▶ biomechanical problems such as poor form;

▶ tight muscle-tendon units, especially during rapid bone growth;

▶ imbalance between muscle groups;

▶ misalignment of the lower extremities;

▶ inadequate footwear; and

▶ exercising on a hard surface.

Preventing overuse injuries may require modifying exercise training during the months of peak growth. Changes to technique, surface, mode or training intensity should be introduced gradually. In addition, early detection and correction of muscle imbalance, poor technique and lower limb misalignment is vital. Exercises to improve muscle-tendon flexibility, joint ROM and muscular strength and endurance should be incorporated into the training regime throughout the season.

Exercise Capacity and Exercise Prescription for Children With Disease

Up to 10% of all children have some chronic illness or health concern that may affect exercise capacity and the ability to participate in regular physical activity. Although many conditions may cause long-term or permanent impairment, there is much to be gained in terms of social development, enhanced self-esteem and self-efficacy, and prevention of other chronic diseases (e.g., cardiovascular disease) by encouraging regular physical activity among children. Regular physical activity is highly recommended for nearly all children with chronic disease or impairment as long as the exercise prescription is individualised to the child's disease or disability, interests and physical capacity. Despite the many benefits of physical activity for children with disease, parents and educators may be reluctant to allow children with disease to fully participate in sports or physical education programs.

A number of diseases or impairments influence exercise capacity and the ability to maintain an active lifestyle. For example, severe asthma that is poorly controlled may prevent a child from participating in competitive sports or even regular exercise. Progressive muscle wasting caused by muscular dystrophy (degenerative disease of the skeletal muscles) inhibits muscle strength and performance of many activities requiring strength and coordination. Moreover, sometimes the disease treatment has long-term implications for growth, physical capac-

ity and the ability to undertake regular exercise. Some drugs used to treat childhood cancers or leukaemia interfere with protein synthesis, growth and various organ functions. Many diseases or treatments cause fatigue or pain, making regular exercise difficult. In juvenile rheumatoid arthritis (inflammation of the joints), pain may limit participation in weight-bearing or high-impact sports. This section very briefly outlines some of the diseases or conditions affecting children and general recommendations for physical activity. The diseases addressed are meant to be a representative rather than a comprehensive listing. A summary of exercise prescription guidelines for children with disease is presented in table 9.1.

Childhood and Adolescent Obesity

Although there is currently no clear definition of childhood and adolescent obesity, it is obvious that the relative proportion of overweight and obese children is increasing in most developed countries. Following are some of the current definitions of obesity in children and adolescents:

▶ Body weight >120% of that predicted for height from standard growth curves

▶ Body mass index (BMI) >85th percentile for age

▶ Triceps skinfolds >85th percentile for age and gender

▶ Body fat >25% for boys and >30% for girls

Since the late-1960s to mid-1970s, obesity has been increasing in prevalence. It is now estimated that more than 20% (and as many as 30%, depending on the definition) of children and adolescents are overweight or obese in Australia; this trend is similar to that observed in adults. This increasing incidence of obesity has alarmed health professionals because the major killers of adults, such as CAD, hypertension and type 2 diabetes, may have their origins in childhood. Childhood obesity is associated with dyslipidaemia, high blood pressure and high insulin levels (a precursor of type 2 diabetes). The clustering of metabolic syndrome risk factors (obesity, hypertension, dyslipidaemia, insulin resistance; refer to chapter 8) may start as early as age 5 in obese children. Moreover, atherosclerotic changes in the heart and blood vessels are apparent in children who are obese. In addition to the physiological consequences of obesity in childhood, there are social and psychological aspects as well. Obesity in childhood and adolescence is associated with negative self-perception, lower self-worth, depression and

TABLE 9.1—Summary of Exercise Recommendations for Paediatric Diseases

Disease/condition	Exercise recommendations	Reason for recommendation
Cardiovascular disease	Clinical program may be needed	Safety—monitor for symptoms
	Variety of activities	Train endurance, strength
	Low to moderate intensity, gradual progression	Safety, restore functional capacity
Type 1 diabetes	Regular and consistent	Better metabolic control
	Monitor blood glucose	Prevent hypoglycaemia
	With partner, group	Help if hypoglycaemia occurs
Obesity	Frequent, regular, high energy expenditure	Sufficient energy expenditure to reduce body fat and weight
	Variety, appropriate intensity	Enhance compliance
	Games, sports	Social interaction
Asthma	Interval, aquatic	Less asthmagenic
	Maintain fitness	Onset of EIB is predictable
	Warm-up important	Refractory period to prevent EIB
	Use preventer and reliever medications	Prevent, relieve EIB
Cystic fibrosis	Maintain cardiorespiratory fitness	Related to prognosis
	Variety of activities	Enhance compliance, social interaction, general physical fitness
Juvenile rheumatoid arthritis	Variety of activities	Train endurance, strength
	Stretching, resistance exercise	Avoid contractures, strengthen muscles around joints
	Avoid excessive use of affected joints	Prevent joint inflammation
Spina bifida	Wheelchair sports	Social interaction, fitness
	Upper body resistance	Maintain posture
Muscular dystrophies	Variety of activities	Train endurance, strength
	Wheelchair sports	Social interaction, fitness
Intellectual impairment (e.g., Down syndrome)	Team sports, group activities	Social interaction
	Variety of activities	Train endurance and strength, prevent obesity

Abbreviations: EIB = exercise-induced bronchospasm.

Compiled from American College of Sports Medicine, 2000, *ACSM's guidelines for exercise testing and prescription*, 6th ed. (Philadelphia: Lippincott, Williams & Wilkins); ACSM, 1997, *Exercise management for persons with chronic diseases and disabilities*. (Champaign, IL: Human Kinetics); P. Reaburn and D. Jenkins, 2000, *Guiding the young athlete*. (St Leonards, NSW: Allen and Unwin); T.L. Tomassoni, 1996, "Role of exercise in the management of cardiovascular disease in children and youth," *Medicine and Science in Sports and Exercise* 28: 406-413; B. Goldberg (ed.), 1995, *Sports and exercise for children with chronic health conditions*. (Champaign, IL: Human Kinetics).

negative perceptions of obese children by their peers. Thus, the high incidence of obesity in young people is cause for significant concern.

As in adult obesity, the causes of childhood obesity are a complex interaction of genetic and environmental influences. It is clear that obesity is at least partially genetically determined, as evidenced by studies revealing that BMI of adopted children is more closely related to BMI of biological rather than adoptive parents. However, the increasing prevalence of obesity in young people over the past 20 years has happened too quickly to be explained by genetic influence alone. Obesity does not appear to be caused simply by overeating, since during this same time frame the average total daily intake of energy has declined in both young people and adults. It is generally accepted that the most likely cause of obesity in children is the combination of a high-fat diet and sedentary lifestyle. Actual medical causes account for less than 10% of childhood obesity.

This increased incidence of obesity is paralleled by a decline in physical activity patterns in young people. Obese children tend to participate in less physical activity than children of normal weight. Inactivity as early as the pre-school years (ages 4-5) increases risk of obesity later in childhood and adulthood. Moreover, overseas studies show a strong dose relationship between television watching and obesity—the risk of obesity is five times higher in children watching 5 h compared with 2 h of television per day. Thus, the key to preventing obesity throughout the lifespan is to reduce the number of children (and adults) leading sedentary lifestyles.

It is now recommended that intervention is warranted even in early childhood when both a child and his or her parents are overweight or obese. (In contrast, no action is recommended if a child under age 3 is overweight but his or her parents are not.) Dieting alone is ineffective for inducing long-term weight loss in children (as in adults; refer to chapter 8) because of the concomitant decrease in lean body mass and resting metabolic rate. Well-controlled studies show that exercise alone is effective for inducing only modest loss of total body weight and fat mass. Significant loss of body weight and fat requires a combination of diet, behaviour modification and physical activity. Family-based interventions appear to be most effective, especially when the focus is on healthy eating rather than dieting and on reducing sedentary behaviour.

Total energy expenditure is important for body weight loss. Exercise prescription for overweight or obese children should incorporate exercise guidelines for children (discussed earlier in the chapter) and obese adults (refer to chapter 8). Although high-intensity exercise is most effective for reducing fat mass, it may not be feasible for unfit and overweight children. Exercise programs that have been effective for long-term weight loss in children and adolescents include 15 to 50 min of exercise (about 250 kcal per session) using a variety of modes, at self-selected pace or 60 to 80% APMHR, three to five times per week. Lifestyle exercise incorporated into the daily routine seems to be more effective for long-term weight loss than structured exercise programs. For example, in one study, children who increased lifestyle activities by cycling to school or exercising in shorter, multiple sessions at self-selected pace exhibited larger and longer lasting loss of body mass than those in a structured exercise program (Epstein, Coleman and Myers 1996). Although moderate exercise (e.g., 30 min cycling at 80% peak heart rate, three times per week) may result in only modest changes in body mass, it has been shown to favourably alter disease risk factors such as blood lipids (Tolfrey, Campbell and Batterham 1998). Physical training may also reduce visceral fat in obese children (Owens et al. 1999).

Because obesity is a predictor of poor adherence, adherence issues are important for long-term maintenance of weight loss. The most effective programs combine reduced support for sedentary behaviour (e.g., discouraging television watching) with opportunities and incentives for active behaviour (e.g., organised sport and local infrastructure designed specifically for children, such as skateboard parks).

Cardiovascular Disease

Cardiovascular disease may be structural, caused by congenital defects of the heart or blood vessels, or acquired through infection or drug abuse. The child with cardiovascular disease will have impaired exercise tolerance and physical fitness because of the pathology and the inactivity imposed by disease. Unless there are contraindications to physical activity, regular exercise is recommended for these children. Because there is a small risk of sudden death during exercise in some cardiovascular diseases of childhood such as Marfan's syndrome or hypertrophic cardiomyopathy, medical clearance and clinical exercise testing are first needed to determine if there are contraindications to participation. Exercise programs should be scientifically based and individualised to the child's needs and condition. Clinical, supervised programs are recommended in North America, although there are few such programs in Australia at present.

Juvenile Rheumatoid Arthritis

Juvenile rheumatoid arthritis (JRA) may first present with fever, rash, joint inflammation and pain, fluid around the heart or in the lungs, and anaemia. Most of these symptoms disappear eventually and only joint inflammation and pain remain. JRA is an autoimmune disorder in which substances produced by the body's immune system accumulate within the joints, causing chronic inflammation of the synovial lining and tendons. Only a few joints or multiple joints may be affected.

Children with JRA are advised to maintain as much physical activity as possible to avoid detraining and loss of bone density and to enable normal participation in school life. For the child with JRA, it is essential to balance the need and desire for physical activity with joint pain and inflammation. Exercise should aim to increase muscular strength and endurance in order to reduce stress on affected joints and enhance joint ROM. Exercise that does not stress affected joints, yet provides a training effect, is recommended. Examples include aquatic sports, low-intensity circuit training, cycling, walking and low-impact exercise to music (aerobics). Contact and collision sports may need to be avoided, along with activities involving impact of the affected joints. For example, gymnastics and volleyball would not be recommended when JRA involves the shoulder, wrist or elbow. Proper warm-up and stretching exercises should be included before any activity.

Muscular Dystrophy (MD)

Muscular dystrophy is a family of inherited diseases, appearing mostly in males, in which the main defect occurs within skeletal muscle, causing progressive deterioration of muscle strength and function. The child with MD may develop normally through about age 3 to 4, with muscle weakness appearing around age 6. Exercise capacity is limited by muscle weakness; mechanical efficiency is low because of weakness and gait problems, leading to early fatigue during exercise. The more severe forms of MD usually cause death by age 30, although patients with milder forms have a longer life expectancy. MD may be accompanied by obesity and cardiac and pulmonary complications.

There are few studies on exercise training for MD patients, although physical activity seems important for a sense of well-being and perception of control over the disease. Resistance training may slow or reverse the decline in muscle function, especially in the slower progressing forms of disease. The main aim of exercise prescription should be to increase muscular strength and endurance and to prevent joint contracture due to inactivity. General guidelines for exercise prescription for children apply, especially with regard to choosing fun, game-type activities whenever possible. Also, the program should focus on muscle function rather than just CRF. Fatigue is common for MD patients, and exercise intensity will need to be adjusted according to fatigue levels. The child with MD will normally have low functional capacity to start, perhaps as low as 10 to 20 W of anaerobic power output in a cycle ergom-

eter test. Arm and leg ergometry and walking are suitable exercises for developing CRF and controlling body mass. Resistance exercise should use the body mass as resistance (calisthenics such as push-ups, sit-ups), small hand-held weights, or machines that provide only light resistance. As in programs for healthy children, 1 to 3 sets of 8 to 12 repetitions of 8 to 10 exercises should be included. Stretching and cardiovascular conditioning should be performed daily if possible and resistance exercise three times per week.

Childhood Cancers

Recent advancements in the treatment of childhood cancers have led to a high rate of long-term survival, as high as 80 to 90% for some forms of cancer. There appear to be long-term effects of treatment, however, that may influence exercise capacity and patterns of physical activity in survivors. Compared with healthy children, survivors of childhood cancer exhibit impaired physical fitness and exercise tolerance, possibly due to cardiac abnormalities and lower physical activity patterns. Survivors of some types of cancer, such as acute lymphoblastic leukaemia, also tend to become obese. Cytotoxic drugs or radiation used to treat cancer may cause cardiac dysfunction or changes in hormone levels that influence exercise capacity (e.g., cardiac output), growth and body composition (e.g., growth hormone). These may persist for several years after treatment and remission.

In a recent study of 13-year-old survivors who had been in remission for 7 years, cancer survivors were shorter and lighter than healthy children and exhibited a 30 to 50% reduction in $\dot{V}O_2$max even when scaled to body size (Johnson et al. 1997). Despite no differences in resting cardiac parameters such as stroke volume or heart rate, stroke volume and cardiac output were lower and heart rate higher at given submaximal work rates in survivors compared with healthy children. It was concluded that the reduction in physical work capacity resulted from long-term effects of drugs used to treat cancer on the ability to increase cardiac output during exercise. Low functional capacity secondary to drug treatment and inactivity during treatment may initiate a sedentary lifestyle in the surviving child, especially if coupled with feelings of over-protection by parents and schools. Although there are few, if any, specific studies on exercise prescription for child survivors of cancer, a case can be made that regular physical activity may be particularly beneficial for restoring functional capacity in these children. Exercise prescription should incorporate the general principles of exercise testing and prescription for healthy children and for those with disease, as discussed previously in the chapter.

Exercise prescription for adult cancer patients is discussed later in this chapter. Exercise prescription for other diseases affecting children are discussed elsewhere, in particular diabetes, cystic fibrosis (CF) and asthma in chapter 8 and cerebral palsy (CP) in chapter 10.

Aging

Aging is associated with declines in many physiological factors that influence physical capacity, including aerobic power ($\dot{V}O_2$max); maximum heart rate (HRmax), cardiac output and stroke volume; total blood, plasma and red blood cell volumes; and skeletal muscle mass and strength (see table 9.2). Decreases in HRmax and muscle mass are the major contributors to declines in both aerobic exercise capacity and muscular strength. In addition, participation in physical activity decreases with age, contributing to declining muscle mass and CRF. The combined effect of inactivity and decreasing physical function may eventually compromise the ability to perform simple activities of daily living (ADLs) such as walking or housekeeping. Although some of these age-related changes are inevitable, such as the decline in HRmax, other changes such as loss of muscle mass may be attenuated through regular exercise.

Average lifespan and the relative proportion of older people are continuing to increase in most developed nations. It is important to find non-medical

TABLE 9.2—Physiological Changes During Aging and Implications for Exercise Capacity or Prescription

Physiological change	Implications for exercise capacity or prescription
↓ HRmax, cardiac output, $\dot{V}O_2$max	↓ endurance exercise capacity
↓ muscle mass + ↑ fat mass	↓ muscular strength and endurance, $\dot{V}O_2$max ↑ risk of falling
↑ resting and exercise blood pressure	Low-moderate exercise to avoid excessive rise in BP and to lower BP over long term
↓ bone mass	↑ risk of fracture; avoid orthopaedic stress Use combination of weight-bearing and muscular strength exercises
↓ motor control and biomechanical factors (e.g., gait, balance, posture, reaction time)	↓ ability for quick movement, agility and coordination ↑ risk of falling Use clear demonstration, simple movements and slow pace
↓ muscle flexibility, joint ROM	↓ agility ↑ risk of injury
↓ glucose tolerance	Exercise prescription to enhance glucose uptake and tolerance
↓ protein synthesis	↓ ability for muscle hypertrophy and tissue repair after damage; longer to adapt to exercise training Use gradual progression ↑ exercise duration rather than intensity

Abbreviations: BP = blood pressure; HRmax = maximum heart rate; ROM = range of motion.

interventions that enhance quality of life and functional capacity, ensuring that older individuals can maintain an independent lifestyle for as long as practical. Society as a whole bears the economic and social cost of the inability of the elderly to maintain an independent lifestyle. Because of recent recommendations that regular physical activity is an important component of a healthy lifestyle at all ages, there is an increasing need for physical activity prescription guidelines aimed specifically at the elderly population. The American College of Sports Medicine has published recommendations for exercise prescription for the elderly (ACSM 1998a, 2000). Regular physical activity has been shown to offer many potential benefits for the older population (see table 9.3).

Aging is also associated with increased individual variability in physical function; that is, people age at different rates with regard to changes in physical function. Spirduso (1995) developed five levels of classification of physical function in older adults (65 years and over), ranging from the physically dependent to the physically elite:

▶ Physically dependent individuals are debilitated by disease and dependent on others for at least some, and sometimes many, of the basic ADLs, such as getting into and out of bed, dressing, rising from a chair and walking.

▶ Physically frail are individuals with disease or conditions, such as stroke, diabetes, arthritis, heart disease, hypertension or cancer, that affect their functional capacity on a daily basis.

These people may be homebound for the most part but may be able to perform some ADLs such as shopping, food preparation or light housekeeping.

▶ Physically independent describes the majority of older adults, who are generally healthy and free of debilitating disease. They remain mobile and independent but are not regularly physically active. Although healthy, they may be vulnerable to unexpected stresses such as illnesses or falls.

▶ Physically fit are those who are physically active at least twice per week and who are active to achieve health benefits. They generally exercise moderately and have above average $\dot{V}O_2$max and muscular strength compared with their sedentary peers.

▶ Physically elite is an unusual and small group of very active individuals who participate in competitive sports or adventure recreation. Their fitness levels are much higher than others their own age and may be comparable to levels in younger adults.

Because of the potentially large variability in physical function and physical activity levels, fitness testing and exercise prescription for older adults should be individualised even more so than for younger populations.

The following sections discuss age-related changes in physiological factors such as aerobic power, muscular strength, endurance and flexibil-

TABLE 9.3—Benefits of Regular Physical Activity During Aging

Benefit	Relevant disease or condition prevented or managed through physical activity
Slow the decline in $\dot{V}O_2$max	CAD, type 2 diabetes
Maintain muscle mass and strength	Arthritis, type 2 diabetes, obesity, LBP, osteoporosis, falls
Prevent increase in body fat	Obesity, CAD, hypertension, stroke, type 2 diabetes, dyslipidaemia, falls
Maintain bone mass	Osteoporosis, falls
Maintain joint ROM and muscle flexibility	Arthritis, LBP, falls
Enhance well-being, self-confidence, QOL reduce anxiety, depression, social isolation	Depression, neurological disease, falls
Maintain glucose tolerance	Type 2 diabetes

Abbreviations: CAD = coronary artery disease; LBP = low back pain; QOL = quality of life; ROM = range of motion.

ity, and balance and gait. In light of the previous discussion on individual variability in physical function, it should be noted that, for the most part, this is a general discussion of physiological changes in the average healthy population (i.e., physically independent and physically fit).

Aerobic Exercise Capacity and Training Effects in the Elderly (Over Age 65 Years)

In sedentary individuals, maximal aerobic power ($\dot{V}O_2$max) declines about 0.5 to 1.0% per year after about age 25 to 30 years. The major reasons for the progressive decrease in aerobic power include central cardiovascular factors such as declining HRmax, stroke volume, cardiac output and blood volume and peripheral factors such as reduced skeletal muscle mass, oxygen extraction and oxidative metabolism. Decreases in HRmax and skeletal muscle mass are the two most important factors. The rate of all these changes accelerates after about age 70 to 75 years. The decrease in aerobic power is reflected in a decrease in physical work capacity. Although older individuals may exhibit peak work capacity of 7 METs or higher before age 75, it is not unusual for maximal work capacity to fall below 4 METs after age 75 years. Thus, even routine ADLs such as cleaning, cooking or shopping (~2.5-5 METs) may be physically demanding for older individuals.

Genetics, physical activity patterns, and environmental and social factors all influence the rate and magnitude of these changes. Although the decreased HRmax may be inevitable, regular physical activity may attenuate declining functional capacity in later years by maintaining or lessening the declines in skeletal muscle mass, oxidative metabolism, maximum cardiac output and stroke volume. Both cross-sectional and longitudinal studies show that the rate of decline in $\dot{V}O_2$max is halved in physically active compared with sedentary individuals. There is also evidence suggesting that regular exercise lessens the age-related decline in HRmax. Genetics influence not only the highest $\dot{V}O_2$max achieved in a person's lifetime (usually around age 20-25) but also the rate of decline in $\dot{V}O_2$max and other exercise-related variables (e.g., muscular strength). For example, older distance runners who have maintained endurance training throughout their lives exhibit $\dot{V}O_2$max values lower than young distance runners (aging effect) but higher than untrained young adults (combined genetic and training effects).

Older people exhibit similar training adaptations to young adults when expressed relative to initial values, that is, as percentage improvement from starting levels. Thus, provided an appropriate training stimulus is used, $\dot{V}O_2$max may increase by 20 to 30% in the elderly, although the absolute $\dot{V}O_2$max will generally be lower because it starts from a lower value. Adaptations require a longer time in older individuals, however, possibly because of the reduced rate of protein synthesis. Beneficial training adaptations documented in the elderly include increased $\dot{V}O_2$max and physical work capacity, decreased resting and submaximal exercise HR and blood pressure, increased lean body mass and reduced body fat mass, enhanced glucose tolerance and improved blood lipid profile.

Anaerobic Exercise Capacity and Muscular Strength in the Elderly

Muscular strength and anaerobic capacity peak around age 20 years but may be maintained with continued training until the late-30s to mid-40s. In sedentary individuals, there is an accelerated loss of skeletal muscle mass after the mid-40s, with resultant declines in muscular strength, endurance, power and anaerobic capacity. Muscular strength may decrease by 25% by age 65 and 40% by age 80 years; anaerobic capacity and power decline even more, up to 60% between ages 25 and 65 years. Skeletal muscle mass decreases in size, and consequently strength, because of declines in muscle fibre cross-sectional area and number, impaired excitation-contraction coupling and lower motor unit number. A selective loss of the larger, faster type II (fast twitch) muscle fibres, especially after age 70 years, has significant impact on both strength and power. In addition, anaerobic capacity and power are influenced by age-related changes in neuromuscular coordination and mechanical efficiency and by reduced motivation to perform a high-intensity task to maximum capacity, possibly for fear of injury. Elderly women seem to lose lean body mass more than men do, but it is unclear whether this is related to true physiological sex differences or simply to different physical activity patterns (i.e., compared with men, women are generally less active and are less likely to engage in vigorous exercise).

As with aerobic capacity, the elderly are capable of improving muscular strength, endurance, power and anaerobic capacity with appropriate training. High-intensity strength training (e.g., >80% 1 RM) has been shown to induce large improvements in muscular strength without injury, provided it is undertaken in a controlled environment (Rall, Meydani et al. 1996; Rall, Roubenoff et al. 1996). Early studies suggested that neural adaptations were primarily responsible for gains in muscular strength in the elderly, but recent studies using more sensitive imaging technology show that elderly skeletal muscle is capable of hypertrophy in response to high-intensity resistance training. This has obvious implications for using resistance training to help prevent age-related declines in skeletal muscle mass and strength. Increases in muscular strength after resistance training are also linked to enhanced motor control skills, such as balance and coordination, and improvements in gait (Rall, Meydani et al. 1996; Rall, Roubenoff et al. 1996). Theoretically, maintenance of muscle mass during aging would have far-reaching benefits including

▶ helping to maintain aerobic power, physical work capacity, muscular strength and endurance, the ability to perform ADLs and thus an independent lifestyle;

▶ helping to maintain healthy body composition (recall from chapter 8 that BMR is related to lean body mass);

▶ enhancing glucose tolerance and thus preventing or helping to manage type 2 diabetes (refer to chapter 8);

▶ preventing falls in the elderly and thus reducing the risk of fracture (refer to chapter 10); and

▶ enhancing the load-bearing ability of muscles around joints, thus helping to manage arthritis (refer to chapter 10).

In addition, lack of muscular strength and endurance is often a limiting factor for the elderly performing regular physical activity. Increasing muscle mass and strength through resistance training may enhance the ability of the elderly to participate in regular endurance exercise, with its myriad health benefits.

Flexibility

Flexibility of the muscles and around joints also declines with age for a number of reasons, including disuse, joint deterioration and less distensible connective tissue caused by degeneration of collagen. These changes occur in connective tissue within skeletal muscle, tendons, fascia and ligaments, ultimately affecting muscle flexibility and joint ROM. It is unclear whether such changes are an inevitable

part of the aging process or if they are due to disuse or pathology or some combination of factors. Certainly, the incidence of osteoarthritis (refer to chapter 10) increases with age; the pain associated with arthritis may also limit ROM and the ability or desire to be physically active, leading to a vicious cycle of disuse, further loss of ROM and muscle flexibility, and inability to perform ADLs. Muscle flexibility and joint ROM can be improved in the elderly through an appropriate stretching regime, although a relatively longer period of time is needed to achieve results compared with younger individuals.

Balance, Posture, Gait and Risk of Falling in the Elderly

The risk of falling increases with age, with potentially devastating consequences for long-term health: one in three people over 65 years will fall each year, and of those who fall and break a hip, about 50% will never be functional walkers again. The risk of falling reflects a combination of physical, perceptive and cognitive factors. Physical factors include the loss of balance and inability to correct disturbances in balance. Weak lower limb muscular strength, especially of the hip adductors, knee extensors and knee flexors, is related to increased chance of falling. Cognitive and visual impairments, as well as some medications that affect balance, also contribute to the risk of falling.

Balance is the ability to maintain the body's position over its base of support (generally the feet). **Static balance** involves control of postural sway during standing and is important for preventing falls. Compared with younger adults, the elderly display greater postural sway when standing; this is more pronounced in women than men and in a one-foot compared with a two-foot stance. **Dynamic balance** involves maintaining postural control during movement (e.g., when reaching for objects or opening doors) or regaining balance after a sudden disturbance (e.g., an unexpected lurch when standing on a bus). Older people require a longer time to recover when stability is slightly disturbed. Posture is the alignment of body parts in relation to each other. Age-related changes in the spinal column, in particular the structure of the vertebrae and intervertebral discs, affect posture by increasing the curve of the thoracic spine. Walking, rising from a chair, stair climbing and bending stress the spine, possibly leading to pain that may in turn limit movement. The elderly individual may then try to avoid these activities if they cause discomfort; however, inactivity and too much sitting exacerbate spinal curvature and weaken postural muscles, resulting in a vicious cycle of more pain and further decreases in mobility.

Gait, or walking movement pattern, also changes during aging. In the elderly, gait is characterised by slower velocity, or walking pace (more so in women than in men), higher cadence (step rate), shorter stride length and increased time with both feet on the ground. Walking velocity is a good predictor of mobility in elderly individuals. Faster walking speed is accomplished by increasing stride rate rather than length (as in younger adults). The elderly also have a tendency to adopt a flexed position when walking, leaning slightly forward because of fear of falling backward, resulting in a stiffening of the body and contraction of major muscles; this is less economical and more fatiguing than a relaxed posture. The combination of limited muscle flexibility, strength and ROM, possible pain from arthritis, and fear of falling often leads to avoidance of walking or other physical activity. The end result is a further decrease in physical fitness and confidence about physical activity.

Both theoretical and empirical evidence suggests that appropriate regular physical activity decreases the risk of falling in the elderly (recently reviewed by Carter, Kannus and Khan 2001). Figure 9.3 describes the means by which regular physical activity may help prevent such falls. Although the optimal amount and type of exercise to prevent falls is not currently known, research suggests that an individualised program of exercise to improve balance and lower limb muscular strength and endurance, three times per week, coupled with regular moderate walking is effective for reducing the incidence of falls in elderly

women (Carter, Kannus and Khan 2001). Exercises emphasising balance, muscular flexibility and strength seem to work better for reducing the risk of falls than simple endurance training alone.

Exercise and Fitness Testing for the Elderly

Since aging is associated with increased prevalence of cardiovascular, neurological and musculoskeletal impairments, pre-program screening is essential. Many older individuals will need prior exercise testing or medical clearance before fitness testing and exercise prescription (refer to chapter 5). Although fitness testing may be helpful for programming, the need for such information should be balanced by consideration of the client's health, goals, exercise history and motivation. That is, fitness testing may not be warranted for the older client interested only in moderate activity or for someone who may be uncomfortable with the procedures. Moreover, some older people may not be physically capable of performing fitness tests, for example, the physically dependent and physically frail, as described previously (Spirduso 1995). Conditions common among the elderly (e.g., musculoskeletal or neurological impairments) may also require modification of standard testing protocols (see table 9.4).

Spirduso (1995) suggests that the choice and extent of fitness testing should be appropriate for the level of physical function. Thus, assessment of individuals classed as physically dependent or physically frail would focus on ADLs, strength, balance, gait and mobility. In contrast, assessment of individuals with

---

▶ Increases leg and back muscle strength and endurance

▶ Improves gait

▶ Enhances confidence in movement and lessens fear of falling

▶ Reduces body weight and fat, enhancing balance

▶ Decreases risk of postural hypotension

▶ Enhances joint ROM and muscle flexibility

▶ Reduces stiffness and pain associated with arthritis

▶ Improves reaction time

Compiled from W.W. Spirduso, 1995, *Physical dimensions of aging.* (Champaign, IL: Human Kinetics); N.D. Carter, P. Kannus, K.M. Khan, 2001, "Exercise in the prevention of falls in older people: A systematic literature review examining the rationale and the evidence," *Sports Medicine* 31: 427-438.

FIGURE 9.3   Means by which regular physical activity may prevent falls in the elderly.

TABLE 9.4—Recommendations for Cardiorespiratory Fitness Testing in the Elderly

	Recommendations[a]	Reasons
Test mode	Weight supported or low impact (e.g., walking, cycle ergometry)	High incidence of musculoskeletal disorders
	Submax test preferred	Avoid risk of injury or cardiac event
		Generally no need for precise measurements
Test protocol	Longer warm-up	Longer time for cardiorespiratory adjustment
	Lower initial work rate	Low functional capacity
	Smaller increments	Balance, gait problems
	Discontinuous protocol	
	Avoid high treadmill speeds	
Monitor	HR, BP, RPE	HR, BP and RPE as basis for exercise prescription
		BP to identify abnormal responses
		RPE to avoid perception of too intense exercise and to avoid early discomfort

Fitness testing means assessment of general physical fitness for exercise prescription purposes; it does not include use of test data for diagnostic or clinical purposes.

[a]Recommendations compared with standard tests for younger individuals.

Abbreviations: HR = heart rate; BP = blood presure; RPE = rating of perceived exertion.

a higher functional capacity (physically independent, fit or elite) could focus more on physical fitness and performance. Many standard assessment protocols have been developed specifically for older individuals or those with movement impairments (discussed in detail in Spirduso 1995), including the following:

PHYSICALLY DEPENDENT AND PHYSICALLY FRAIL

▶ Self-report inventories of ADLs and regular physical activity

▶ Gait analysis

▶ Measurement of joint ROM

▶ Performance tests of hand control (e.g., grip strength) and leg muscular strength (using a dynamometer or tensiometer)

▶ Tests of balance and mobility, such as the get-up-and-go test (time to rise from a chair, walk 3 m, turn, walk back to chair and sit)

▶ Timed Physical Performance Test of diverse physical activities related to ADLs (e.g., writing, simulated eating, lifting a book, picking up a coin, walking 16 m, stair climbing)

PHYSICALLY INDEPENDENT

▶ Tests of agility and balance, such as the timed one-leg stance with arms extended laterally

▶ Field tests of walking (12-min test or 800-m timed walk) or submaximal predictive tests (e.g., cycle ergometry) to measure aerobic power

▶ Tests of muscle flexibility, such as the sit-and-reach test

▶ Performance tests of leg muscle strength (e.g., 30-s sit-and-stand test) or using dynamometry or weight machines

▶ Williams-Greene physical function tests (an extensive battery of tests of mobility, strength, balance, flexibility, gait and agility) or Tinetti Gait and Balance Evaluation (scale of gait, balance and flexibility)

PHYSICALLY FIT AND PHYSICALLY ELITE

▶ $\dot{V}O_2$max using cycle ergometry, treadmill or submaximal predictive tests

- Muscular strength of major muscle groups using dynamometry or weight machines
- Standard tests of muscle flexibility and joint ROM (e.g., sit-and-reach test)
- Standard tests of gait, balance and agility (sport specific for elite)

If fitness testing is warranted and clearance for exercise has been obtained from a medical practitioner, there are several precautions to take with elderly clients. Fitness testing using weight-supported exercise, such as a cycle ergometer, is preferable to the treadmill to accommodate possible problems with gait, balance or coordination among some untrained elderly clients. If the treadmill is used, the incline rather than speed should be increased because fast walking may cause falls, and the client is more likely to end the test prematurely because of unease. A handrail may be used to assist those with balance or coordination problems. Because of the low functional capacity in untrained older clients and the longer time to achieve steady state, tests should begin at a low intensity (2-3 METs) and progress with small increments (0.5-1 METs). The intervals should be relatively long (>3 min), but the test should aim to conclude within 8 to 12 min to avoid undue fatigue. A familiarisation session is recommended to acquaint the client with the equipment and protocol and to ensure that the client is comfortable with the procedure and can thus exercise to the desired end-point. A longer warm-up may be beneficial to increase circulation and avoid early discomfort, especially for those with arthritis (refer to chapter 10).

If precise measures of fitness are not needed, submaximal testing using a bicycle ergometer is preferable to maximal testing. Field tests such as the 12-min walk or timed 800-m walk are appropriate for those without gait or balance problems. Heart rate and blood pressure should be monitored during and after the fitness test to identify any abnormal responses (refer to chapter 6); if any occur, the exercise threshold at which the abnormal response appeared should be noted. The elderly client should also be observed for any other irregular responses, such as heat illness, dizziness, joint or muscle pain, or discomfort. Monitoring RPE (refer to chapter 6) during fitness testing is useful for exercise prescription for clients who do not wish to monitor heart rate during regular exercise or for those on medication that affects the heart rate response to exercise.

Assessment of muscular fitness may include simple tests such as grip strength, sit-ups or modified push-ups. If additional measures of muscular strength are needed for prescription purposes, say for a resistance training program, it is preferable to use dynamometers or weight machines rather than free weights. Testing maximum strength using the 1 RM method may be contraindicated because of risk of injury or unwillingness of older clients to exert such force. One alternative is to test 3 RM, which requires less force (and resistance) and is less likely to cause injury or discomfort. All assessment of muscular strength should be preceded by an appropriate cardiovascular and muscular warm-up that includes stretching and total body exercises (to increase circulation and warm the muscles). Flexibility and ROM testing is also useful, given the high incidence of arthritis among the elderly (refer to chapters 6 and 10).

Assessment of gait, balance and coordination is recommended, especially for older individuals who are unaccustomed to regular physical activity or who may have problems with walking or balance. A number of mobility, gait, balance and coordination tests (see Spirduso 1995 for details) are often used in the clinical context with specific diseases or conditions affecting mobility, such as neurological disease. The Tinetti Gait and Balance Evaluation is a simple, comprehensive means to assess gait, balance and flexibility; scores on this test correlate with the incidence of falls in the elderly. Briefly this evaluation includes the following:

MEASURES OF BALANCE

- Sitting balance
- Rising from a seated position and sitting down from a standing position
- Two-leg standing balance with eyes open and closed
- Light nudge to subject's chest while standing
- 360° turn
- One-leg standing balance
- Reaching, bending and back extension

MEASURES OF GAIT

- Initiation of walking
- Step characteristics (length, height, symmetry, continuity, heel position)
- Straightness of path
- Trunk position and sway
- Acceleration of walking speed

Exercise Prescription for Elderly Clients

The same general guidelines for healthy adults apply to prescribing exercise for the elderly, along with a greater emphasis on safety and moderation (ACSM 1998a). Many cardiovascular and metabolic adaptations to exercise training are qualitatively similar in older and younger adults. For example, resting and submaximal heart rates decline after endurance training. When expressed relative to starting levels, older healthy individuals show similar improvements in aerobic power and muscular strength compared with younger adults (i.e., improvements of 20-30% in $\dot{V}O_2$max or muscular strength). However, although muscular strength and endurance may improve considerably, a longer time is needed to see such changes. The important point is that regular physical activity is capable of modifying disease risk factors such as blood lipid profile, insulin sensitivity, blood pressure and adiposity in older individuals.

For the elderly, the goals of regular physical activity are to improve functional capacity, muscular strength and endurance, quality of life and functional independence and to slow or prevent the onset of disease. Consequently, the exercise prescription should focus on developing cardiorespiratory fitness, muscular strength and endurance, flexibility and range of motion, and other variables such as balance and coordination. The elderly are also attracted by the social interactions of physical activity programs, and group- or community-based programs may be especially effective.

Because of the wide variability of health, functional capacity and physical activity habits among the elderly, individualisation of exercise prescription should be based on health status and functional capacity. For example, the needs, interests and capacity of a physically dependent individual are very different from the needs of a healthy, physically independent or physically fit elderly person. For simplicity, using Spirduso's (1995) classifications, the following groups are considered together: (a) physically independent, fit and elite and (b) physically dependent and frail.

Endurance Exercise Training for the Physically Independent, Fit and Elite Elderly

Given the increasing prevalence of disease and the wide individual variability in health and fitness with aging, individualised exercise prescription is crucial for a safe program and long-term compliance. Aerobic exercise modes that are less likely to induce orthopaedic stress should be considered. Examples include activities that are low-impact (e.g., walking, low-impact aerobics) or weight-supported (e.g., cycling, swimming or water-based)(see figure 9.4). Exercise intensity may vary but is generally recommended in the range of 50 to 70% HRR for older healthy individuals, although lower intensities (40-50% HRR) may be appropriate at the onset or for those with low functional capacity (ACSM 1998a, 2000). Target heart rates should be based on actual measured HRmax when available (from a clinical exercise test); simple age-predicted maximum heart rate is of limited value given the wide variability of HRmax and the fact that many older individuals take medications that affect heart rate. Older people may not wish to monitor heart rate during exercise, so RPE or the simple "talk test" may be appropriate for setting exercise intensity. Self-selected pace may be preferable because aging is associated with decreased mechanical efficiency.

From the public health perspective, the elderly are advised to exercise moderately at least three times per week and on most days, if possible. If vigorous exercise is included, it should be performed on alternate days to allow recovery and minimise risk of overuse injury. Older, previously inactive clients may find it difficult to exercise continuously for any length of time and may better tolerate interval training (alternating 3- to 5-min periods of work and rest) or 10-min exercise sessions performed at different times throughout the day. The ability to thermoregulate is somewhat compromised in the elderly, and general precautions to avoid heat illness should be taken. These include monitoring clients for signs of heat illness and encouraging clients to wear light and loose-fitting clothes, to exercise during cool times or in controlled environments (e.g., water, air-conditioned gym) and to replace fluids during and after exercise.

Resistance Training for the Physically Independent, Fit and Elite Elderly

As noted previously, aging is associated with significant loss of muscle mass and strength, which may adversely affect functional capacity and the ability to perform ADLs. Recent research suggests that older individuals can improve muscular strength and endurance through appropriately designed resistance training (Taafe and Marcus 2000), although progress will generally be slower than that expected in younger adults. The goals of resistance training for the elderly are to develop and maintain muscular fitness (strength and endurance), to maintain lean body mass and to enhance general well-being and the ability to perform ADLs.

MODE

▶ Load-bearing activity whenever possible to maintain bone density

▶ Low impact (e.g., walking, aquatic, cycle ergometry) if there are orthopaedic concerns

▶ Accessible, convenient, economic

▶ Group activities to allow social interaction

INTENSITY

▶ Low-moderate intensity (RPE 11-13; <60% HRR or $\dot{V}O_2$max) unless already fit and interested in performance or higher intensity exercise

▶ Increase duration before intensity for progressive program

▶ If increasing intensity, do so gradually

▶ Use actual HRmax rather than APMHR or use RPE to set intensity

DURATION

▶ ≥30 min per session

▶ Interval exercise often better tolerated

▶ Can use short sessions spaced throughout day

▶ Increase duration rather than intensity to accommodate increased fitness

FREQUENCY

▶ Most days if possible but at least 3 to 5 days per week

▶ If vigorous exercise, ≤3 days per week

PRECAUTIONS

▶ Screening and appropriate medical clearance essential

▶ Consider potential problems with gait, balance and coordination

---

Abbreviations: RPE = rating of perceived exertion; HRR = heart rate reserve; HRmax = maximum heart rate; APMHR = age-predicted maximum heart rate.

Compiled from American College of Sports Medicine, 2000, *ACSM's guidelines for exercise testing and prescription*, 6th ed. (Philadelphia: Lippincott, Williams & Wilkins); ACSM, 1997, *Exercise management for persons with chronic diseases and disabilities*. (Champaign, IL: Human Kinetics); D.E. Forman, C.T. Pu, and C.E. Garber, 1999, Exercise counselling in the elderly. In *Lifestyle Medicine*, edited by J.M. Rippe (Malden, MA: Blackwell Scientific); American College of Sports Medicine Position Stand, 1998a, "Exercise and physical activity for older adults," *Medicine and Science in Sports and Exercise* 30: 992-1008.

FIGURE 9.4 Guidelines for exercise prescription for the previously inactive elderly: Cardiorespiratory conditioning.

Individualised resistance training that takes into account fitness test data and any impairments (e.g., arthritis, hypertension, diabetes) is strongly recommended. Gentle exercise such as tai chi and yoga is often attractive to many elderly, especially those just beginning a program. These activities have the added benefit of simultaneously training muscular strength and endurance, ROM, flexibility, balance and coordination. If weight training is appropriate and desired, circuit resistance training using ma-chines rather than free weights is preferred because it can improve muscular endurance while requiring less skill and minimising risk of injury (see figure 9.5). There is some debate over recommended frequency of resistance training for the elderly. The U.S. Surgeon General and ACSM recommendations are that resistance training should be performed two to three times per week with at least 48 h rest between sessions (USDHHS and CDC 1996; ACSM 1998a, 2000). On the other hand, a recent paper suggests

MODE

▶ Machine weights, hand-held weights and flexible bands preferred over free weights

▶ Multi-joint using large muscle groups

▶ Related to ADLs

▶ Circuit training also enhances cardiorespiratory fitness

INTENSITY

▶ 12-13 RPE unless contraindicated

▶ Increase number of repetitions or sets before increasing resistance

DURATION/VOLUME

▶ 1 to 3 sets

▶ 8 to 15 repetitions per set

▶ 8 to 10 exercises over entire body

▶ 20 to 30 min per session recommended

FREQUENCY

▶ 1 to 3 days per week with ≥48 h rest between sessions

PRECAUTIONS

▶ Supervised at onset

▶ Normal breathing, no breath holding

▶ Avoid maximal lifts (use 3 RM rather than 1 RM for testing)

▶ Gradual progression, especially during first 8 weeks

▶ Pain-free lift over entire ROM

▶ Avoid during joint inflammation (refer to chapter 10)

▶ Blood pressure is unlikely to rise dramatically in low- to moderate-intensity resistance exercise

---

Abbreviations: ADLs = activities of daily living; RPE = rating of perceived exertion; RM = repetition maximum; ROM = range of motion.

Compiled from American College of Sports Medicine, 2000, *ACSM's guidelines for exercise testing and prescription*, 6th ed. (Philadelphia: Lippincott, Williams & Wilkins); ACSM's *Exercise management for persons with chronic diseases and disabilities*. (Champaign, IL: Human Kinetics); D.R. Taaffe, R. Marcus, 2000, Musculoskeletal health and the older adult," *Journal of Rehabilitation Research and Development* 37: 245-254.

FIGURE 9.5   Guidelines for exercise prescription for the previously inactive elderly: Muscular conditioning.

that once-weekly high-intensity resistance training (8 repetitions at 80% 1 RM) induces the same effects as two to three times per week (Taafe et al. 1999). Training should include 8 to 10 exercises involving the major muscle groups, each performed 8 to 15 times (repetitions). Since multi-joint movements are less likely to cause orthopaedic stress, they are preferable to those involving single joints. The older individual should aim to work at an RPE of 12 to 13 and should not perform any exercise more intense than 8 RM (i.e., avoid maximal or near maximal lifts). Exhaustive resistance training is more likely to cause musculoskeletal injury and to excessively increase blood pressure.

Because of the potential for injury to bones or soft tissues, attention to personal safety is essential. Programs must be closely supervised at the onset, focusing on correct posture, breathing and lifting techniques. It is important to instruct clients to breathe normally, usually exhaling during the force-generating movement to avoid the Valsalva manoeuvre. The first 6 to 8 weeks should be performed with minimal resistance to allow neural and connective tissue adaptations and to ensure that proper form is learned. Speed of movement should be slow and controlled at all times, especially during the eccentric phase (muscle lengthening) of each movement. For individuals with musculoskeletal impairments such as arthritis or low back pain, all movements should be performed within a pain-free range of motion (discussed further in chapter 10).

Flexibility and Range of Motion (ROM)

Stretching exercises should also be included to maintain or improve flexibility and ROM; the same general guidelines as for younger adults apply (refer to chapter 7). Stretching should be incorporated into the warm-up and cool-down, before and after any aerobic or muscular conditioning session, that is, at least three times per week and preferably daily. Low-level, whole body exercise such as a gentle walk or cycle before each stretching session increases circulation and body temperature and thus increases muscle distensibility. Exercises should cover all the major muscle groups, with particular attention to the back, hip and thigh muscles, which are important for posture and basic movements. For the frail elderly or those with low functional capacity, several weeks of stretching exercises may be appropriate before beginning aerobic and muscular conditioning. It is important to emphasise controlled movement through a pain-free ROM. Some stretches may need to be modified to accommodate specific impairments such as arthritis. For example, low back and hamstring stretching should be performed in a way that does not stress the low back or hips, such as from a seated or supine position rather than standing. Similarly, arm, trunk and shoulder stretching may be performed in a seated position. Elderly people at risk of osteoporosis should avoid excessive flexion or extension of the spine.

Exercise Prescription for the Very Old and Physically Dependent or Frail Elderly

Recent research has dispelled the myth that the very old (>80 years) or frail elderly (weak or with very low functional capacity) should avoid exercise (ACSM 1998a). Regular physical activity is now encouraged, although at a lower level than might be expected for a healthy elderly individual. The main focus of activity should be to improve muscular strength and endurance, mobility and functional capacity (see figure 9.6). Contraindications to activity among the frail elderly include unstable or uncontrolled disease, acute illness, weight loss, musculoskeletal pain and frequent falls. For some frail elderly, resistance and balance training should precede other physical activity programs since a certain level of muscular strength and balance is required for movements such as walking. Seated activities or exercises using support (e.g., a chair or bar for support while standing) may be needed to improve muscular strength and endurance in those with balance problems. Resistance should be provided by light hand-held weights, weight machines or elastic bands or by using the body as resistance (e.g., calisthenics). Exercise should focus on enhancing movement required for daily activities:

▶ Develop muscular strength and mass (especially in lower limbs) before beginning aerobic program.

▶ Gentle stretching and ROM exercises may be needed before beginning strength program.

▶ Include strength and movement exercises related to ADLs (e.g., rising from chair).

▶ Mode should be appropriate to disability, gait or musculoskeletal disorders.

▶ Incorporate specific gait, balance and coordination exercises.

▶ Progression should be very gradual.

▶ Low intensity (e.g., 40-60% $\dot{V}O_2$max or HRR, RPE <12) may be appropriate at all times.

▶ Consider social and environmental barriers to participation.

▶ Consider other diseases and disabilities (e.g., CHD, PVD, Parkinson's, osteoporosis, arthritis; refer to chapters 8 and 10).

Compiled from American College of Sports Medicine, 1998a, "Exercise and physical activity for older adults," *Medicine and Science in Sports and Exercise* 30: 992-1008.

FIGURE 9.6   Special guidelines for exercise in the frail elderly (>80 years).

▶ Standing from a seated position and vice versa

▶ Walking and turning

▶ Upper body strength

▶ ROM of the hips, feet, ankles and shoulders

▶ Maintaining posture and balance

▶ Hand function

For example, in a frail elderly client, simply rising from a seated to standing position may require nearly 100% of maximum strength in the hip and knee extensors (in contrast, this task requires <50% maximum strength in a younger person). For such an individual, increasing muscular strength and endurance so that simple movements require a much lower percentage of maximum strength may significantly enhance quality of life and the capacity for independent living.

For those who are relatively mobile but unable to walk for any distance, weight-supported activities such as stationary cycling, water-based exercises and arm ergometry may help improve cardiovascular fitness and muscular endurance. For others with more profound mobility problems, many exercises can be performed from a seated position, for example, upper body muscular strength and endurance work with hand-held weights; hand strength and function exercises; ankle, foot and knee mobility and strength exercises; and upper body stretching. Once sufficient muscular strength, endurance and fitness levels are achieved, the program should aim for exercise at least three times each week, for at least 20 min in duration (in 10-min sessions repeated throughout the day if needed), at 40 to 60% HRR or 11 to 13 on the RPE scale. Mobility and stretching exercises may be performed daily.

Exercise Motivation and Adherence in the Elderly

Exercise motivation and adherence issues are slightly different in older compared with younger populations (refer to chapter 4 for discussion of exercise adherence principles). Older people are motivated to begin a physical activity program by the opportunity to enhance functional capacity, health, well-being and quality of life and by encouragement from a physician. The elderly are more attracted to low- to moderate-intensity exercise that focuses on health, well-being and functional capacity for ADLs rather than performance (except, of course, veteran athletes). Group programs are popular with older individuals because of the social interaction and support. Once older people begin physical activity, they are more likely to continue if they perceive the program is of appropriate intensity, meets their specific needs and has led to improvements in health, well-being, mobility, functional capacity or fitness. Enjoyment and a feeling of belonging to a group are also predictors of continued participation. Barriers to participation include the perception that frailty or poor health limits mobility required of exercise,

Case Study 9.3

Elizabeth is 60 years old and lives on a rural property near a small town of 500 people. Until recently, she was physically active most of her life in the daily management of the property, which has now been taken over by her grown children and their families. She has noticed that in the past few years she has become weaker, especially in her upper body and back, and that many daily tasks, such as lifting, carrying and walking, are becoming more demanding. Elizabeth wishes to remain physically active and to regain her physical capacity. Over the years, she has been very involved in many regional community groups. Although she is not averse to group activity, she would like a home-based program that is not entirely dependent on driving to town. Develop a 6-month physical activity program for Elizabeth.

Key Issues

1. What are the factors motivating Elizabeth to begin an exercise program?

2. What precautions are necessary before Elizabeth begins a program?

3. What aspects of physical fitness are important to address in her program?

4. How will you combine Elizabeth's specific request for a home-based program with her previous experience in community groups?

5. What factors will likely enhance or interfere with her continued participation?

fear of pain or injury, concerns about the safety of the exercise environment and lack of support from the physician, family or peers. In addition, most retired people live on fixed incomes and many rely on public transport, so cost and access are important factors.

Exercise During Pregnancy

Given that regular physical activity is now recommended as part of a healthy lifestyle for all individuals, it seems logical that a woman would wish to maintain some level of activity throughout pregnancy. In terms of exercise prescription, pregnancy presents a unique challenge in that the needs of both the mother and the developing foetus must be considered. There are several potential benefits, and few risks, associated with a scientifically based exercise program continued throughout pregnancy, provided that medical clearance is first obtained and contraindications to exercise are heeded.

Anatomical and Physiological Changes During Pregnancy

Many anatomical and physiological changes occur during pregnancy that may influence exercise capacity or increase risk of injury during physical activity (summarised in table 9.5). During pregnancy, resting blood volume, hematocrit, heart rate, cardiac output and oxygen consumption all increase, ensuring adequate oxygen delivery to the foetus. Tidal volume and minute ventilation also increase to maintain arterial oxygen saturation. Resting metabolic rate increases, requiring an additional 300 kcal (1260 kJ)/day energy consumption. Release of the hormone relaxin causes joint and ligament laxity, especially in the pelvis, which may predispose the pregnant woman to joint injury or pain. As pregnancy progresses, increasing maternal body mass and forward displacement of the centre of gravity will influence economy of movement and oxygen cost of activity in weight-bearing activities such as walking or aerobics.

TABLE 9.5—Anatomical and Physiological Changes During Pregnancy and Potential Influence on Physical Work Capacity

Physiological change	Influence on physical work capacity	Modification to exercise program
Joint laxity	Increases joint flexibility; may increase risk of injury and back pain	Avoid high-impact activities or contact sports; include light resistance and postural exercises to strengthen back muscles
Maternal weight gain, mainly in abdominal and pelvic regions	Alters balance by moving centre of gravity; alters biomechanics and energy cost of activity	Avoid activities requiring balance (skiing, road cycling), depending on amount of weight gain
Increased resting and submaximal heart rate and cardiac output; changes in heart rate-$\dot{V}O_2$ relationship	Maximum values achieved at lower exercise intensity; less room to increase above resting levels	Use RPE rather than HR to monitor exercise intensity; submaximal predictive fitness tests are invalid
Increased resting and submaximal minute ventilation	Higher energy cost of breathing; discomfort during intense exercise (especially in third trimester)	Use RPE or comfort level to monitor exercise intensity; avoid intense exercise
Gestational diabetes (only in some women)	Alters substrate utilisation at rest and during intense exercise	Regular moderate activity may help limit gain in body mass, improve glucose tolerance and prevent need for insulin

Abbreviations: HR = heart rate; RPE = rating of perceived exertion.

Exercise Responses During Pregnancy

The increases in resting metabolic rate, heart rate, oxygen consumption and minute ventilation mean there is less room for increases in these variables during exercise. The submaximal heart rate of a pregnant woman is higher than that of a non-pregnant woman at an equivalent work rate. During pregnancy, resting blood glucose level is lower, and there is increased reliance on carbohydrates as a fuel source. The higher minute ventilation increases the metabolic cost of breathing. Upward growth of the foetus into the abdominal region elevates the diaphragm, especially in the third trimester. These changes result in decreased physical work capacity (by as much as 50%), hyperventilation and possibly dyspnoea at high work rates.

Concern is sometimes raised that, during exercise, increased oxygen demand by the mother's working muscles together with decreased uterine blood flow may limit oxygen availability to the foetus. However, this is not a serious concern during most forms of exercise because foetal oxygen delivery is generally maintained by hemoconcentration, increased oxygen extraction and redistribution of blood flow favouring the placenta. Maternal hyperthermia, as caused by fever, during the first trimester has been associated with neural tube defects, but there is no evidence linking exercise-induced changes in maternal core temperature and birth defects in humans. It appears that in most exercise situations, thermoregulatory mechanisms are sufficient to keep maternal core temperature below the critical 39° C threshold associated with these defects. The exception may be very vigorous, prolonged exercise in the heat (e.g., a marathon) in which dehydration may contribute to an increase in core temperature above this threshold.

Some women develop diabetes during pregnancy (called gestational diabetes) that usually resolves after delivery. In non-insulin-dependent (type 2) gestational diabetes, regular moderate exercise (e.g., two to four times per week at 50% $\dot{V}O_2$max) may stimulate glucose uptake and may possibly prevent the need for exogenous insulin. Women with insulin-dependent (type 1) gestational diabetes should exercise only on advice of the physician and preferably in a supervised setting.

There are few effects of exercise, either positive or negative, on the outcome of pregnancy. There is generally no effect on birth weight or likelihood of pre-term delivery, although birth weight may be reduced by heavy exertion (as in a very physically demanding job). Recent data show that 30 to 60 min of moderate exercise on 3 to 6 days per week does not compromise maternal weight gain or birth weight (Clapp and Little 1995; Marquez-Sterling et al. 2000). There is some suggestion that the second stage of labour may be shortened in physically active women. Exercise throughout pregnancy is associated with less maternal weight gain; reduction of symptoms such as fatigue, nausea, back pain and leg swelling; and enhanced quality of sleep, self-esteem and body image in the mother (Marquez-Sterling et al. 2000). Moreover, maintaining physical fitness during pregnancy will help the woman return to normal activity patterns sooner after delivery.

Recommendations for Exercise During Pregnancy

Physical activity is recommended throughout an uncomplicated pregnancy. Regardless of exercise history or fitness level (i.e., even for athletes), it is essential that a pregnant woman first obtains approval from her physician for any intended program. Because of dramatic changes in a variety of physiological factors as listed previously, fitness testing is of limited value during pregnancy. For reasons of safety, it is recommended that pregnant women do not participate in a fitness assessment requiring maximal effort (aerobic power, anaerobic capacity, muscular strength).

According to the American College of Obstetricians and Gynecologists (ACOG 1994), exercise is contraindicated during high-risk pregnancies. Contraindications to, or reasons for stopping, exercise during pregnancy include the following:

- ▶ Risk of pre-term delivery
- ▶ Pregnancy-induced hypertension
- ▶ Multiple gestations (e.g., twins, triplets)
- ▶ Growth retardation of foetus
- ▶ Persistent bleeding or large fluid discharge from the vagina
- ▶ Sudden swelling of hands, face or ankles or pain in one calf
- ▶ Excessive fatigue
- ▶ Abdominal pain
- ▶ Persistent contractions
- ▶ Severe headache, visual disturbance or unexplained dizziness

There are three general groups of women who undertake exercise during pregnancy:

- Normally inactive women who wish to become physically active
- Recreationally active women who wish to maintain fitness during pregnancy and who wish to return to similar levels of activity soon after delivery
- Athletes who intend to return to competitive sport at some point after pregnancy

The exercise prescription should thus reflect previous exercise history and future plans of the expectant mother.

In 1985, the ACOG issued recommendations regarding exercise during pregnancy that limited exercise to <15 min at a heart rate of 140 beats · min⁻¹. In light of subsequent research showing few if any adverse effects of exercise during pregnancy, these guidelines were revised in 1994 to be less conservative and prescriptive (ACOG 1994). A summary of the ACOG recommendations for exercise during pregnancy is presented in figure 9.7. Some women develop supine hypotension due to compression of the inferior vena cava by the foetus when lying in a supine position (e.g., bench presses, sit-ups). Thus, the ACOG guidelines recommend avoiding such exercise after the first trimester. Energy intake must account for the increased energy cost of pregnancy (300 kcal [1260 kJ]/day) and exercise (an additional 200-500 kcal [840-2100kJ]/day of exercise). As mentioned previously, it is important to ensure adequate

thermoregulation during exercise. To maintain core temperature within a safe level during exercise, the pregnant woman should

- exercise during cooler parts of the day or in a controlled environment,
- avoid prolonged intense exercise especially in the heat,
- wear appropriate clothing to allow sweating and heat dissipation,
- ensure adequate fluid intake during and after exercise, and
- avoid prolonged immersion in heated spa baths or saunas.

Previously inactive women are advised to begin and maintain low-intensity and low-impact exercise such as walking, swimming, other water-based activities (e.g., water walking, aquaerobics), using exercise equipment (e.g., cycle ergometer) or a supervised low-impact aerobic program designed for pregnant women. The previously inactive woman is not advised to begin a strenuous exercise program once pregnant.

Most previously active women spontaneously decrease exercise intensity and duration as pregnancy progresses, and it is not deemed necessary to closely monitor exercise intensity provided there are no complications or contraindications. As pregnancy progresses, physical and biomechanical factors (e.g.,

---

- Mild to moderate activity is preferable to intense activity.
- Regular activity (>3 days per week) is recommended.
- Avoid exercise in supine position after first trimester.
- Athletes should reduce exercise intensity as pregnancy continues.
- Avoid exercise to exhaustion, exercise in hot environments and prolonged intense exercise.
- Avoid activity that increases risk of abdominal trauma (e.g., contact sports).
- Modify (or avoid) activities requiring balance (e.g., skiing, road cycling, dancing) as mother's shape (and centre of gravity) change.
- Ensure adequate diet to cover additional 300 kcal [1260 kJ]/day required of pregnancy (independent of physical activity).
- Ensure heat dissipation (especially during the first trimester) with fluid replacement and appropriate clothing and by choosing cooler exercise environments.
- Gradually resume activity over 4 to 6 weeks post-partum.

Compiled from American College of Obstetricians and Gynecologists, 1994, *Exercise during pregnancy and the postpartum period.* Technical Bulletin 189. (Washington, DC).

FIGURE 9.7 Summary of recommendations by the American College of Obstetricians and Gynecologists (ACOG) for exercise in pregnancy and postpartum.

increased maternal body mass, change of centre of gravity) and safety considerations (e.g., the desire to avoid falling) may require altering mode of exercise, for example, changing from jogging to walking or from road to stationary cycling. A resistance training program to strengthen postural and supporting muscles and thus minimise back pain can be continued if certain precautions are taken: supine exercise is not performed after the first trimester; higher repetition, lower resistance exercise (e.g., 8-12 RM) is used; and safety is considered (e.g., using weight machines rather than free weights).

Competitive athletes or women who normally perform high-volume exercise need to alter training at some point in the pregnancy, usually by the fifth month. There is a case to be made for avoiding exercise in a competitive setting at all stages of pregnancy because prolonged intense exercise at any stage may compromise blood flow and thus delivery of oxygen and other nutrients to the foetus. Prolonged intense exercise in the heat may raise core temperature to a point that may increase the risk of developmental defects in the first trimester. In addition, joint laxity and changes in body shape, size and centre of gravity alter the mechanics of movement and increase the risk of musculoskeletal injury during intense weight-bearing exercise. A general recommendation is that no more than 30 min of intense exercise should be performed at any given session; longer duration exercise is possible if exercise intensity is reduced accordingly.

Contact and High-Risk Sports

Participation in contact and collision sports presents particular concerns for the pregnant athlete and, from a legal perspective, for sports clubs. According to the 1994 Sports Medicine Australia (SMA 1994) guidelines, sports may be classified as

- ▶ non-contact (e.g., swimming, low-impact aerobics),
- ▶ limited contact in which contact may occur or there is a slight risk of falling (e.g., netball, touch football, racquet sports), and
- ▶ unlimited contact and collision (e.g., soccer, baseball, football, martial arts, gymnastics).

As already indicated, participation in non-contact sports throughout pregnancy should not be limited as long as there are no contraindications, medical approval is obtained and the ACOG guidelines are met. During the first trimester of pregnancy (first 3 months), the developing foetus is placed well within the pelvic girdle, which provides protection from blows to the abdomen. With advancing pregnancy, the foetus and placenta move progressively higher into the abdominal region, where they may be vulnerable to damage from blows or falls. During normal pregnancies, SMA states that limited contact sports may be continued during the first and possibly into the second trimester, but participation in unlimited contact and collision sports should be

Case Study 9.4

Kara is 27 years old and a nationally ranked triathlete over the Olympic distance (2-km swim, 30-km cycle, 10-km run). She has just learned she is 5 weeks pregnant. She was intending to compete in a World Cup race in 4 weeks' time. The race will take place on the Gold Coast in April.

Kara asks you if she should compete in this event. She also asks you to write a training program to maintain her fitness throughout her pregnancy so she can resume competing soon after her baby is born. Kara believes she has not yet achieved her best performance, and she is not willing to consider the possibility of retiring for several years.

Key Issues

1. Should Kara compete in 4 weeks? What are the reasons for and against her competing?
2. What modifications to her usual training should be made during her pregnancy? What precautions should be taken?
3. How soon after delivery will Kara be able to resume competition?
4. How will Kara be able to combine the responsibilities of motherhood with maintaining her sporting career?

restricted to the first trimester only (and only with physician approval). For reasons of safety for both mother and developing foetus, certain activities are excluded throughout pregnancy including scuba diving, mountain climbing or trekking, novice downhill skiing, ice-skating and horseback riding. A woman should stop participating in these activities as soon as she knows or suspects she is pregnant.

Cancer

Cancer is the first or second leading cause of death in most developed countries, accounting for approximately 25% of all deaths each year in Australia. Cancer is a complex group of diseases, depending on type and location, arising from the progressive and uncontrolled growth of the descendants of a single transformed cell. The contributing factors to cancer are multifaceted, involving genetic influences, environmental exposure (e.g., to radiation or toxic chemicals) and lifestyle (e.g., diet, smoking, physical activity). A tumour may grow slowly, taking years before causing symptoms, or may be aggressive, leading to death within weeks or months of diagnosis. The most common forms are lung, bowel and prostate cancers in men and breast, reproductive system and lung cancers in women. Australia has the highest rate of skin cancer in the world, and its incidence is also increasing.

Epidemiological evidence shows lower rates of some types of cancer in physically active groups. At present, the strongest evidence linking reduced risk of cancer and physical activity is for all-cause (i.e., not delineating different sites) and colon cancers. There is moderately strong evidence that exercise protects against breast cancer in women and prostate cancer in men and limited evidence suggesting a link for ovarian and endometrial cancers in women and lung cancer in men. Physical activity appears to reduce the risk of cancer by about 20 to 50% in a dose-dependent manner (i.e., the more activity, the lower the risk of cancer). Moderate physical activity, as generally recommended for good health, is associated with reduced risk of cancer, although more intense exercise appears to give additional benefits.

Physical Activity and Cancer Patients

Regular physical activity is now recommended as an adjunct therapy for many cancer patients to enhance functional capacity, psychological adjustment and quality of life. With recent advancements in chemotherapy and surgery, many cancer patients are surviving for many years after initial diagnosis and treatment. Although the minimum and optimum types of exercise have not yet been determined, regular moderate activity has been shown to alter a number of important variables in cancer patients. A vast majority of cancer patients undergoing chemotherapy report significant fatigue, and moderate exercise training has been shown to reduce subjective feelings of fatigue in such patients (Dimeo, Fetscher et al. 1997; Dimeo, Tilmann et al. 1997; Mock et al. 1997). Moreover, cancer-related fatigue has been linked to psychological factors such as mood state, anxiety and depression (Dimeo, Fetscher et al. 1997), and these factors appear to be beneficially modified in physically active cancer patients and survivors (Dimeo, Fetscher et al. 1997; Mock et al. 1997).

Moderate exercise counteracts the loss of, and may even increase, functional capacity and $\dot{V}O_2max$ in cancer patients undergoing chemotherapy (Dimeo, Fetscher et al. 1997; Dimeo, Tilmann et al. 1997; Mock et al. 1997). By increasing energy expenditure, regular exercise also appears to counteract the normal gain of body mass and fat associated with breast cancer treatment. This is important because excess body fat is associated with decreased life expectancy of breast cancer patients. In addition, interval exercise training by hospitalised patients undergoing high-dose chemotherapy has been reported to decrease pain, diarrhoea and disturbances of blood cell counts (common complaints during chemotherapy) and lead to shorter stays in hospital compared with patients who did not exercise (Dimeo, Fetscher et al. 1997; Dimeo, Tilmann et al. 1997).

Exercise Capacity in Cancer Patients

Cancer patients undergoing treatment or recovering post-surgery will have low functional capacity and muscle wasting or deconditioning secondary to enforced rest. More than 80% experience fatigue, and many experience nausea as a side effect of treatment. Fitness testing may be inappropriate or of little value for cancer patients during treatment regimes. On the other hand, a cancer patient who has completed treatment and is in remission may be tested as for a healthy adult if desired (and approved by the medical practitioner). A clinical exercise test is essential for any cancer patient over age 65 years or with cardiovascular disease risk factors (refer to chapters 2 and 8). Several issues concerning fitness testing and exercise prescription for the cancer patient must be addressed. For example, some forms of chemotherapy may cause cardiomyopathy, arrhythmia or alterations in the cardiorespiratory responses to exercise. Radiation therapy may cause neuropathy and permanent scarring, which may affect gait, coordination, muscular strength or ROM. Surgery involving amputation or organ removal (e.g., breast, lung) may result in permanent disability specific to that site (e.g., loss of underlying muscle after mastectomy, reduced lung capacity after removal of a lung). Anaemia, a common side effect of chemotherapy, reduces aerobic exercise capacity and causes early fatigue during exercise.

Exercise Prescription for Cancer Patients

The minimum and optimum levels of exercise for cancer patients are not known at present, primarily because this is a new area of study. The highly variable nature of the disease, individual responses to cancer and treatment, and difficulty recruiting sufficient subject numbers to achieve good statistical power make it difficult to perform empirical research. Improvements in fatigue, physical work capacity, body fat and psychological variables have generally occurred in studies using moderate exercise. In the absence of any clear guidelines, most investigators err on the side of caution when prescribing exercise for cancer patients. Recent research shows that exercise such as 30 min of walking three to five times per week is well tolerated and leads to improvements. However, this is achieved only after a gradual progression starting with shorter intervals (e.g., 5×3 min per day in the 1st week, 3×10 min per day in the 4th week, and so on). This level of exercise is consistent with recommendations for physical activity for healthy adults, and at present, there is little empirical evidence to warrant more intense aerobic exercise for these patients. There are many possibilities for future research regarding the inclusion of resistance exercise for non-athlete cancer patients and more intense exercise for the cancer patient wishing to participate in sport.

Although moderate exercise may be beneficial for most cancer patients and has few adverse side effects, there are, naturally, some situations in which exercise is inappropriate. Contraindications to exercise for cancer patients are summarised in table 9.6. Exercise is not recommended if there is evidence of infection, fever above 37.5°C, low platelet count, abnormalities of cardiac function (e.g., atrial fibrillation) or severe fatigue, weakness or nausea. Because of risk of cardiac arrhythmia, exercise is generally not recommended for 24 h before and after chemotherapy. In some cases, the cancer may have spread (metastasised) to the bone, thus weakening the bone tissues; these patients must avoid heavy weightlifting, high-impact activities and stretching involving spinal compression.

Case Study 9.5

Sally is 44 years old. She was diagnosed with breast cancer 10 months ago and had a mastectomy of her right breast 9 months ago. Having recently completed chemotherapy and radiation therapy, she has experienced considerable weight gain (8 kg). She is 165 cm tall, now weighs 72 kg, and wishes to lose as much of the 8 kg as possible. Sally played competitive netball for 30 years, and she would like to eventually return to her team. Recognising that her current upper body strength, range of motion and overall fitness are insufficient to resume competitive netball, she asks you for a training program to enable her to return to her team within the next 5 months. Sally has access to a fitness centre at work and is prepared to exercise up to 5 days per week to achieve her goal of returning to the team.

Key Issues

1. What are Sally's main goals for her program? How achievable are these in 5 months?

2. Why did she gain weight during the treatment?

3. How will you balance the need to lose weight with the goal of improving range of motion, muscular strength and cardiovascular fitness in her program?

4. Are there any precautions needed in prescribing exercise for Sally?

TABLE 9.6—Contraindications to Exercise or Fitness Testing in Cancer Patients

Contraindication	Reason
Unusual fatigue or shortness of breath	Discomfort during exercise
Acute nausea during exercise	Fatigue and dyspnoea may be exacerbated
Vomiting or diarrhoea within the previous 24 h	Discomfort Exercise may cause further dehydration Chance of hypoglycaemia
Intravenous chemotherapy within the previous or next 24 h	Risk of arrhythmia
Infection or fever	Immune system may be suppressed Exercise can increase core temperature
Low blood cell counts: platelets $<50 \times 10^9 \cdot L^{-1}$ leukocytes $<3 \times 10^9 \cdot L^{-1}$ haemoglobin $<12 \ g \cdot dL^{-1}$	Compromised immune function or clotting

Compiled from G. Selby, 1997, Cancer. In *ACSM's exercise management for persons with chronic diseases and disabilities*. (Champaign, IL: Human Kinetics), 121-124; J.E. Hicks, 1990, Exercise for cancer patients. In J.V. Basmajian and S.L. Wolf (eds.), *Therapeutic exercise*. (Baltimore: Williams & Wilkins), 351-367; M.L. Winningham, M.G. MacVicar, and C.A. Burke, 1986, "Exercise for cancer patients: guidelines and precautions," *The Physician and Sportsmedicine* 14: 125-134.

In addition to general recommendations for improving physical work capacity, there are special concerns for cancer patients recovering from surgery. The exercise prescription must be individualised to address specific needs of surgical patients and may also need to incorporate guidelines for other conditions. For example, a radical mastectomy may involve loss of muscle in the chest and shoulder, and if lymph nodes have been removed, there may also be adhesions and swelling (lymphoedema). These will result in loss of range of motion and muscular strength in the affected shoulder and arm. Specific exercises to increase muscular strength and joint range of motion are essential for regaining normal function at the onset of any exercise program. To give another example, lung cancer surgery involves removal of part of the lung or possibly the entire organ, which may adversely alter the cardiorespiratory response to exercise (e.g., decreased tidal volume). Recent research suggests that the degree of impairment of functional capacity and $\dot{V}O_2$max is related to the amount of lung removed (Nezu et al. 1998) and exercise capacity may be limited by dyspnoea. In this case, exercise prescription following guidelines for the COPD patient (refer to chapter 8) using either the RPE or dyspnoea scales would be recommended.

Summary

Regular physical activity is recommended for individuals of all ages. The basic principles of exercise prescription apply, with modifications to accommodate goals, needs, interests, physical capacity, health concerns and factors influencing adherence. Children should not be treated as miniature adults when prescribing exercise. The physical limitations on exercise capacity, the role of physical activity and sport in physical and social development, the interests of children and the need to develop lifelong skills are important considerations for physical activity for youth. Children with chronic disease or impairment should also be encouraged to become physically active through appropriate exercise prescription. The elderly make up an increasing proportion of the population, and society can derive many social and economic benefits by promoting physical activity among the elderly. The declining functional capacity and skeletal muscle mass associated with aging may require adaptation of the general guidelines for physical activity. Regular physical activity helps attenuate loss of functional capacity, aerobic power, muscular strength and lean body mass and assists in maintaining glucose tolerance, ADLs and quality of life. Even the very old or frail elderly can benefit from appropriate physical activity.

Pregnancy requires alteration of the usual physical activity program. Women with uncomplicated pregnancies may continue to participate, and they usually self-select more moderate exercise intensity and duration as pregnancy progresses. Moderate exercise is not associated with adverse outcomes, may enhance maternal well-being and prevent excessive weight gain during pregnancy, and increases the likelihood the woman will continue to be active after delivery. Pregnant women are advised to avoid contact or collision sports and other potentially dangerous activities. Regular moderate physical activity is also associated with beneficial effects in cancer patients, including less muscle wasting and weakness, reduced fatigue and nausea, enhanced functional capacity, feelings of well-being and prevention of weight gain (in breast cancer patients).

Selected Glossary Terms

anaerobic capacity—Average work output over 30 to 60 s in an all-out exercise test, often using cycle ergometry.

anaerobic glycolysis—The capacity of muscle cells to produce energy (ATP) and the body to perform exercise using the anaerobic glycolytic metabolic pathway.

anaerobic power (or peak power)—The highest power output generated during the first 3 to 5 s of an all-out exercise test, often using cycle ergometry.

dynamic balance—Maintaining postural control during movement, as in reaching while standing or regaining balance after a sudden disturbance.

juvenile rheumatoid arthritis (JRA)—An autoimmune disorder in which substances produced by the body's immune system accumulate within the joints, causing inflammation and pain.

muscle hypertrophy—Growth of a muscle or muscle group, generally as a result of resistance training; individual muscle fibres increase in diameter by adding new contractile and connective tissue proteins.

muscular dystrophy (MD)—An inherited disease mostly in males causing progressive deterioration of muscle cells, muscle wasting, weakness and loss of muscle function.

overuse injuries—Exercise-induced repetitive microtrauma causing an inflammatory response, and possibly chronic inflammation, leading to structural changes in tissues such as bone, tendons, ligaments or joints.

static balance—Control of postural sway during standing; is important for preventing falls especially in the elderly.

Student Activities and Study Questions

1. Describe the changes in body size, composition and neural development that occur with growth and development during childhood and adolescence. How would these changes influence endurance exercise capacity? Anaerobic exercise capacity? Muscular strength and power? How would you incorporate this information into training programs for children in various sports—swimming, rowing, track and field, soccer?

2. Attend and observe at least one (more, if possible) sport training session for children in various age groups (from 6 to 16 years). Note any differences in the training of children of different ages (e.g., duration, intensity, skill work). What reasons are there for such differences?

3. Attend and observe at least one (more, if possible) physical activity program for elderly people in your city/region. What is the main focus of these programs? Try to talk with the instructor/leader and some participants. Find out what motivates them to lead or attend these programs. What benefits do they see happening as a result of the program?

4. Find and read some recent research studies on exercise capacity and training in the elderly (try to focus on endurance exercise, anaerobic capacity or muscular strength). What factors seem to limit the ability of older people to increase exercise capacity? Can older people train as hard as younger people (not elite athletes but average people)?

5. Attend and observe an exercise class/program for pregnant women or cancer patients. Alternatively, see if you can attend a public lecture on either of these topics. What types of physical activity are advocated? What are the scientific rationales behind these recommendations? Discuss with a participant in one of these programs (a pregnant woman or a cancer patient) his or her particular physical activity program. What are the perceived benefits of the program? What motivates him or her to be physically active?

CHAPTER 10

Exercise Prescription for People With Musculoskeletal, Neurological and Neuromuscular Impairment

There are myriad diseases or conditions affecting the nervous, muscular or skeletal systems that may influence the capacity for movement, physical activity and exercise. These diseases or conditions may be congenital (e.g., muscular dystrophy) or acquired at or soon after birth (e.g., cerebral palsy), while others may occur later in life as a result of injury or trauma (e.g., osteoarthritis, acquired brain injury), disease processes (e.g., stroke), reasons unknown (e.g., multiple sclerosis, chronic fatigue syndrome) or aging (e.g., osteoporosis). Some of these diseases or conditions may be quite mild and intermittent (e.g., mild forms of arthritis), others may be transitory (e.g., low back pain, chronic fatigue syndrome), while still others are debilitating and possibly life threatening (e.g., stroke, acquired brain injury). Impairment of physical capacity may affect the ability to lead an independent lifestyle, may reduce quality of life and may also increase the risk of diseases associated with physical inactivity.

Recent national initiatives to promote physical activity, such as Active Australia, encourage a physically active lifestyle for all people, including those with disability or impairment. Exercise managers are often employed in clinical settings to apply and extend the basic principles of exercise prescription toward rehabilitation of motor function and the capacity for physical activity in those with musculoskeletal and neuromuscular impairment. This chapter addresses basic information about physical activity prescription for those with more common musculoskeletal and neuromuscular disorders that the exercise manager may encounter in professional practice.

Musculoskeletal Disorders

The term *musculoskeletal disorder* includes conditions and diseases, such as arthritis, osteoporosis and low back pain, that involve the major muscle groups or the skeletal system. Musculoskeletal disorders are a major source of chronic pain and among the most common complaints requiring medical attention. Osteoarthritis, the most common form of arthritis, is the 10th leading cause of disability-adjusted life years (DALYs;

described in chapter 2). Low back pain is estimated to affect up to 80% of the population at some point. Osteoporosis, which causes loss of bone integrity, is increasing in prevalence with the lengthening of the average lifespan. Besides the direct costs of medical care and medication for these disorders, there are significant social and other costs associated with reduced quality of life and employment opportunities and resultant workers' compensation, loss of wages and decreased work productivity.

Regular physical activity may be useful for both primary and secondary prevention of musculoskeletal disorders. For many individuals with these conditions, a vicious cycle of physical inactivity in reaction to chronic pain leads to further impairment and loss of physical function. The key is to develop appropriate exercise prescriptions that accommodate the particular impairment and avoid pain while at the same time improve physical function. Table 10.1 gives a brief summary of general concerns and guidelines for fitness testing and exercise prescription for musculoskeletal disorders.

Low Back Pain

Although not a life-threatening disorder, low back pain (LBP) is a major health concern because of its high prevalence, costs and impact on quality of life. About 80% of Australians will experience LBP at some point in their lives. Because of the pain associated with untreated LBP, individuals may become physically inactive, leading to loss of functional capacity and increased risk of major diseases such as cardiovascular disease or osteoporosis. The social and psychological costs of living with constant pain cannot be quantified but should not be overlooked.

Regular physical activity and maintaining physical fitness may protect against LBP. There is good evidence that the risk of low back injury increases in physically inactive or unfit individuals, and aerobic exercise training hastens recovery after an incident of LBP. Obesity, especially abdominal obesity, contributes to LBP by shifting the centre of gravity and increasing stress on the spine; physical activity helps prevent this situation by regulating body mass.

TABLE 10.1—Summary of Assessment Recommendations for Musculoskeletal Disorders

Disease or condition	Exercise/fitness test recommended	Other useful tests or information	Contraindications or precautions to consider for assessment
Low back pain	Weight supported (e.g., cycling) Avoid modes that stress the spine (e.g., rowing, stepping, running)	Muscular strength, flexibility, joint ROM (especially hips, back, hamstrings) Muscular endurance more important than strength	Avoid assessment until 4 wk after pain onset No maximum lifts if pain present Avoid flexion or hyperextension of spine
Arthritis	Standard if possible May need to change mode or protocol depending on joints affected	Muscular strength, flexibility, joint ROM, agility	Warm-up required Avoid during active disease/ inflammation
Osteoporosis	Body weight supported (e.g., cycle ergometry)	Muscular strength, gait, balance	Avoid in frail elderly Avoid compression, flexion or hyperextension of spine Use 3 RM not 1 RM to assess strength

Assuming the client has been pre-screened and cleared for testing by a medical practitioner, if needed, according to the 2000 ACSM guidelines (see chapter 5).

Abbreviations: ROM = range of motion; RM = repetition maximum.

Although exercise is now recommended for most individuals with LBP, prescription of inappropriate exercises or improper performance of suitable exercises may cause or exacerbate back injuries (recently reviewed by McGill 2001). Strengthening the spine stabilisers seems to provide some protection against development of LBP.

LBP may result from a single traumatic event such as an automobile accident or a collision in sport or, more commonly, as the accumulation of repeated minor trauma or excessive loading. Injury may involve disc **herniation** or **prolapse** caused by repetitive combined compression, flexion and torsion of the spine, as in repeated lifting while bending or twisting. Bony failure or injury to ligaments or tendons may result from acute trauma (e.g., auto accident), collision (e.g., sport injury) or a fall involving landing on the buttocks. During lifting, ligaments rarely tear as a result of a single event; rather, a ligament tears during a lift usually because it has been weakened or damaged by a prior traumatic event. Thus, effective rehabilitation of acute injuries to the back is essential for preventing further injury and disability.

Although not all back injuries can be prevented, the likelihood can be lessened by maintaining a neutral spine position during lifting (i.e., avoiding bending or twisting); twisting while lifting imposes a far greater compression on the spine than development of an equal force in simple flexion/extension (McGill 2001). Regular participation in physical activity that enhances cardiovascular and muscular endurance, especially of the trunk and abdominal musculature, also seems to lessen the risk of low back injury.

Exercise Capacity and LBP

Exercise capacity will not be directly altered by LBP, but it may be impossible to accurately assess cardiovascular fitness if exercise tolerance is limited by pain. Thus, diagnostic exercise testing may not provide useful information since the patient may stop exercise because of pain well before the appearance of symptoms or signs of cardiovascular disease (e.g., ECG irregularities). It is recommended that a person experiencing LBP not be tested for at least 4 weeks after the onset of pain. The choice of cardiovascular fitness test may be dictated by the location and severity of pain, and tests involving treadmill walking or stationary cycling are preferable to those requiring running or other forms of exercise that stress the spine (e.g., stepping, rowing). An extensive muscular warm-up before testing is recommended. Assessment should include measures of

joint range of motion (ROM) and muscular strength, endurance and flexibility, provided this can be accomplished without pain. Because lack of flexibility in the hips, back and hamstring muscle groups contributes to LBP, assessment should include ROM of these areas. Maximal strength testing is contraindicated during the acute phase after an injury and may be contraindicated at any time if pain occurs.

Exercise Prescription for LBP

The aim of an exercise program should be to promote tissue regeneration and to strengthen supporting tissues while avoiding excessive loading and further damage to the lower back. The exercise prescription should include programs for gaining and maintaining general fitness, as well as specific exercises aimed at strengthening the back and other supporting tissues. These must be accomplished while minimising spine loading, and emphasis should be on maintaining neutral lordosis, or the natural back curve (i.e., avoiding arching the back), throughout all forms of activity. Because LBP is highly variable between people, the exercise prescription must be individualised, taking into account current fitness level, exercise history, site and severity of injury, and goals of the client. Some general guidelines for exercise for people with LBP are given in figure 10.1.

There are three main phases of an exercise program for LBP. The first phase, which can begin almost immediately, focuses on motor control and muscle coordination exercises that train the spine stabilisers to provide support for the back without stress. Calisthenics and other postural exercises (e.g., with a Swiss Ball) may be performed daily. A recently developed concept is that of **core stability**—performing exercises specifically to improve muscular endurance of the trunk and abdominal musculature, which is integral to spine stability. The second phase, which can begin within the first 2 weeks after onset of pain, aims to build cardiovascular endurance through low-impact or weight-supported moderate-intensity aerobic exercise. Suitable exercises include walking, water-based activities (e.g., swimming, aquaerobics, water walking) and stationary cycling. The program should begin at low intensity and progress gradually. Daily exercises of the spine stabilisers should be continued.

The third phase includes exercises for muscular strength, endurance and flexibility but should not begin until at least 2 weeks after the onset of pain. Exercises to enhance muscle flexibility and joint

---

EXERCISE MODE

▶ Aerobic fitness lessens risk of LBP and enhances recovery after injury.

▶ A variety of abdominal exercises is suggested.

▶ Muscular warm-up before and cool-down after exercise is essential.

EXERCISE FREQUENCY AND INTENSITY

▶ Daily exercise of spine stabilisers, muscle flexibility and joint ROM is recommended.

▶ Muscular endurance is more important than muscular strength.

▶ Individualise program by nature of injury, fitness level, exercise history and goals.

▶ Start at low intensity and progress gradually.

PRECAUTIONS

▶ Emphasis should be placed on developing or regaining functional capacity and on injury prevention.

▶ Avoid compression (e.g., hyperextension, free weights).

▶ Avoid twisting in flexed or extended positions.

▶ Maintain neutral lordosis (natural curve of spine) during all exercises.

▶ Stop exercise if pain is present.

▶ Consult a medical practitioner or physiotherapist for persistent pain.

FIGURE 10.1   General recommendations for exercise for low back pain.

ROM should focus on maintaining trunk stabilisation (to protect the spine from excessive loading) while improving hip and knee mobility (since these may contribute to LBP). Stretching exercises that do not load the spine (e.g., the "cat-camel" stretch, figure 10.2a, or seated stretch, figure 10.2b) or that are performed lying down (see figure 10.3) are recommended. Muscular endurance is more important than pure strength for rehabilitation and prevention of LBP. Both dynamic and isometric muscular endurance exercises are recommended, for example, higher repetitions at lower resistance such as ≥10 RM. Use of free weights such as barbells, especially lifts requiring twisting or hyperextension of the back, should be discouraged for most individuals except when required by particular athletes (e.g., gymnasts, divers). In addition, abdominal strength is important for stabilisation of the lower back. A variety of abdominal exercises should be prescribed because no single exercise works all abdominal muscles. Variations of abdominal curl-ups are preferable to sit-ups since they induce less stress on the spine (McGill 2001).

Specific exercises of the spine stabilisers to enhance muscle flexibility and joint ROM are most effective if performed daily. Exercises to improve cardiovascular and muscular endurance may be performed less frequently, as recommended for general health (e.g., ≥3 days per week for cardiovascular and ≥2 days per week for muscular conditioning).

Exercise by itself may not be effective for alleviating chronic LBP. Other treatments may include bed rest (although this should be minimal to avoid detraining effects), medication (e.g., anti-inflammatory drugs or pain killers), massage, manipulation, weight loss, postural retraining and surgery.

Arthritis

The term *arthritis* represents a constellation of over 100 diseases with differing aetiologies but all characterised by inflammation of the joints. The two most prevalent forms are **osteoarthritis (OA)** and **rheumatoid arthritis (RA);** OA is the more common form. The prevalence of arthritis increases with age, affecting 12% of the Australian population over-

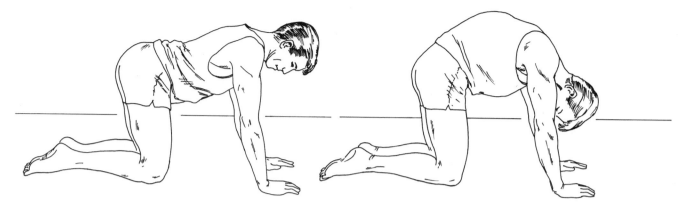

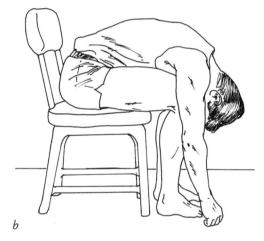

FIGURE 10.2 *(a)* "Cat-camel" stretch for the lower back and *(b)* seated stretch for the lower back.

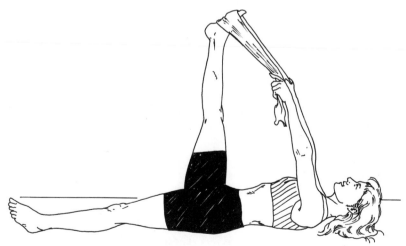

FIGURE 10.3 Hamstring and lower back muscle stretch.

all and most people at some point in their lives. Arthritis is the major form of musculoskeletal disease and the second most common reason for visiting the doctor in Australia; it is estimated to cost the Australian community $4.5 billion each year in medical, rehabilitation and disability costs. Moreover, an inactive lifestyle often imposed by joint pain increases the risk of other diseases such as cardiovascular disease, type 2 diabetes and osteoporosis.

OA is characterised by joint inflammation that is secondary to mechanical changes, leading to structural changes in the joint and degradation of articular cartilage and underlying bone; it often results from trauma (e.g., joint injury) or as a consequence of excessive load bearing (e.g., in obesity). OA presents as joint pain, most frequently in the hip and knee, and may occur unilaterally (only one joint) or bilaterally (both joints simultaneously). There has been much debate over the role of physical activity in causing this form of arthritis. It is now believed that the prevalence of OA is increased in athletes only when associated with joint injury/stress and that in the absence of joint injury, physical activity and sport do not increase the risk of its development. Non-steroidal anti-inflammatory drugs (NSAIDs) are often used to provide pain relief and reduce inflammation of OA.

RA is an autoimmune disorder in which substances produced by the body's immune system accumulate within the joints, causing chronic inflammation of the synovial lining and tendons; it occurs symmetrically (i.e., both sides) and in several joints simultaneously, especially in the hands and feet. About 75% of those with RA are women. RA generally has an earlier onset than OA and develops mainly between the ages of 20 and 40, although there is a juvenile form that appears earlier (discussed in chapter 9). This form of arthritis is characterised by alternating periods of active disease (flare-ups) and remission; flare-ups may last several weeks. RA is classified into four categories according to severity of symptoms. Symptoms include early morning joint stiffness, joint pain and swelling, low-grade fever, fatigue and possibly weight loss. NSAIDs may provide pain relief, but antirheumatic drugs are more effective because they slow the progress of disease.

Exercise Capacity and Arthritis

Arthritis patients often avoid exercise for perhaps years because of joint pain and stiffness. As a result, they often have low functional capacity and muscular strength and may be overweight or obese (OA,

mainly). Poor range of motion and pain within certain joints may preclude the use of some fitness testing modalities (e.g., treadmill for those with lower limb involvement). Thus, assessment of cardiovascular fitness may not be possible or alternative testing modes (e.g., arm ergometry; refer to chapter 6) may be needed for some individuals with arthritis. Careful pre-program screening (and possible referral for a medical examination and exercise stress test; refer to chapter 5) is essential, however, because a history of inactivity and low functional capacity along with the older age of patients with OA may predispose them to cardiovascular or metabolic diseases. Assessing flexibility, joint range of motion and muscular strength of affected and unaffected joints can yield important information for exercise prescription. Any fitness/exercise testing requires extensive warm-up to protect the muscles and joints from injury and to ensure a good effort by the client.

Exercise Prescription for Arthritis

Regular exercise is now advocated for the treatment of arthritis, provided that the program maintains a careful balance between rest and exercise, protection and activity of joints, and aerobic and muscular conditioning. Since RA, and to a lesser extent OA, involves alternating periods of active inflammation and remission, the program must be adaptable to allow rest, reduced levels of activity or change of exercise mode when required. For example, walking may be the preferred exercise mode during remission, but during active disease affecting the hips or knees, the client may find aquatic or upper body exercise more comfortable.

In addition to the usual goals of physical activity (e.g., prevention of cardiovascular or metabolic diseases, enhancement of quality of life), programs should aim to

▶ increase or maintain joint range of motion and stability,

▶ improve muscular strength and endurance,

▶ enhance endurance exercise capacity,

▶ induce body weight loss or maintain optimum body mass, and

▶ decrease joint pain.

Consequently, the exercise program should focus on three main areas: joint mobility (e.g., stretching muscles around joints, especially those affected by disease), muscular strength (e.g., isometric or dynamic exercise, with or without weights) and aerobic conditioning (e.g., walking, swimming, cycling). To avoid stress on the joints, weight-supported or low-impact activities such as swimming, cycling, walking and water-based or low-impact aerobics are preferable, especially when lower limb joints are affected by disease. Specific guidelines for exercise prescription are given in figure 10.4. All exercise sessions should include a warm-up and should ensure that exercise mode and intensity are well within the client's exercise capacity and limits of pain. To prevent injury and increase joint ROM and muscle flexibility, the warm-up should include both cardiovascular and muscular components; a warm-up performed in warm water (28° C) may be especially effective. Since arthritis is often accompanied by early morning stiffness, exercise should be scheduled for a later time of day when stiffness and pain are less likely to limit movement and medication is most effective.

Resistance training can be an important part of an exercise program for both OA and RA because increased muscular mass and strength attenuate shock around the affected joints, especially those involved in weight bearing (e.g., hips, knees). Recent research shows that in well-controlled RA, patients are capable of relatively high-intensity muscular strength training (e.g., 6-8 repetitions at 80% of 1 RM) without exacerbation of disease and often with reductions in self-reported joint pain (Rall, Roubenoff, et al. 1996; van den Ende et al. 1998). Such training was shown to improve aerobic capacity, muscular strength and joint mobility more than standard ROM exercises. In RA, whole body protein breakdown may increase in the inactive individual, which may be reflected in loss of body mass and especially muscle mass during active disease. Recent research suggests, however, that this may be prevented by muscular strength training (Rall, Rosen, et al. 1996). It is important to note that in these studies, patients were closely supervised and performed resistance exercise only after 10 min of warm-up exercises in a heated pool.

EXERCISE MODE

▶ Include a variety of activities to increase joint mobility, muscular strength and cardiovascular fitness.

▶ Use weight-supported or low-impact exercise such as cycling, swimming or aquatic activities whenever possible to reduce stress on the joints.

▶ Muscular strengthening exercises using weights should at first be supervised for proper form and technique.

▶ Use isometric and dynamic resistance exercise to strengthen muscles around affected joints.

EXERCISE FREQUENCY AND INTENSITY

▶ Maintain a regular program, daily if possible but at least three to four times per week.

▶ Exercise when stiffness, pain and fatigue are lowest and when medications are most effective.

▶ Use appropriate exercise intensity to provide health benefits without stressing affected joints.

PRECAUTIONS

▶ Always warm up before exercise with a warm bath/shower or light activity that increases temperature in the muscles.

▶ Move joints smoothly and slowly, especially when performing stretching and strengthening exercises.

▶ Modify or delete an activity or movement if pain or swelling is present in a particular joint.

▶ Stop exercise if severe pain is present.

▶ Supportive footwear is important for weight-bearing activities.

FIGURE 10.4   Guidelines for exercise for the client with arthritis.

Case Study 10.1

Rebecca is 49 years old and works full time as a researcher. She was a nationally ranked gymnast in her youth and has remained active through aerobics, jogging and triathlon training. Over the past several years, however, she has been forced to gradually reduce her physical activity level because of rheumatoid arthritis in her knees, ankles and occasionally hips. She feels she has reached a point where her fitness program seems inadequate to maintain her fitness during flare-ups. Flare-ups occur about every 3 to 4 months and usually last 1 to 2 weeks each time.

She seeks your advice on resuming a more active lifestyle. Write a long-term adaptable exercise program that can be used during both flare-ups and remissions to help Rebecca regain and maintain her fitness.

Key Issues

1. Can Rebecca remain physically active despite the arthritis? What are the potential benefits and risks of exercise for her?

2. What modes of exercise are best suited to her condition?

3. What specific aspects of physical fitness need to be addressed in the exercise prescription? How will these be incorporated into the program?

4. How will the program accommodate exercise during flare-ups?

Osteoporosis

Osteoporosis is a disorder of the skeleton characterised by low bone mass (or **bone mineral density**) and structural deterioration of bone, causing bone fragility and increased risk of fracture. The prevalence of osteoporosis increases with age and, given the rising average life expectancy in developed countries such as Australia, is expected to continue increasing over the next 20 to 30 years. While a vast majority (about 80%) of those with osteoporosis are women, there is now an increasing prevalence in men as their life expectancy rises. Osteoporotic fractures occur more frequently in women than do most major life-threatening disorders such as myocardial infarction, stroke or cancer. Although a bone fracture may appear insignificant for a younger individual, statistics on the long-term deleterious effects of bone fractures in the elderly are staggering: Half of all older people who suffer hip fractures will be disabled, nearly 20% of women with hip fractures will require long-term nursing home care and 20% of hip fracture victims die within 1 year of the fracture. The 1992 estimated direct cost of osteoporotic fractures in Australia was $780 million.

The causes of osteoporosis are multifactorial, reflecting both genetics and lifestyle. Genetic factors include race/ethnicity (higher incidence in Caucasians of European descent), family history, thin build and early menopause or hormonal deficiency.

Lifestyle factors include physical inactivity, diet (low calcium intake, anorexia), alcoholism, smoking and exercise-associated amenorrhoea. Other diseases (e.g., endocrine disorders, cancer) or drugs (e.g., corticosteroids) may also induce secondary osteoporosis by their negative effects on bone deposition. Bone is a metabolically active tissue, constantly undergoing remodelling in which osteoclastic bone resorption is balanced by osteoblastic bone formation. However, during aging, the rate of bone resorption exceeds that of formation, leading to net loss of bone mineral density and strength. Postmenopausal women are most affected because of declining levels of oestrogen, which stimulates bone formation; endocrine disorders (e.g., amenorrhoea) or other factors (e.g., smoking) that lower oestrogen levels may also cause net bone loss at younger ages.

In addition to adequate dietary intake of calcium and other nutrients (and avoidance of smoking), recent evidence strongly suggests that physical activity begun early in and continued throughout life is important for preventing osteoporosis. Peak bone mass is achieved early in life (by early 20s in both sexes) and begins to decline after about age 30 to 35 years. It is thought that the risk of fracture increases as bone density falls below a critical threshold. The "calcium bank" analogy suggests that a higher bone density achieved in early adulthood (higher bank balance) guards against bone density declining below this critical threshold because of resorption (withdrawals) later in life (Bailey, Faulkner and McKay 1996). Thus, regular physical activity should be encouraged among children and adolescents to maximise peak bone mass (deposits), and activity should be continued throughout adulthood and old age to help maintain bone density (bank balance). A healthy diet, also essential for achieving and maintaining bone density, should include adequate protein, total energy and calcium, with moderate fat levels.

There is compelling evidence that bone mass is influenced by physical activity: Bone mass decreases during immobilisation (e.g., paraplegia, limb casting) or in the absence of load-bearing activity (e.g., spaceflight, bed rest). Asymmetries in bone mass between limbs have been demonstrated in athletes from sports requiring unilateral movement (e.g., tennis) or in children with unilateral conditions or diseases (e.g., fracture in one leg or Legg-Calvé-Perthes disease). Cross-sectional studies show higher bone mineral density in athletes involved in load-bearing or high-impact sports (e.g., gymnastics, running, weightlifting); the effects are most pronounced at the load-bearing sites. High-impact activity (e.g., gymnastics, ballet) even appears to somewhat counteract the harmful effect of menstrual disorders, characterised by low oestrogen levels, on bone density of load-bearing sites.

While physical activity is important for achieving peak bone mass in childhood to early adulthood, exercise has a minimal effect on bone mass later in life. Rather, exercise benefits later in life relate more to maintaining or slowing the decline in bone mass and preventing falls. Studies typically show less than 1% increase in bone mass after 6 to 12 months exercise training such as running or weightlifting. Although a small increase, its beneficial effects are magnified when contrasted with the typical *loss* of bone mass of approximately 1 to 2% over the same period in non-exercising women (Taafe and Marcus 2000). It is generally accepted that hormone replacement therapy (HRT, i.e., replacing oestrogen and progesterone in postmenopausal women or those whose ovaries have been removed) provides a greater stimulus (around 2%) to bone deposition in that same time frame. More important, HRT and exercise are synergistic; that is, the combination of HRT and exercise causes additive increases in bone mass (up to 4% over 12 months). Thus, exercise seems most effective for preventing osteoporosis when combined with HRT. (There are, however, side effects and possible long-term consequences of HRT, and the physician's decision to prescribe HRT is

made after balancing the potential benefits and risks for each woman.)

The importance of physical activity for preventing other adverse outcomes of declining bone mass in older individuals (e.g., poor posture due to structural changes in the vertebrae causing pain when sitting or moving, and compromised breathing) is often overlooked. Also, although it does not necessarily influence bone mass, an appropriate program to increase muscular strength and enhance coordination and balance may have significant value by preventing falls that could cause fractures in the elderly (Taafe et al. 1999).

Exercise Capacity and Osteoporosis

Osteoporosis by itself does not limit exercise capacity. However, since low bone density and osteoporosis occur most commonly in elderly inactive women, low functional capacity may be expected. Pre-program screening for cardiovascular and metabolic diseases is essential, and fitness testing should follow guidelines for older individuals as discussed in chapter 9. Testing for balance and gait (refer to chapter 9) may also be warranted. Maximal fitness testing using the treadmill may be contraindicated to avoid injuries from falls; once the client has been cleared by medical examination, submaximal testing using a cycle or arm ergometer may be preferable. In those with advanced osteoporosis, kyphosis (curvature of the spine) may limit pulmonary function and thus exercise tolerance; seated exercise using a cycle ergometer may be necessary. Maximal strength testing (i.e., 1 RM) may be contraindicated because of the higher risk of injury and prevalence of hypertension among older women. Use of 3 RM may be advisable since it will require a lower resistance (refer to chapter 6). Forward flexion and hyperextension of the spine should also be avoided to prevent excessive compression of possibly weakened vertebrae.

Exercise Prescription for Osteoporosis

Now that physical activity has been widely accepted as an important determinant of bone mineral density, the best prevention of osteoporosis in future generations lies in convincing people at an early age to adopt a lifetime of physical activity. Bailey, Faulkner and McKay (1996) made several suggestions for optimising bone mineral acquisition during growth and development, with the underlying assumption that increased peak bone mineral density early in life will help guard against pathologically low levels in old age. Because the ability of bone to adapt to mechanical loading is greatest in the growing skeleton, there should be an early commitment to a lifetime of physical activity begun in childhood and continued throughout life. Vigorous daily activity of shorter duration and from a variety of sports/activities will ensure beneficial effects on bones throughout the body.

Preferred activities to maximise bone density in children and adolescents are those that enhance bone acquisition: weight-bearing movements, exercises requiring the whole body or large muscle groups, and exercises that increase muscular strength. Most forms of youth sport or normal physical activity would satisfy these recommendations, and the important point is that children develop a lifelong habit of varied and regular physical activity. Inactivity and immobilisation should be avoided as much as possible, and when inactivity is necessary (e.g., because of injury), some form of brief weight-bearing exercise should still be performed daily. In addition, development of healthy bones is further enhanced by a well-balanced diet and avoidance of smoking and disordered eating patterns.

Once achieved, peak bone mass is less influenced by physical activity; that is, physical activity is less effective at increasing bone mass in adulthood. Both load-bearing and resistance exercises are important in older age groups because maintenance of bone integrity is specific to the area loaded. Thus, load-bearing activities such as jogging or aerobics help maintain (or slightly increase) bone density in the ankle, leg and hip, whereas upper body resistance exercise (weight training) acts on bone density in the spine, shoulder and upper limbs. Exercises to improve dynamic balance and coordination, in addition to muscular strength, reduce the risk of falling and thus the risk of fracture in older individuals (Taafe et al. 1999).

An effective exercise program includes both aerobic (cardiovascular) and muscular strength conditioning that incorporates load-bearing activity without excessively stressing the musculoskeletal system. The program should also include flexibility, agility, coordination and balance exercises and simple recreational activities to minimise the risk of falling. Walking, jogging, exercise machines (e.g., stair climbers), circuit resistance training, aerobic dance or exercise to music, and calisthenics are all appropriate. Although swimming, other water-based activities and weight-supported activities such as cycling may increase cardiovascular fitness and muscular strength (and may be preferred in some conditions, such as arthritis), they are not generally associated with increased bone mass and should be supplemented with weight-bearing activity whenever pos-

sible. Stretching exercises should be performed with caution by clients with known low bone density or by those on long-term medication that influences bone density (e.g., corticosteroids). It is especially important that these individuals avoid excessive loading or compression of the spine (e.g., avoid hyperextension or hyperflexion of the spine, avoid lifting free weights in a standing position).

Neurological and Neuromuscular Disorders

Myriad neurological and neuromuscular disorders affect movement, exercise capacity and the ability to maintain a physically active lifestyle. Because many of these conditions are genetic, are caused by trauma or have unknown causes, physical activity cannot be considered a means of primary prevention. However, physical activity has tremendous potential benefits for rehabilitation by enhancing quality of life, self-efficacy and sense of well-being, and the ability to lead a more independent lifestyle. In addition, physical inactivity often imposed by disease or impairment increases the risk of other conditions (e.g., CVD, osteoporosis), with further adverse consequences for health. It is beyond the scope of a single chapter to discuss all of the neurological and neuromuscular disorders. To illustrate the basic principles for prescribing exercise for individuals with neurological/neuromuscular impairment, this section focuses on representative disorders that occur at various stages in the lifespan (e.g., cerebral palsy at birth, spinal cord or acquired brain injury at any time, multiple sclerosis in early to midadulthood and Parkinson's disease in old age).

Table 10.2 provides a brief summary of exercise recommendations for the neurological and neuromuscular disorders discussed in the following sections.

Cerebral Palsy

Cerebral palsy (CP) is a non-progressive neurological disorder of movement or posture caused by lesions in the upper motor neurons of the brain occurring before, at or soon after birth. CP may arise during the first or second trimester of foetal development because of disturbances to normal development of the motor regions of the brain, or it may develop during or after birth as a result of brain injury secondary to factors such as trauma, lack of oxygen or infection. Since the upper motor neurons

TABLE 10.2—Summary of Fitness Assessment Recommendations for Neurological and Neuromuscular Disorders

Disease or condition	Exercise/fitness test recommended	Other useful tests or information	Contraindications or precautions to consider for assessment
Cerebral palsy	Cycle ergometry (arms, legs, both) or wheelchair on treadmill	Joint ROM, muscle flexibility, gait analysis, balance	May need to strap hands or feet to pedals Spasticity may not permit safe assessment of muscular strength
Spinal cord injury	Mode appropriate to level of impairment Discontinuous protocol Low initial work rate, gradual increments	Joint ROM, muscle flexibility, muscular strength and endurance	Monitor HR, BP, thermoregulation May need strapping, abdominal binding to maintain grip or posture Padded supports (seat) Empty bladder/leg bag before testing
Stroke, acquired brain injury (ABI)	Cognitive impairment may prevent effective testing Low initial work rate, gradual increments Mode appropriate to injury and impairment	Balance, gait analysis, joint ROM, muscular strength and flexibility	Spasticity may require one-sided testing Seizures may occur during intense exercise in ABI patients
Multiple sclerosis	Avoid treadmill Use upright or recumbent cycle ergometry Low initial work rate, gradual increments	Joint ROM, muscle flexibility, gait analysis, balance	Monitor HR, BP, thermoregulation May need to strap hands or feet to pedals Test when fatigue is lowest
Parkinson's disease	Avoid treadmill Use cycle ergometry	Gait analysis, coordination, balance, joint ROM, muscle flexibility, muscular strength and endurance	Test at peak activity of medication Familiarisation session helpful Monitor HR, BP, RPE
Chronic fatigue syndrome	Submax preferred, but prediction based on HR may not be valid Interval exercise test better tolerated	Previous test data before onset of CFS	1-3 days rest before Avoid if excessive fatigue or active illness Subject may not achieve predicted maximum work rate or HR

Assuming the client has been pre-screened and cleared for testing by a medical practitioner, if needed, according to the ACSM guidelines (see chapter 5).

Abbreviations: ROM = range of motion; HR = heart rate; BP = blood pressure; RPE = rating of perceived exertion; submax = submaximal fitness testing.

Compiled from American College of Sports Medicine, 1997, *ACSM's exercise management for persons with chronic diseases and disabilities*. (Champaign, IL: Human Kinetics); K.F. Lockette and A.M. Keyes, 1994, *Conditioning with physical disabilities*. (Champaign: Human Kinetics).

of the brain are involved, the main impairment involves loss of control of muscle tone and spinal reflexes, specifically the ability to move, balance and maintain postural control. CP is among the most common physical disabilities occurring in children.

Cerebral palsy may be described according to the extent of neuromuscular impairment. Approximately 70% of CP cases exhibit **spasticity** resulting from damage to the motor cortex. Spasticity reflects increased muscle tone, or **hypertonicity,** which may range from mild to severe and usually involves flexors of the upper body and extensors of the lower extremities. The "scissors" gait and toe-walking movement patterns are typical examples (see figure 10.5). Spasticity causes weakness and underdevelopment of the **antagonist muscle** groups (i.e., muscle groups not affected by hypertonicity). Within each individual with CP, spasticity may fluctuate according to many factors. In general, spasticity is better (i.e., decreased muscle tone) after gentle, slow static stretching but may be worsened by fatigue, quick movement, cold or emotional stress. Athetoid CP, which involves the basal ganglia, occurs in about 20 to 30% of cases and is characterised by writhing, involuntary movement primarily of the trunk and extremities. Ataxic CP involves the cerebellar or cerebral pathways and occurs less often. It results in unsteadiness and involuntary movement of the trunk and extremities; the ability to balance and maintain control of trunk movements is impaired.

Approximately 25% of people with CP exhibit convulsive disorders, most often in **hemiplegia** (involvement of one side), and some may be on anticonvulsive medication. Up to 50% of children and adults with CP have perceptual motor disorders affecting their ability to perceive spatial relationships between themselves and various objects. Most individuals with CP are of normal intelligence, and only a small percentage (10-15%) exhibit intellectual impairment. Regardless of whether or not there is intellectual impairment, visual, speech and language difficulties may arise that could interfere with the ability to communicate clearly. It is therefore important not to automatically assume that communication problems indicate intellectual impairment in the CP client.

Regular physical activity, whether within recreational or sporting venues, is advocated for all individuals with CP. The Cerebral Palsy International Sport and Recreation Association (CP-ISRA) has developed an eight-level system for classifying CP athletes for sport competition, from CP1 to CP8. An important feature of this system is that it classifies athletes by functional ability rather than the actual cause of impairment. It can also be applied to athletes with other forms of non-progressive brain lesions such as stroke, acquired brain injury or brain tumours. Many sports are using this system to classify athletes for competition. Table 10.3 gives a brief summary of the degree of impairment and physical abilities of individuals at each level.

Exercise Capacity and CP

Exercise capacity varies with the extent and severity of disability. CP generally results in a lower physical work capacity because of the combined effects of hypertonicity, inactivity, muscle weakness and mechanical inefficiency caused by poor coordination. The CP client may experience early muscular fatigue, which may limit exercise performance before a true metabolic maximum is achieved. During submaximal exercise, heart rate, blood pressure and minute ventilation are higher than normal because of mechanical inefficiency; that is, the same work rate elicits a higher physiological response. The recommended modes of exercise for assessment of aerobic capacity include cycle ergometry (legs, arms or

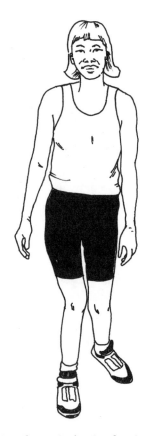

FIGURE 10.5　The typical gait of an individual with cerebral palsy.

TABLE 10.3—Brief Summary of CP-ISRA Classifications and Exercise Prescription Recommendations

Level, severity	Functional ability	Exercise prescription recommendations
CP1 Severe spastic or athetoid quadriplegia	Poor muscle strength, ROM, trunk stability, leg movement Inefficient wheelchair propulsion	From wheelchair, mainly arms Use strapping Functional movement, guided resistance
CP2 Moderate-severe spastic or athetoid quadriplegia	Can walk short distances with assistant device Poor dynamic trunk control Can propel manual wheelchair short distances	As for CP1
CP3 Moderate spastic quadriplegia or severe hemiplegia	Can walk short distances with assistant device Fair trunk control Slow propulsion of wheelchair with one or two arms	From wheelchair or lying position Strapping for heavy lifting Free or machine weights for upper body Stretch lower body spastic muscles Strengthen antagonists to spastic muscles
CP4 Moderate-severe spastic diplegia	Can walk short distances Good dynamic trunk control Uses wheelchair for daily activities and sports Poor balance when standing	From wheelchair, sitting, lying or standing if can balance Weights and stretching as for CP3 Aerobic exercise in wheelchair
CP5 Moderate spastic diplegia	Walks well with assistant device Able to run Good control of upper extremity Fair balance Does not use wheelchair	Position as for CP4 Weights as for CP3 Aerobic exercise without wheelchair
CP6 Moderate athetosis or ataxia	Walks without device Gait/coordination difficulties Good dynamic trunk control and upper extremity strength	From wheelchair, sitting, or lying position Exercise arms and legs Free or machine weights Aerobic exercise, but running may increase spasticity
CP7 True ambulatory hemiplegia	Mild-moderately affected upper extremity Possible spasticity in affected arm Minimal-mildly affected lower extremity	From wheelchair, lying or standing if can balance Free or machine weights Unilateral exercises because of asymmetry in strength or coordination Focus on functional movements
CP8 Minimally affected	Minimal involvement in one arm Minimal to no involvement in trunk, lower extremity	Few limitations Focus on muscular and aerobic conditioning

Abbreviations: CP-ISRA = Cerebral Palsy International Sports & Recreation Association.

Compiled from K.F. Lockette and A.M. Keyes, 1994, *Conditioning with physical disabilities.* (Champaign, IL: Human Kinetics); M. Ferrar and J. Laskin, 1997, Cerebral palsy. In American College of Sport Medicine, 1997, *ACSM's exercise management for persons with chronic diseases and disability.* (Champaign, IL: Human Kinetics), 206-211.

both), wheelchair ergometry or wheelchair pushing on a treadmill. Leg or arm ergometry may require strapping the feet or hands to the pedals. Treadmill walking or field tests (e.g., 6- to 12-min walk) may be used in ambulatory individuals with adequate coordination and balance. If possible, joint range of motion and muscle flexibility should also be assessed. Depending on the severity of disability, gait analysis, balance tests and measures of muscular strength are also useful as a basis for exercise prescription. Muscular strength may be significantly affected by spasticity, and coordination problems may prevent safe assessment of strength.

Exercise Prescription for CP

When prescribing exercise for the individual with CP, it is essential to first understand the extent and severity of physical, cognitive and communication disabilities. A balanced program including conditioning for aerobic fitness, muscular strength and endurance, and flexibility is recommended (refer to table 10.3). Some modification of equipment may be needed, such as bandaging (non-adhesive) or strapping the hands or feet to equipment. Exercise programs should first focus on coordination, control and effective technique. Both cardiovascular and

muscular conditioning should be performed regularly (e.g., two to three times per week) and stretching exercises daily. Because spasticity adversely affects joint ROM and strength of the antagonist muscle groups, daily stretching of tight spastic muscles and resistance exercise to strengthen the antagonists may improve ROM. Strengthening the hypertonic muscles may increase spasticity and thus have a detrimental effect. Resistance exercise may be performed on weight machines while seated in a wheelchair or using other support. Good trunk stability and balance are needed to use free weights. An elastic binder around the trunk and supporting bench may aid stability of this region. Moderate to severe coordination difficulties due to spasticity, athetosis or ataxia may prevent use of free weights or weight machines; flexible bands (Thera-Band®) or guided resistance with a partner may be appropriate.

Duration and intensity of exercise will vary depending on the disability, fitness level and interest of the client. General guidelines as for able-bodied individuals apply (refer to chapters 2 and 7):

▶ For development of cardiorespiratory fitness: 20 to 40 min per session, three to five times per week, at 40 to 85% HRR

Case Study 10.2

Julie is 13 years old and has spastic diplegic cerebral palsy. She walks independently and is an intelligent girl who has generally been compliant with various forms of therapy. Recently, however, she has become rebellious, as many teenagers do. She is sociable and enjoys sports and games but does not currently exercise much. Although she participates in twice-weekly physical education classes at school, involvement in class activities has become difficult of late. Her doctor and parents believe she would benefit from regular physical activity, and she has expressed an interest in exercising at the local, well-appointed gym at which you work.

Write a 6-week progressive exercise program for Julie that incorporates the gym equipment and programs and at least one session per week outside the gym. The gym has a heated 25-m pool, pin weights designed for women, free weights, aerobics programs and exercise equipment such as electronic treadmills, bikes, rowing and stair climbing machines.

Key Issues

1. Will you ask Julie to complete a physical fitness assessment? Why or why not? If yes, which tests would be helpful?

2. What combination of endurance and resistance exercise will you prescribe? Why?

3. What types of resistance exercise program will you prescribe? Why?

4. What types of exercise will you recommend for her session outside the gym? What precautions, if any, are needed?

5. Are there any organised sports that you might recommend for Julie? Why?

▶ For development of muscular strength: 2 to 3 sets of 8 to 12 repetitions of 8 to 10 exercises performed two to three times per week

There are specific safety concerns when prescribing exercise for individuals with CP. A routine of slow static stretching is needed at the start and end of each session to reduce muscle tone, especially in spastic muscles. Good body alignment, particularly during resistance training, is essential to prevent injury and enhance the effectiveness of each exercise. Some individuals may experience convulsive seizures, although these are less likely to occur during exercise than at rest. If a seizure occurs, remove potentially hazardous objects, gently lower the person to the ground if needed and do not intervene. Because the CP client may have a perceptual motor disorder, exercises using implements (e.g., balls) or with complex movement patterns may be difficult but should nevertheless be encouraged. Slow and clear demonstrations, simple movement patterns and an uncluttered exercise environment are beneficial. Close monitoring, including spotting during resistance training, is recommended at the onset of any activity program.

Spinal Cord Injury

Spinal cord injury (SCI) involves impairment or loss of motor or sensory function in the trunk or limbs resulting from damage to neurological tissues within the spinal canal. The degree of impairment and loss of function is related to the level of injury—in general, the higher the level of injury, the greater the impairment. Injury to the spinal cord at the cervical or upper thoracic levels (C1-8, T1) results in **quadriplegia,** or impaired neurological function in all four extremities, trunk and pelvic organs, although some use of the arms may remain. C4 is the highest level of injury in which the patient can live without artificial breathing support. Injury to the thoracic region (T2-12) results in **paraplegia,** or neural impairment of the lower extremities and possibly part of the trunk or pelvic organs, with retention of function in the upper extremities. Both quadriplegia and paraplegia can be partial or complete, depending on the extent of damage. Injury to the lower spine (L1-5, S1-4) may cause impairment in the legs or pelvic organs.

The loss of neural integrity in the spinal cord results in muscular paralysis (loss of voluntary movement), loss of sensation, and impairment of the sympathetic nervous system (SNS) below the level of injury. A complete injury is one in which there is no muscle or sensory function at least three vertebral segments below the neural level of damage. When some neural transmission still occurs through the damaged area or some sensory function is retained below the level of injury, it is classified as an incomplete injury. The injury classification is based on the lowest muscular and neurological functional level remaining, not the actual anatomical site of injury. Impairment of the sympathetic nervous system affects regulation of heart rate, blood pressure, sweating and thermoregulation, and blood flow distribution.

SCI most commonly occurs after trauma, such as motor vehicle accidents, or severe injury in sport or recreation (e.g., football, diving, cycling accidents). As such, many SCI patients are young adult males with previously active lifestyles. Given recent advances in acute medical treatment and rehabilitation, an individual with SCI may live for many years after the initial injury. SCI is estimated to cost between $300 to $500 million each year in health and welfare expenditure. In contrast to many years ago when most SCI patients died as a result of the initial injuries or related dysfunction, the most prevalent cause of death in SCI patients is now cardiovascular disease. Inactivity imposed by the loss of motor function is thought to be a major contributor to development of cardiovascular diseases in these individuals; for example, dyslipidaemia (refer to chapter 8), especially low HDL-C concentration, is a common feature of SCI. Regular physical activity may thus play an important role in preventing cardiovascular disease and improving quality of life in people with SCI. Regular physical activity may be beneficial by helping to

▶ control body weight, body fat and blood lipid levels;

▶ increase muscle mass, strength and functional capacity (e.g., ability to transfer into and out of a wheelchair);

▶ enhance quality of life and sense of well-being;

▶ prevent joint contractures and pressure sores; and

▶ maintain postural control in the wheelchair.

Exercise Capacity and SCI

As mentioned in the previous section, risk of cardiovascular disease may be high in individuals with SCI, and medical screening and clinical exercise testing may be needed before testing fitness levels or prescribing exercise (refer to chapters 5 and 6). Because oxygen consumption is directly related to the amount of active musculature, exercise capacity is limited by the extent of injury and musculature involved. In addition, impaired sympathetic nervous system regulation of heart rate and blood pressure limits cardiac output and thus oxygen delivery to working tissues. Consequently, exercise capacity is considerably lower in individuals with SCI compared with the able-bodied.

The mode of exercise test is obviously influenced by the extent of impairment and muscular function retained. Some people with SCI may be able to walk or cycle, some can use wheelchairs and some may need to use upper body exercise, such as arm ergometry, to assess aerobic exercise capacity. Sometimes assessment of cardiorespiratory fitness is not possible. For clients capable of wheelchair pushing, field tests or wheelchair ergometry may be preferable to arm ergometry since it involves higher O_2 uptake and is more related to activities of daily living. Appropriate tests to estimate peak $\dot{V}O_2$ include a 12-min wheel-distance test based on the relationship between distance covered and O_2 uptake or tests at progressive submaximal work rates based on the relationship between exercise heart rate and O_2 uptake using arm ergometry (Steadward 1998). In arm ergometry, peak power output is low, about 50 W in quadriplegia and 50 to 120 W in paraplegia. Discontinuous protocols using small increments (e.g., 5-20 W) are better tolerated than continuous protocols. Peak heart rate is less than 130 beats · min^{-1} in quadriplegia and slightly higher in paraplegia. Both hypotensive and hypertensive responses may occur in quadriplegia—hypotensive because of the lack of a leg muscle pump to aid venous return in upright exercise and hypertensive from impairment of SNS function. Blood pressure and heart rate should be monitored throughout testing, and the test should be stopped if systolic blood pressure exceeds 200 mmHg in the quadriplegic or 260 mmHg in any individual with SCI.

Assessing upper extremity muscular strength and overall flexibility, especially of the shoulder, elbow, wrist, hip and knee, provides additional useful information for the exercise prescription. It may be necessary to strap the trunk or abdomen to ensure good posture or to strap the hands or use holding gloves to ensure a firm grip on arm cranks. Individuals with SCI are susceptible to pressure sores because of loss of sensation, and the skin should be protected and cushioned (e.g., padded seat cushion on ergometer). The bladder (or leg bag) should be emptied before any testing to prevent autonomic hyperreflexia (discussed in the following section). Since thermoregulation is compromised in SCI, all assessment should be performed in a controlled environment and the client closely monitored for signs of heat intolerance.

Exercise Prescription for SCI

Table 10.4 gives some general guidelines for choice of exercise mode and body position for people with SCI. The exercise prescription must be individualised to accommodate the extent of disability, functional capacity, client's goals and needs, and access to facilities. The general recommendations for able-bodied individuals also apply to clients with SCI: To improve cardiorespiratory function, perform three to five exercise sessions per week, for 20 to 60 min per session, at 50 to 80% peak heart rate (as tested, not predicted); and to enhance muscular function, perform two sessions per week of 3 sets of 8 to 12 repetitions of resistance exercise. Stretching should be performed daily.

Exercise prescription should focus on preventing disease (e.g., lowering risk of cardiovascular disease) and enhancing functional capacity (e.g., activities used in daily living such as transferring into and out of a wheelchair). Obviously, mode of exercise must be tailored to the client's capability, but it should also be varied to prevent overuse of the upper body musculature. Depending on the extent of disability, suitable modes include arm crank ergometry, weightlifting (machines, barbells, free weights) (see figure 10.6), wheelchair pushing (treadmill, track, road), boxacise, aquatic exercise or, when possible, walking (treadmill, free). Strengthening and stretching the shoulder girdle and other upper body muscles, especially back extensors and rotator cuff muscles, are important for maintaining good posture during exercise as well as during activities of daily living. In addition, the program should include exercises to stretch shortened or spastic muscles (e.g., lower body flexors) that result from sitting in a wheelchair.

Since functional capacity is often low (except in trained wheelchair athletes), intensity should start low and progress gradually. Interval exercise will be better tolerated, especially at the start. Strapping or binding with non-adhesive material may be needed to maintain posture or grip on the equipment. For example, strapping spastic lower limbs will enhance performance of upper body resistance exercise; abdominal binding or support if these muscles are not active will enhance performance of arm ergometry.

It is recommended to monitor heart rate, blood pressure, posture/balance and signs of heat intolerance and autonomic hyperreflexia. As mentioned previously, thermoregulation is impaired in SCI, so

TABLE 10.4—General Recommendations for Exercise for People With Spinal Cord Injury

Level of impairment	Mobility	Muscular conditioning
C4-6	Mainly in wheelchair Trunk support and splints often needed	Multi-joint exercises of back and shoulder extensors, rotator cuffs, scapular stability
C7-8	Mainly in wheelchair; some may be able to transfer out of wheelchair to bench or to propel wheelchair Abdominal binder may be needed	Weight machines Multi-joint exercises of back and shoulder extensors, rotator cuffs, scapular stability
T1-5	Can propel wheelchair Some may stand with leg braces and upper extremity support	Weight machines Multi-joint exercises of back and shoulder extensors, rotator cuffs, scapular stability
T6-10	Normal upper extremity function Can propel wheelchair Some may walk with leg braces and forearm crutches	Free and machine weights Back and shoulder extension, rotator cuffs, abdominal, trunk rotation
T11-14	Use wheelchair or walk with leg braces and forearm crutches	Free and machine weights Upper extremity extensors, abdominal, trunk rotation, hip flexion, knee extension
L5-S5	Can walk with or without braces Some may use wheelchair for long distances	Free and machine weights Multi- and single-joint exercises of trunk, back, shoulder extension and rotation, abdominal, knee flexion and extension

Compiled from K.F. Lockette and A.M. Keyes, 1994, *Conditioning with physical disabilities.* (Champaign, IL: Human Kinetics); S.F. Figoni, 1997, Spinal cord injury. In American College of Sports Medicine, 1997, *ACSM's exercise management for persons with chronic diseases and disabilities.* (Champaign, IL: Human Kinetics), 175-179.

clients should exercise in a controlled environment (e.g., pool, air-conditioned gym) and wear minimal, loose-fitting clothes. Autonomic hyperreflexia involves an exaggerated autonomic response to irritation of the skin or viscera below the level of injury. Commonly triggered by a distended bladder or tight clothing, autonomic hyperreflexia may cause an excessive rise in blood pressure, headache, sweating above the level of injury and paleness below, nasal obstruction and depressed heart rate. If left unchecked, it can become serious and possibly life threatening. Should this condition occur, the first action is to have the individual sit up because lying down increases blood pressure (by enhancing venous return). Remove or remedy the irritating stimulus (e.g., loosen clothing or abdominal binder, empty leg bag). If symptoms persist, seek emergency medical care. Autonomic hyperreflexia may be prevented by emptying the bladder or leg bag before exercise and wearing loose clothing.

Stroke and Acquired Brain Injury

The brain may be permanently injured by a single event in which blood flow to the brain is impaired (as in bleeding within the brain) or by direct physical trauma (as in a blow to the head). A **stroke,** or **cerebrovascular accident (CVA),** is caused by vascular insufficiency to the brain as a result of thrombosis (blood clot), haemorrhage (bleeding) or embolism (clot moving through the circulation). **Acquired brain injury (ABI)** has a different cause, but the pathology and outcome may be similar to stroke. ABI most often occurs as a result of severe trauma to the head, for example, in a motor vehicle accident. Regardless of the initial event, in both

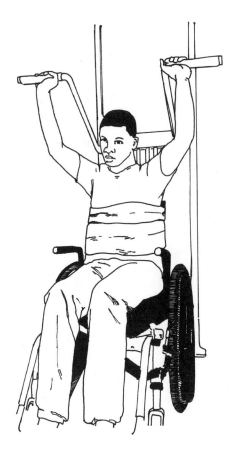

FIGURE 10.6   An individual with SCI lifting weights from a wheelchair.

stroke and ABI ischaemic neural tissue dies, resulting in permanent damage to that area of the brain. This may involve cognitive or physical impairments, depending on the extent of damage and the area of the brain affected.

Stroke is the third leading cause of death in most developed countries and a significant cause of disability among the elderly. Stroke may occur at any age, although about 80% of stroke victims are older than 65 years. Risk factors for stroke include hypertension, smoking, diabetes, alcoholism and coronary artery disease; obesity and dyslipidaemia may also contribute to the risk of stroke by increasing blood pressure and by promoting atherosclerosis. Although the evidence is inconclusive, regular exercise may prevent stroke by helping to control risk factors (e.g., lowering blood pressure, improving glucose tolerance) and by reducing blood viscosity (thereby lessening the risk of a clot). There is, at present, inconclusive evidence to support the role of exercise in secondary prevention of stroke (i.e., reducing risk of further events in the stroke survivor). ABI can occur at any age, but it is most prevalent in young adult men (mainly aged 15-24 years). Exercise may play a role in management of ABI because of its positive effects on quality of life and physical function.

Brain damage resulting from stroke or ABI may cause a variety of impairments of cognitive or physical function, including

Case Study 10.3

Victor is 28 years old. Three years ago, he had a complete spinal cord injury at T7-8. Victor regularly participated in athletics (middle distance), cross country running and triathlons before his injury, and he has recently decided to start road racing (5 km and over). His initial goal is to improve his fitness, but he would eventually like to compete in this sport. Victor has access to an old racing chair through the Sporting Wheelies and Disabled Association. He is at present apparently healthy except for a decubitus ulcer on his upper left buttock.

Key Issues

1. Is distance training appropriate or feasible for Victor in the long term? Give reasons for your answer. What factors must be considered in making this decision?

2. How will the ulcer influence his beginning a training program? What is the time course of recovery for this ulcer? What types/modes of training are appropriate alternatives for him during this time?

3. Describe when and how wheelchair pushing might be introduced to Victor's training routine.

4. What aspects of chair design, seating and training will be important for preventing a recurrence of the ulcer?

▶ impairments of motor or sensory function in the affected extremities,

▶ defects in visual processing,

▶ impairments of speech and communication,

▶ confusion and memory loss, and

▶ impairments of learning new voluntary movement patterns.

Compared with stroke, ABI tends to result in more cognitive dysfunction, and it may also significantly affect social and behavioural factors, such as increased aggression. In addition, there may be permanent physical disability resulting from the original trauma that caused the injury. ABI is also associated with muscle wasting during the first several months. These physical and cognitive impairments influence exercise capacity and the choice of appropriate exercise for stroke/ABI patients.

Exercise Capacity and Stroke and ABI

Most stroke patients are elderly, and they are often affected by hypertension, CAD and musculoskeletal problems such as arthritis, necessitating proper screening and medical clearance. Moreover, functional capacity may be low because of deconditioning after the initial event. Cognitive impairments such as confusion and aphasia (impaired speech and communication) may make it difficult for the stroke patient to fully understand the requirements of exercise testing. Many stroke patients also take medications (e.g., beta-blockers) that may affect test results.

Exercise capacity depends on the nature and severity of injury and the degree of neural impairment. In stroke patients, flaccidity, spasticity or weakness on one side, or in one set of extremities, may interfere with coordinated movement, as in maintaining pedal cadence in cycle or arm ergometry. Impairment of balance will affect walking gait and possibly the ability to maintain sitting posture, such that assessment of cardiorespiratory fitness may be difficult. Arm and leg ergometry using the unaffected side may be necessary. Impairments of neural and motor function may limit exercise capacity, and few stroke patients achieve predicted maximal exercise values (e.g., age-predicted maximum heart rate). Measurement of muscular strength and flexibility, ROM, coordination, balance and gait is useful for subsequent exercise prescription and as a benchmark for assessing progress during rehabilitation (as discussed in the section on aging in the previous chapter).

Most of these principles apply to exercise testing for people with ABI. However, ABI clients may also have cognitive disorders or permanent orthopaedic injuries (e.g., amputation after a motor vehicle accident) as a result of the initial trauma, which may influence exercise capacity and possibly the ability of the client to comply with testing procedures. Muscle wasting may occur during the first several months after traumatic injury such as ABI, leading to loss of muscular strength. ABI may also be associated with seizures, discussed in the section on cerebral palsy.

For those who experience seizures, the risk of seizure is somewhat higher during exercise that induces hyperventilation (i.e., intense exercise) compared with rest; personnel testing ABI patients should be prepared to ensure client safety if a seizure occurs.

Exercise Prescription for Stroke and ABI

The classification system developed for individuals with CP is also used to describe the degree of impairment and ability of those recovering from stroke or with ABI (refer to table 10.3). For the client who has had a stroke, 6 to 12 months may be needed for recovery, during which time the focus is on medical and physical rehabilitation to restore basic physical function and ADLs. Shoulder pain is common, due to "frozen shoulders" (hypertonic muscles around the shoulder), subluxation or tendonitis, and specific exercises are needed. Respiratory muscle impairment may also occur, which will limit ventilation and exercise capacity, requiring very low intensity and possibly interval exercise to start. It may be necessary to first regain muscular strength and endurance through resistance training before progressing to cardiovascular conditioning.

After ABI, cognitive impairments may cause confusion and memory deficit, and patience may be required when teaching the client new skills. ABI is also associated with other cognitive and social effects including irritability and aggression, which may influence the choice of setting or mode of activity. When developing an activity program for the client with ABI, choose simple tasks, provide clear verbal instructions and demonstrations, and offer convenient visual cues such as wall charts and written exercise plans.

For clients with ABI or recovering from a stroke, the mode of exercise is dictated by the extent of impairment, both physical and cognitive. Many patients need a supervised program to monitor balance, coordination and comprehension, at least at the start. Seated or weight-supported exercises are generally safest. Preferred modes include cycle ergometry rather than road cycling, treadmill walking (with a handrail and emergency stop) instead of free walking, and weight machines or elastic bands rather than free weights. If there is significant weakness or paralysis on the affected side, unilateral exercise (e.g., arm and leg ergometry) of the unaffected side may be necessary; specific stretching, strengthening and ROM exercises may be needed to regain function on the affected side. Exercises should consist of relatively simple movements if there are cognitive or coordination impairments.

For cardiovascular conditioning and disease prevention, the same general recommendations for physical activity for the general populace apply to clients with stroke or ABI, such as 30 min of moderate-intensity exercise on most days. The age difference between stroke and ABI clients (generally older and younger adults, respectively) must be considered when developing specific exercise prescriptions based on these recommendations. If the individual is taking medication known to affect HR, exercise intensity should be assessed with RPE rather than HR. Also, as recommended for general health, muscular strength and endurance exercise should include 1 to 3 sets of 8 to 12 repetitions of 8 to 10 exercises focusing on the major muscle groups, performed at least twice per week. Maximal lifts should be avoided by the stroke patient because of risk of excessively high blood pressure, and regular breathing must be emphasised to avoid the Valsalva manoeuvre. Coordination, gait and balance exercises can be included in the muscular conditioning session. Stretching, ROM and specific therapeutic exercises to improve functional movement should be performed daily.

Multiple Sclerosis

Multiple sclerosis (MS) is an autoimmune neurological disease in which the body's immune cells (T lymphocytes) breach the blood-brain barrier and attack myelin. The resulting demyelination of nerves disrupts smooth conduction along the neuron, causing disorders of movement and coordination. One of the most common neurological diseases affecting young adults, MS begins in the late 20s through to middle age. Physical characteristics of MS include spasticity of some muscles, poor coordination, impaired balance, fatigue and muscle weakness, partial or full paralysis, numbness or loss of sensation, and tremor. In addition, MS may also affect autonomic function, causing dysfunction in regulation of heart rate, blood pressure and thermoregulation.

MS is a progressive disease, but the severity and pattern of progression may be unpredictable and highly variable between individuals. Three main patterns of progression have been identified:

▶ Alternating periods of exacerbation and remission, with full or partial recovery during remission

▶ Slow progression without remission

▶ Combination of the first two patterns, but with incomplete recovery during remission and progressive worsening during successive exacerbations and remissions

The third pattern of MS progression occurs most frequently.

Exercise Capacity and MS

Because MS is often associated with inactivity, obesity and hypertension, medical screening is needed before beginning an exercise program (refer to chapter 5). Specific features of MS may limit exercise capacity. Ataxia, or loss of coordination in the trunk and limbs, can impair balance and cause shakiness in the affected limbs. Spasticity or muscle weakness may be asymmetrical, decreasing mechanical efficiency and causing early fatigue. Foot drag and muscle stiffness are common features of spasticity and weakness, and loss of sensation in the limbs may impair balance and the ability to perform upright exercise such as walking or running. In addition, heat intolerance may cause an excessive and potentially dangerous rise in core temperature during exercise. All of these factors must be considered during exercise testing or when prescribing physical activity for individuals with MS.

Upright or recumbent cycling is recommended for exercise testing because problems with balance make treadmill testing impractical. If the patient has use of all extremities, arm and leg ergometry may be used. Toe clips, heel straps and hand strapping may be needed to maintain grip on hand and foot pedals. As always, warm-up before any exercise is important. Exercise testing should begin at a very low level and progress gradually by 10- to 20-W increments during cycle ergometry. Interval or discontinuous protocols and testing over 2 days rather than 1 day may induce less fatigue and be better tolerated. To prevent heat stress, the test should take place in a cool environment. Heart rate and blood pressure should be monitored and the test stopped if SBP rises above 200 mmHg or DBP above 115 mmHg or a hypotensive response (i.e., drop in systolic blood pressure) occurs. Other tests such as gait analysis and measures of joint range of motion and muscular strength and endurance are helpful for exercise prescription. Because mechanical efficiency is low, oxygen uptake is generally higher at any given work rate in MS patients compared with normal values; low mechanical efficiency contributes to early fatigue during exertion.

Exercise Prescription for MS

The vast majority of MS patients (70-85%) exhibit fatigue, often debilitating, that adversely affects the ability to perform ADLs and ultimately influences quality of life. Since fatigue is often exacerbated by physical exertion, many MS patients are inactive, and the most severely affected patients tend to be the least active. Although regular exercise cannot alter the progression of disease, recent evidence suggests that appropriate physical activity may help maintain functional capacity and thus enhance quality of life (reviewed by Petajan and White 1999).

An exercise program must be individualised for the MS patient, taking into account the pattern of progression, severity and type of disability, and other factors such as obesity or hypertension (see table 10.5). The prescription should be adaptable, allowing for periods of exacerbation and remission (if this pattern is exhibited) and daily variations in fatigue. The client should exercise at a time of day when fatigue is lowest; fatigue is often at its worst in mid- to late afternoon. Low-intensity exercise is preferred because it is less likely to cause undue fatigue, increase core temperature dangerously or increase spasticity. The exercise prescription should focus on improving functional capacity and ADLs (e.g., upper body muscular strength and endurance for transfers into and out of a wheelchair). Whenever possible, aerobic exercise should involve a large muscle mass to provide a training effect while preventing or lessening local muscle fatigue. For patients with problems of balance and coordination, support, strapping or assistance may be necessary. Heat-intolerant clients should wear

---

TABLE 10.5—Examples of Exercise Training Components for People With Multiple Sclerosis

Type of conditioning	Examples of exercises
Aerobic	Interval to avoid fatigue
	Cycle ergometry, walking, aquatic
	Seated if balance is impaired
	Low to moderate intensity to avoid increased core temperature
	3-5 d/wk
Muscular strength and endurance	Multi-joint, bilateral exercises
	Strengthen muscles opposing spastic muscles
	Weight machines if balance is impaired
	Calisthenics with body weight as resistance
	Elastic bands (e.g., Thera-Band®)
	2-3 d/wk on alternate days to aerobic
Muscular flexibility and joint ROM	Active or passive (partner assisted)
	Stretch hip flexors, knee flexors, plantar flexors if in wheelchair or exhibit spasticity
	Daily and before/after muscular strength exercises

Compiled from K.F. Lockette and A.M. Keyes, 1994, *Conditioning with physical disabilities.* (Champaign, IL: Human Kinetics); J.A. Mulcare, 1997, Multiple sclerosis. In American College of Sports Medicine, 1997, *ACSM's exercise management for persons with chronic diseases and disabilities.* (Champaign, IL: Human Kinetics), 189-193.

light, loose-fitting clothes and exercise in a cool environment (e.g., air-conditioned gym, pool) or at cooler times of the day; these clients should be monitored for signs of heat intolerance. Recommended air and water temperatures for exercise are 22 to 24° C and 27 to 29° C, respectively. Heart rate and blood pressure should also be monitored during exercise to ensure these values remain within the recommended ranges.

Low-intensity aerobic activities should be performed three to five times per week to increase cardiorespiratory fitness and control body weight and blood pressure. Suitable modes include stationary cycling (arm or leg), walking, wheelchair rolling, swimming or other aquatic exercise. Interval exercise is better tolerated than continuous exercise; appropriate work and rest intervals are 2 to 5 min work and 1 to 2 min rest. To avoid excessive fatigue, resistance training should be included two to three times per week on days when aerobic exercise is not performed. Resistance training should focus on trunk, shoulder and pelvic stabilisers and on postural muscles such as extensors of the knee, hip and low back. Achieving good postural control will enhance mechanical efficiency for ADLs and other activities. In general, spastic muscles should not be strengthened; rather, the focus should be on strengthening the opposing muscle groups. Weight machines are preferable to free weights if there are problems with balance, coordination or trunk stability. For clients with stability or balance problems, seated exercise or strapping may be helpful (see figure 10.7). Visual cues such as exercising in front of a mirror will help the client maintain posture and balance. Large muscle as opposed to isolated muscle group exercises and multi-joint rather than single joint exercises are recommended as a time-efficient way to improve muscular strength without causing undue fatigue. Stretching exercises should be performed daily and before and after each exercise session, emphasising the spastic muscles. If the client uses a wheelchair, the hip flexors, knee flexors and plantar flexors should also be stretched daily to prevent contractures.

Some MS patients exhibit cognitive effects such as memory loss or depression. Written instructions are helpful, and clear demonstrations and visual cues may need to be repeated regularly. RPE may not be appropriate for some clients with cognitive deficits. The client should avoid prolonged exercise during periods of exacerbation (worsening of symptoms), perhaps maintaining only the stretching components and then gradually resuming the exercise program once remission begins; medical clearance

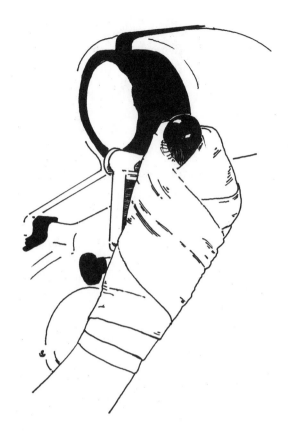

FIGURE 10.7   Proper hand strapping for use in arm ergometry.

should first be obtained before the exercise program is resumed.

Parkinson's Disease

Parkinson's disease (PD) is a progressive neurological condition involving the extrapyramidal system that results in a variety of movement disorders such as tremor, akinesia (freezing during movement), muscle rigidity and dyskinesia (involuntary movements). In PD, death of dopamine-producing cells in the basal ganglia causes a deficiency of the neurotransmitter dopamine causing disruption in function of this area of the brain involved in control of movement. The most common form of PD, called idiopathic, usually occurs after the age of 50, progresses slowly and is mainly characterised by tremor. A less common form begins at an earlier age, is generally associated with rapid progression and poor prognosis, and is mainly characterised by akinesia.

PD causes noticeable changes in muscle function and strength, posture, gait and other movement patterns. Muscle rigidity begins in the neck and shoulders, progressing to the trunk and extremities. Posture is characterised by kyphosis (curvature of the spine), flexed knees and elbows, and adducted shoulders. Walking is characterised by a hesitant start, a slow, shuffling gait with short, hurried steps and an increased duration of the double-limb support phase (i.e., longer time with both feet on the ground). PD patients exhibit decreased ability for rapid movement and change of pace, as well as decreased postural righting reflexes, making them vulnerable to falling. These movement decrements significantly affect the ability to carry out ADLs such as walking, stair climbing, food preparation and bathing. Dementia is sometimes present, as are loss of facial expressions and volume and clarity of speech. Symptoms may fluctuate from day to day. Most PD patients take multiple medications, some of which may contribute to cardiac arrhythmia and dyskinesia.

Although PD adversely affects quality of life, the major causes of death are cardiovascular and pulmonary diseases. Most patients have obstructive pulmonary dysfunction resulting from rigidity of thoracic, vertebral, cervical and facial muscles. The PD patient may also exhibit cardiac abnormalities such as arrhythmia and fixed pulse rate, the inability of heart rate to increase in response to physiological stress. Physical inactivity, often forced on the patient because of movement disorders, increases risk of cardiovascular disease, muscular atrophy, loss of muscular strength and reduced bone mineral density. Some studies suggest reduced mortality in physically active PD patients, although since patients self-select to be physically active, it is difficult to know whether exercise reduces mortality or whether those able to exercise are healthier in general. Regardless of whether physical activity reduces mortality in individuals with PD, recent evidence strongly suggests that a well-structured exercise program can enhance quality of life and decrease symptoms of disability.

Exercise Capacity and PD

Because most PD patients are inactive, elderly, at risk of cardiovascular diseases and may exhibit cardiac and pulmonary abnormalities, medical screening and exercise testing are essential before beginning any exercise program (refer to chapters 5, 6, 8, and 9). Assessment should be performed at peak activity of medication, usually about 45 min after the medication has been taken. Because of difficulties

with gait and balance, a cycle ergometer rather than a treadmill should be used for testing. Muscle rigidity causes mechanical inefficiency, and familiarisation sessions before testing to allow the patient to practice cycling will yield more accurate data. The PD patient will exhibit reduced muscular strength and size (because of atrophy), decreased ability for hip extension and knee extension/flexion, and inability to quickly alter movement pace. Thus, the test should begin at a low work rate and progress gradually, avoiding rapid changes in pace or resistance.

The fitness assessment should include measures of cardiorespiratory fitness, muscular strength and flexibility, joint range of motion, balance and coordination (refer to chapters 6 and 9). Heart rate, blood pressure, RPE, maximum work rate, exercise time and, if possible, $\dot{V}O_2$max should be recorded. For example, a recent study using cycle ergometry found similar $\dot{V}O_2$max values in male and female PD patients and matched healthy control subjects (Stanley, Protas and Jankovic 1999). However, compared with controls, the PD patients exercised for a shorter time and had higher oxygen uptake values at each submaximal work rate, suggesting reduced exercise tolerance and mechanical efficiency. It was concluded that a wide range of variables should be measured to accurately assess physical fitness in PD patients.

Exercise Prescription for PD

The aims of physical therapy and exercise are to prevent joint contractures in bed-ridden or inactive patients, modify risk factors for cardiovascular disease, increase range of motion and muscular strength, and enhance QOL and the capacity for ADLs. The exercise prescription should include five general categories of exercise:

▶ Aerobic conditioning

▶ Muscular strength and endurance

▶ Flexibility and range of motion

▶ Functional ability

▶ Balance and motor control

These were discussed in further detail in the section on aging in the previous chapter.

Because patients experience frequent fluctuations in symptom severity and response to medication, the program should be individualised and adaptable. Each exercise session should be performed at a consistent time after taking medication.

Table 10.6 summarises general recommendations for exercise prescription for PD. Recommended

---

TABLE 10.6—Examples of Exercise Training Components for People With Parkinson's Disease

Type of conditioning	Examples of exercises
Aerobic	Cycle ergometry, water walking, swimming
Balance, initiation of movement	Walking forward, backward
	Swiss Ball exercises
	Start-and-stop movements, changing direction on external cues
Coordination	Bouncing balls
	More complex walking patterns coordinating arms and legs
Muscular strength	Water-based (aqua) aerobics using water as resistance
	Roll exercises on padded mats
	Calisthenics using body weight or resistive bands

Compiled from I. Reuter, M. Engelhardt, K. Stecker, and H. Baas, 1999, "Therapeutic value of exercise training in Parkinson's disease," *Medicine and Science in Sports and Exercise* 31: 1544-1549; E.J. Protas, R.K. Stanley, J. Jankovic, 1997, Parkinson's disease. In American College of Sports Medicine, 1997, *ACSM's exercise management for persons with chronic diseases and disabilities.* (Champaign, IL: Human Kinetics).

---

modes of exercise include weight-supported activities such as cycle or rowing ergometry, water-based activities, and circuit resistance training on weight machines. Short interval walking (20-30 m) forward and backward will help improve coordination. Because the PD patient is generally physically inactive with low functional capacity, low-intensity exercise (<11-13 RPE) is recommended. Aerobic and resistance exercise and stretching should be performed at least two to three times per week, and postural or functional activities (e.g., rising from a chair) should be performed daily. In a recent study, idiopathic PD patients who exercised twice per week for 14 weeks demonstrated significant improvements in ratings of motor disability, ADLs, subjective ratings of well-being and symptoms of dyskinesia that lasted for 6 weeks after the program ended (Reuter et al. 1999). The exercise program included one session per week of muscle-strengthening exercises in the pool using water as resistance and one session per week of gym-based exercise to music concentrating on flexibility, balance and gait. Exercise in water is beneficial because the water provides gentle resistance and decreases rigidity of muscles, and movements may be performed without fear of injury from falls.

Group exercise may help overcome the social isolation often experienced by PD patients. Because of the inability to change pace rapidly and difficulty with balance, complex movements requiring frequent changes in pace or direction of movement should be avoided. Movements should therefore be simple, at a constant pace and clearly demonstrated. External cues such as music, visual and voice prompts, and repeated directions will help, since the PD patient is better able to respond to external rather than internal cues. PD is also associated with autonomic system dysfunction, which alters the heart rate, blood pressure and sweating responses to exercise. In some PD clients, HR does not increase in response to physical stress such as exercise, so RPE is more useful than heart rate to monitor intensity. Blood pressure should be monitored when possible. Because sweating is reduced, the PD patient may have problems with thermoregulation during exercise. Low-intensity exercise in a cool environment is recommended, and patients should be advised to wear light clothing and reminded to drink frequently.

Chronic Fatigue Syndrome

Chronic fatigue syndrome (CFS) is a debilitating condition characterised by excessive fatigue persisting for more than 6 months for which there is no other identifiable clinical cause. Symptoms include cognitive and sleep disturbances, generalised muscle weakness and soreness, fever, and swollen or painful lymph nodes. CFS tends to occur mainly in adults in their late 20s to early 40s. No clear association

Case Study 10.4

As an exercise scientist specialising in musculoskeletal rehabilitation, you are approached by the medical director of a large nursing home. The staff is interested in applying for a community grant to provide physical activity facilities and programs for their residents.

Of the home's residents, about 20% have some type of neurological disorder, mainly Parkinson's disease, a vast majority (>85%) have some form of arthritis, 20% are considered "frail" elderly (refer to chapter 9) and 80% are over 70 years of age.

The home has a large multi-purpose room (7 × 12 m), also used for social functions, that can be used for the program. A large nearby storeroom can house any exercise equipment when not in use. The community grant will fund up to $5,000 of equipment or facility modification.

Design the room layout, indicating the type of equipment you would recommend. Write an adaptable program that can accommodate the needs of all residents (after medical clearance by their doctors, of course).

Key Issues

1. How much, and what type of, exercise equipment would be suitable for this program? Is cost a major factor? Can you organise a suitable program without equipment?

2. What do you think will be priorities for the residents in this activity program? How would you find out about their goals and preferences? What can you do to make the program attractive to the residents?

3. What educational support would you want to include in the program(s) for the home's residents? What organisations might you contact to provide such support or where would you find the information needed?

4. What specific types/modes of activity will you incorporate into the program(s)? Why?

has been established between socio-economic class or educational level and prevalence of CFS. Some studies suggest that women are more likely than men to experience CFS, but this could relate more to sampling and health care settings from which data are obtained than to the actual prevalence (Cox 2000). Symptoms of CFS may persist for up to several years, with periods of relapse, before complete recovery. While the aetiology of the condition is unknown, there appears to be predisposing and precipitating factors common to most cases, and two main current theories attribute the syndrome to a previous viral infection or to immune dysfunction (or to some combination of the two). CFS patients tend to have been high achievers with busy lifestyles in the months to years leading up to the onset of symptoms. Many patients report that symptoms developed after a period of high stress coupled with an acute, usually viral, infection. Main precipitating factors seem to be a combination of high psychosocial stress levels, overwork and viral infection, the latter of which may be the trigger for appearance of symptoms. A tendency for high achievement often means that the individual continues to work, and sometimes exercise, through the infection without allowing adequate recovery from the illness.

Post-exertion fatigue, sometimes lasting days after intense exercise, is frequently reported by CFS patients. CFS shares some similarities of symptoms with depression and the overtraining syndrome (response to excessive exercise training in the high-performance athlete; refer to chapter 11). However, CFS is associated with less mood state disturbance and more physical complaints compared with depression, suggesting different pathophysiological processes (Cox 2000). Athletes experiencing CFS often cite a previous viral infection as the trigger for the onset of symptoms. CFS is unique as a neuromuscular disorder in that it is generally transitory and not permanent or progressive. Patients usually recover without permanent impairment, although this may take months to years

It is currently debated whether CFS is a dysfunction primarily originating in the central nervous system or in peripheral tissues such as skeletal muscle. In some patients, there is evidence that both may contribute, although recent studies strongly suggest a central origin (Freeman and Komaroff 1997). CFS patients appear to exhibit autonomic dysfunction in response to exercise, as evidenced by an inability to achieve age-predicted maximum heart rate (Cordero et al. 1996; De Becker et al. 2000). Because of the muscular weakness and soreness and the post-exertion fatigue experienced by patients with CFS, clinical research has focused on skeletal muscle as a possible site of dysfunction. Some studies suggest impairment of skeletal muscle structure and metabolism, such as abnormalities in mitochondrial structure, increased acidosis upon mild exertion, and alterations in muscle phosphocreatine concentrations and repletion after exercise (McCully et al. 1996). These have not been consistently observed, however. If confirmed by further work, these alterations may indicate significant limitations on the metabolic activity of skeletal muscle, and in turn, the exercise capacity of CFS patients.

Exercise Capacity and CFS

Compared with age-matched healthy individuals and with published norms, CFS patients exhibit low functional capacity, as assessed in an exercise test to volitional fatigue. It is unclear whether such impairment reflects effects of the syndrome itself or results from the detrained state forced on patients as a result of debilitating fatigue. A recent case study assessed exercise capacity in an athlete tested 2 years before the onset of CFS, during the condition and then after recovery (Rowbottom, Keast, Green, et al. 1998). In this athlete, maximum work capacity, $\dot{V}O_2$max and anaerobic threshold remained low even after recovery from CFS. It was concluded that detraining is a major contributor to the low functional capacity, since this remained low even after recovery from illness, and that neurological factors may influence the perception of fatigue. One study using a gradual interval exercise test to volitional fatigue showed nearly normal cardiorespiratory responses (e.g., exercise to 90% of predicted values) with no post-exercise fatigue, suggesting that test format may influence the ability of CFS patients to exercise to maximum (Sisto et al. 1996).

Exercise Prescription for CFS

The low functional capacity, muscular weakness and post-exertion fatigue experienced by CFS patients must be considered when developing the exercise prescription. The general guidelines for moderate-intensity physical activity as discussed in chapter 2 can be used with some modifications. The physical activity program should begin at a relatively low level and should progress gradually. Low functional capacity and alterations in autonomic input to the heart suggest that use of target heart rate may be inappropriate and the RPE scale may provide a better basis for prescribing exercise intensity, especially in the early stages of an exercise program. CFS patients may benefit from interval training with relatively long rests between work intervals. Post-exertion fatigue, when reported, begins within 6 h and may last for 48 h after exercise. Thus, although daily activity may be a long-term goal for the CFS patient, exercise on alternate days may be required in the early stages of a program.

Exercise prescription should also focus on regaining both endurance exercise capacity (e.g., through low-intensity, longer duration interval exercise) and muscular strength (e.g., through circuit-type resistance training with long rest intervals). Resistance training should focus on muscular endurance through high-repetition (>8 reps), lower resistance work. The recommendation given for healthy individuals also applies—start with 1 set and progress to 2 to 3 sets of 8 to 10 exercises of large muscle groups. Gradual progression may help avoid delayed fatigue and muscle soreness. It is important to emphasise gradual progression of exercise intensity and duration because many people with CFS are high achievers who may tend to expect rapid progress or to overdo exercise in the early stages of a program. It is doubtful that the competitive athlete will be able to resume daily high-intensity training until after complete recovery from CFS.

Summary

Musculoskeletal and neuromuscular disorders affect a wide segment of the population at various stages in the lifespan. Some may affect the ability to perform normal movement patterns because of pain (e.g., LBP, arthritis) or neural impairment (e.g., SCI, CP). These conditions may range from being painful and temporarily debilitating but not life threatening (e.g., LBP) to serious permanent impairments caused by severe trauma (e.g., SCI, ABI) to progressive diseases (e.g., MS, PD). In many instances, these conditions are not fatal, and patients often live for extended periods with the disorder or impairment. Physical inactivity imposed by impairment increases the risk of cardiovascular and metabolic diseases. Regular physical activity is recommended for all individuals, including those with physical impairments due to musculoskeletal or neuromuscular disorders. For individuals with musculoskeletal and neuromuscular impairments, there are many potential benefits of a physically active lifestyle—decreased risk of cardiovascular and metabolic diseases and enhanced quality of life, sense of well-being and ability to maintain an independent lifestyle. Because severity of impairment varies widely between individuals, even those with the same disease or condition, it is essential to individualise the physical activity prescription to develop safe and effective programs.

Selected Glossary Terms

acquired brain injury (ABI)—Traumatic brain injury resulting in permanent damage to the affected area of the brain, which may involve cognitive or physical impairment.

antagonist muscle—A muscle or muscle group that opposes the movement of another muscle group.

bone mineral density—Amount of bone tissue (bone mass) per unit volume, reflecting the mineralisation of bone.

cerebral palsy (CP)—A non-progressive neurological disorder of movement or posture caused by lesions in the upper motor neurons of the brain occurring before, at or soon after birth; the main impairment involves loss of control of muscle tone and spinal reflexes, specifically the ability to move, balance and maintain postural control.

chronic fatigue syndrome (CFS)—A debilitating condition characterised by excessive fatigue persisting for more than 6 months for which there is no other identifiable clinical cause. Symptoms include cognitive and sleep disturbances, generalised muscle weakness and soreness, fever, and swollen or painful lymph nodes.

core stability—Muscular endurance and strength of the abdominal and trunk muscles needed for spine stability and postural control.

hemiplegia—Impaired neurological function and movement on one side of the body; occurs in disorders such as cerebral palsy or acquired brain injury.

herniation or **prolapse**—A herniated or "slipped" disk is a protrusion or tearing of the intervertebral disk causing compression of the spinal cord or nerve roots, resulting in back pain and sometimes disability.

multiple sclerosis (MS)—An autoimmune neurological disease in which the body's immune cells breach the blood-brain barrier and attack myelin; the resulting demyelination of nerves disrupts smooth conduction along the neuron, causing disorders of movement and coordination.

osteoarthritis (OA)—The most common form of arthritis in which joint inflammation is caused by structural changes and degradation of articular cartilage in the affected joints, often as a result of injury.

osteoporosis—A disorder of the skeleton characterised by low bone mass (or bone mineral density) and structural deterioration of bone, causing bone fragility and increased risk of fracture.

paraplegia—Impaired neurological function and movement in the lower extremities resulting from injury to the spinal cord in the thoracic region (T2-T12); can be partial or complete.

Parkinson's disease (PD)—A progressive neurological condition involving the extrapyramidal system due to deficiency in the neurotransmitter dopamine that results in a variety of movement disorders such as tremor, akinesia (freezing during movement), muscle rigidity and dyskinesia (involuntary movements).

quadriplegia—Impaired neurological function and movement in all four extremities resulting from injury to the spinal cord in the cervical or upper thoracic region (C1-8, T1); can be partial or complete.

rheumatoid arthritis (RA)—An autoimmune disorder in which substances produced by the body's immune system accumulate within the joints, causing chronic inflammation of the synovial lining and tendons.

spasticity (or hypertonicity)—Increased muscle tone; common in neurological disorders such as cerebral palsy or acquired brain injury; spastic muscles experience a nearly-continual state of contraction, reducing their function and range of motion around nearby joints.

stroke, or **cerebrovascular accident (CVA)**—Caused by vascular insufficiency to the brain as a result of thrombosis (blood clot), haemorrhage (bleeding) or embolism (clot moving through the circulation); often causes permanent loss of physical or cognitive function in the affected part of the brain.

Student Activities and Study Questions

1. In recent years, a technique has been developed using electrical stimulation of skeletal muscles to allow some individuals with SCI to exercise. For which type of people with SCI is this technique suitable? Why? What are the long-term benefits of exercise using electrical stimulation?

2. What particular gait, balance and coordination exercises would you recommend for clients with or at risk of osteoporosis? For those with multiple sclerosis? Parkinson's disease? Explain your answers.

3. Why is chronic fatigue syndrome so difficult to diagnose? Examine the research literature on CFS and exercise/sport. What might be the physiological link between CFS and viral illness in athletes?

4. Locate and attend a public information session on one or more of the diseases/conditions described in this chapter. What are the main concerns of people attending these sessions? Is physical activity mentioned? In what context? Try to discuss physical activity with some of the people attending these sessions. What are their impressions of physical activity for people with impairment? Are they encouraged to become physically active? Why or why not?

5. Attend training sessions and, if possible, sport competitions for athletes with disabilities. What similarities can you see between training programs for able-bodied athletes and those with disabilities in similar sports? What differences (beyond the obvious)? Explain the reasons for any differences you observe.

CHAPTER 11

Optimising Performance of Athletes

So far, this book has focused on promoting physical activity for the wider population and individuals with specific health concerns or impairments who may benefit from physical activity. We now turn our attention to a group of people with other needs—athletes whose primary aim is to enhance performance in sport. Of course, health is still a concern for athletes, but the concern is of a different nature. For the general population and those with impairments, emphasis is placed on the role of physical activity in primary and secondary prevention. In contrast, the main focus for athletes is developing optimal training to enhance performance while keeping the athlete free of illness that might adversely influence performance. Thus, for athletes, both the outcomes (performance rather than health) and methods to achieve these outcomes (intense rather than moderate exercise training) are different.

To fully discuss optimal training for athletes is beyond the scope of a single chapter; there are entire books devoted to assessment and training of high-performance athletes. Rather, this chapter first discusses some general topics related to optimising performance across all sports, such as sport nutrition, **overtraining syndrome, periodisation of training, tapering** and **cross-training.** This is followed by discussion of training techniques for specific types of athletes involved in endurance, speed, strength, power and team sports.

Optimising Nutrition for Athletes

Proper nutrition is an essential component of training the high-performance athlete. In recognition of the importance of proper nutrition, many athletes and teams consult dietitians. Dietary imbalance or deficiency may impair the athlete's performance and health. For example, iron deficiency reduces haemoglobin content in the blood, impairing the ability of blood to deliver oxygen and, ultimately, impairing endurance exercise performance and immunity to infection. Many athletes focus on diet only in the few days before a major competition. In reality, however, attention should be given to diet throughout the season (and even off-season) because of varying dietary needs at different phases of the training cycle.

The competitive athlete's diet must ensure adequate (and optimal) total energy, carbohydrate, protein, water and trace elements such as vitamins and minerals. High-performance athletes train several hours each day, on most if not all days of the week; such training consumes large amounts of energy, and a diet low in energy affects the athlete's ability to maintain a high training load and reduces the quality of work. Low total energy intake has been associated with overtraining syndrome (discussed later in the chapter) and loss of body mass, especially lean tissue. In female athletes, inadequate total energy intake may lead to excessively low body fat levels and hormonal dysfunction, causing menstrual disturbances and loss of bone mass. Protein deficiency interferes with the ability of skeletal muscles to support the increased rate of protein turnover needed for muscle hypertrophy, to repair tissue damaged by intense exercise and to provide metabolic adaptations such as increased enzyme activity. Carbohydrate (CHO) provides an essential substrate (glycogen and glucose) for both endurance and repeated high-intensity sprint/power exercise. A diet low in this nutrient will adversely affect competitive performance and the ability to train at high intensity in endurance, sprint and strength/power sports. Both iron and protein are also required by the immune system; deficiency of either of these factors may increase susceptibility to frequent illness among athletes. Water is an essential, but often neglected, component of a sound diet. Failure to maintain hydration during and after exercise impairs performance and can lead to serious heat illness.

Total Energy Intake

Athletes in heavy training need an estimated 48 to 71 kcal (200-300 kJ) per kg body mass per day to support the energy requirements of training in addition to normal function. The actual value varies by individual, depending on body size (larger athletes need more); age (younger still-growing athletes may need more, veteran athletes less); type, duration and intensity of training; and whether weight gain or loss is required. Often, high-performance athletes training for several hours each day have difficulty simply finding time to consume sufficient energy. The consequences of inadequate total energy consumption include loss of body mass and lean body mass, fatigue, increased risk of overtraining, reduced ability to recover within and between training sessions, and risk of other deficiencies such as **iron-deficiency anaemia** (because a low-energy diet is often low in iron).

To ensure adequate total energy intake, the athlete is advised to eat five to six meals throughout the day. These may need to be deliberately scheduled rather than relying on the athlete to eat when hunger dictates. Many athletes do not feel hungry or cannot tolerate solid meals within a few hours of training (both before and after); liquid meals or supplements can be useful for providing adequate energy and nutrients. Some athletes are required to train intensely while maintaining low body mass (e.g., jockeys, light-weight rowers, gymnasts, wrestlers). These athletes must plan an efficient diet to ensure optimal nutrition in smaller amounts; CHO- and protein-rich foods form an important part of the diet for these athletes.

Carbohydrate

Carbohydrate (CHO) is an essential nutrient for every athlete, regardless of the type of training. Muscle **glycogen** provides a major substrate for both anaerobic glycolysis (used in repeated high-intensity exercise such as sprint, interval or strength training) and oxidative metabolism (as in endurance events or interval exercise with short rest intervals). Muscle glycogen stores may be depleted by repeated high-intensity sprinting, prolonged resistance training, some game activities (such as Australian Rules football) or endurance exercise lasting longer than 40 to 60 min (depending on intensity). The consequences of inadequate CHO intake include general fatigue, inability to complete high-intensity training sessions (because of low muscle glycogen levels) and headache, dizziness or nausea (from low blood glucose levels).

Athletes are advised to consume a CHO-rich diet throughout the training season, providing at least 60% of total daily energy intake. This equates to between 5 and 13 g of CHO per kg body mass per day, depending on the level of activity (see table 11.1) and phase of training or competition cycle. To provide this level of CHO, frequent smaller meals may be needed because many CHO-rich foods are also very filling. CHO-containing fluids, such as sports drinks, and supplements, such as sports bars, may provide sufficient CHO at specific times when solid meals are inconvenient (e.g., in recovery; discussed further later in the chapter).

Simple sugars may make up to 5 to 10% of daily total energy intake during intense prolonged training. Recently, the concept of simple or complex CHO was replaced by the term *glycaemic index (GI)*. The GI of a food indicates the magnitude of increase in blood glucose level after ingestion. To determine GI, blood glucose level is measured 2 h after ingestion of 50 g of a given food. GI is assessed relative to pure glucose (GI = 100), and the lower the GI, the smaller the rise in blood glucose level over the 2 h; table 11.2 lists some low-GI and high-GI foods. If adding high-GI foods to the diet, they should come from low-fat foods such as jams, honey, soft drinks or confection-

TABLE 11.1—Recommended CHO Content of the Diet by Activity Level

Activity level (per day)	Recommended CHO intake
General activity/sport <60 min/day or low-intensity exercise	5-6 g · kg^{-1}
60-120 min high-intensity or >120 min moderate-intensity exercise	6-8 g · kg^{-1}
2-5 h moderate- to high-intensity exercise or during taper before competition	9-10 g · kg^{-1}
Extreme exercise >5 h	12-13 g · kg^{-1}

Compiled from P. Reaburn and D. Jenkins (eds.), 1996, *Training for speed and endurance*. (St. Leonards, NSW: Allen and Unwin), 143.

TABLE 11.2—Examples of Foods With Low and High Glycaemic Index (GI)

Low-GI foods	High-GI foods
Dairy products	Corn flakes
Bran	Potatoes
Beans/legumes	White bread
Nuts	Sweets, confectionery
Pasta	Soft drinks, cordial
Porridge	Watermelon, bananas

Compiled from P. Reaburn and D. Jenkins (eds.), 1996, *Training for speed and endurance*. (St. Leonards, NSW: Allen and Unwin); L. Burke and V. Deakin, 2000, *Clinical sports nutrition*, 2nd ed. (Sydney: McGraw-Hill).

ery and not high-fat items such as chocolate or pastry.

Glycogen synthesis and storage within skeletal muscle are enhanced by a diet high in CHO combined with endurance training. Skeletal muscle glycogen stores are higher in endurance and strength/power athletes than in untrained individuals. CHO ingestion during prolonged exercise (>60 min) delays the onset of fatigue by helping to maintain muscle glycogen and blood glucose levels; CHO ingestion during recovery after intense prolonged exercise enhances muscle glycogen synthesis and replacement of depleted stores. Specific recommendations for CHO intake before, during and in recovery after exercise are discussed in further detail in upcoming sections.

Protein

Exercise increases protein turnover by increasing the rates of both protein degradation and synthesis. When muscle glycogen is depleted during prolonged exercise (whether continuous or interval), protein may be used as a substrate for ATP production; amino acids may provide up to 10% of the energy requirements in glycogen-depleting exercise. Over the long term, a protein-deficient diet may cause impaired immune function and muscle wasting. On an absolute basis, both endurance and strength/speed athletes require extra protein compared with the average non-athlete. The general recommendations are as follows:

► Sedentary individuals: 0.8 g protein per kg body mass per day

► Strength/power/speed athletes: 1.5 to 2.0 g per kg

► Endurance athletes: 1.5 to 1.6 g per kg

Although athletes require additional protein, it can be provided by a well-balanced diet high in CHO and moderate in protein, without the need for protein supplements. Since the athlete consumes more total energy each day because of higher energy demands, a well-balanced diet automatically provides the additional protein needed. For example, a 70-kg athlete consuming 4,800 kcal [20 MJ] per day of total energy, of which the protein content is 12 to 15% (as recommended), would take in 136 to 170 g of protein each day. This equates to 1.9 to 2.4 g of protein per kg body mass, which more than meets the recommended protein intake for an endurance athlete.

Excess protein in the diet or provided through supplements is either excreted in urine or used to synthesise fats. High-protein foods and supplements are expensive, and over the long term, excessive protein intake may cause kidney damage. To provide sufficient protein each day, the athlete should consume up to five meals of about equal protein content, about 35 g of protein at each meal. Low-fat animal protein is generally the best source because it provides all of the essential amino acids and is a good source of other essential nutrients such as iron, calcium and zinc. Strictly vegetarian athletes undertaking intense exercise training may need to make a conscious effort to consume sufficient protein.

Fat

A diet high in CHO (>60% of energy from CHO) and moderate in protein (~15% of energy) generally leaves little chance for too much fat. Moderate fat consumption is recommended for all individuals because of the association between a high-fat diet (especially saturated fat) and obesity, dyslipidaemia and other disorders (discussed in chapter 8). In addition, the athlete needs to consume a relatively low-fat diet to avoid excessive fat deposition. Adipose tissue is not metabolically active (i.e., does not contribute to performing physical work), and any excess requires additional energy for movement. On the other hand, fatty acids provide a major substrate for exercise and are needed for several essential bodily functions such as hormone synthesis and cell growth. A diet containing too little fat (<10% of daily energy) can lead to low levels of the protective HDL-C and excessively low body fat levels, contributing to hormonal dysfunction, especially in female athletes. A moderate-fat diet providing about 20 to 25% of total energy from fats is recommended. Saturated fats (primarily from animal sources) should be minimised by choosing low-fat varieties (e.g., lean cuts of meat, low-fat dairy products) or substituting unsaturated or monounsaturated items (e.g., margarine instead of butter).

In recent years, some have suggested that fat loading (the "Zone diet") enhances endurance performance. This controversial diet is relatively high in fat (40% of total energy), low in CHO (40% of energy) and high in protein (20% of energy). The few studies showing benefits from fat loading have used previously untrained subjects or recreational athletes training at low intensity (~60% $\dot{V}O_2$max). There is at present little scientific evidence to support this diet for the competitive, high-performance athlete training at higher intensity (≥80% $\dot{V}O_2$max) who relies on CHO (glycogen) as a major substrate. In contrast, a wealth of scientific evidence demonstrates the need for a high-CHO diet for endurance athletes. There is also current interest in supplementing the diet with medium chain triglycerides; it is thought that their easy entry into the mitochondria may enhance fuel availability and thus enhance performance. However, there is at best equivocal evidence of enhanced performance with this type of supplement.

Iron

Iron is an essential element (called a *mineral* in the nutrition literature) for synthesis of oxygen-carrying components, such as haemoglobin and myoglobin, and cytochromes of oxidative metabolic pathways (electron transfer chain). Iron deficiency in athletes is caused by increased red blood cell turnover and iron loss in sweat. Intense exercise may also lead to destruction of red blood cells (haemolysis) because of oxidative and mechanical stress and changes in blood pH. Iron deficiency (anaemia) results in fatigue, reduced endurance exercise capacity and increased risk of infection. The level of serum ferritin (an iron storage protein) provides a good indication of total body iron stores. Although iron is contained in many foods, it is best absorbed from animal sources, such as red meat. Thus, vegetarian athletes must be especially careful to avoid iron deficiency. Vitamin C aids in absorption of iron, whereas tea or excess fibre can interfere with iron absorption. An athlete with significant iron deficiency should seek treatment by a doctor and dietitian, and iron supplementation is generally a short-term (weeks) rather than long-term strategy. Supplementation is beneficial only for athletes who are anaemic because of iron deficiency and offers no benefit to performance in athletes who are not deficient. Excessive iron intake is generally not helpful, can interfere with absorption of other elements such as zinc, may cause uncomfortable side effects, such as constipation or intestinal pain, and can be dangerous in those with a genetic disposition toward iron storage disease.

Optimising Nutrition Throughout Training and Competition

Although these general dietary guidelines apply throughout most of the training season, there are particular times when slight alterations are needed to provide an optimal diet. Such times include the few days before competition and during and immediately after exercise (whether in competition or training).

Pre-Competition Diet

Maximising muscle glycogen stores is the main focus during the few days before competition, especially for events in which glycogen depletion may occur. Time to fatigue in intense endurance or repeated interval exercise is related to initial muscle glycogen levels; increasing these levels can delay the time to fatigue and thus enhance performance. Glycogen supercompensation or **carbohydrate loading** diets are recommended for continuous exercise lasting more than 60 min or when multiple games are played over a few days during a tournament. CHO loading is accomplished by consuming a diet containing >10 g CHO per kg body mass for 2 to 3 days before competition. Exercise volume must also be correspondingly reduced during this time (tapered) to allow the muscles to increase glycogen synthesis.

The pre-event meal should be easily digestible to provide CHO and fluid yet minimise discomfort, and foods should be familiar to the athlete. The meal should include foods low in fat (fat takes longer to digest), a mixture of low to high GI (to ensure adequate glucose) and foods low in fibre (to minimise gastric discomfort). Fluids are especially important (discussed in the following section). Table 11.3 lists some commercially available CHO drinks and supplements and their recommended use before, during and after exercise.

A larger meal may be eaten 3 to 4 h before competition and a smaller snack 2 h before. Some athletes are too nervous to comfortably eat a solid meal before competition, and liquid supplements may be better tolerated. Some individuals are sensitive to high-CHO foods within 1 h of competition, exhibiting an insulin-mediated rebound hypoglycaemia, which causes symptoms such as fatigue or headache. These athletes should avoid foods with a high GI such as soft drinks, cordial or confectionery within 1 h of competition.

TABLE 11.3—Commercially Available CHO Supplements

Supplement	CHO composition	Optimal time of ingestion[a] and purpose
Sports drink	5-7% by volume	Before—ensure hydration During—maintain hydration, provide CHO After—replace fluids and electrolytes, enhance glycogen replacement
High CHO drink	>13% by volume	2-5 h before—maximise glycogen levels After—enhance glycogen replacement
Sports bar	>70% of energy	2 h before—pre-event snack During—CHO source when solid food needed After—enhance glycogen replacement
CHO gel	>50% by volume	Before and during (only with additional fluids)—maximise glycogen levels After—enhance glycogen replacement

[a]Before, during or after exercise.

Compiled from H. O'Connor, 1996, "Practical aspects of fluid replacement," *Australian Journal of Nutrition and Dietetics* 53: S27-S34; J. Pearce, 1996, "Nutritional analysis of Australian and New Zealand fluid beverage replacement," *Australian Journal of Nutrition and Dietetics* 53: S35-S42.

Foods During Exercise

Consumption of CHO during exercise prevents hypoglycaemia and delays muscle glycogen depletion, particularly in type I (slow twitch) muscle fibres. Thus, CHO supplementation during exercise enhances performance in events lasting longer than 60 min. The choice of CHO in a liquid or solid form is a matter of preference and may be determined by the sport. For example, only liquids can be easily consumed during distance running, but solid food may be eaten during road cycling. Solid foods should be easily digestible and low in fat and fibre, such as bananas or sports bars. Fluid replacement is essential during prolonged exercise, especially in the heat, and should not be compromised by ingestion of solid foods. CHO-containing liquids, such as sports drinks, may be better tolerated and provide needed fluids as well as CHO. Most sports drinks contain 6% glucose (i.e., 60 g CHO per 1 L fluid), as well as sodium chloride (salt) to enhance fluid uptake. A general guideline is to consume 600 to 1,400 ml of fluid containing 50 g CHO per hour of exercise. The amount of fluid and CHO will vary with the athlete's size and position (in team games), intensity and duration of exercise, mode of exercise, and ambient temperature and humidity. A relatively large volume of fluid ingestion is needed to maintain a high rate of gastric emptying. The GI of a food eaten during exercise is not important because insulin is suppressed during exercise.

Diet to Aid Recovery

Food consumed during recovery after exercise should enhance muscle and liver glycogen replenishment, replace fluids and electrolytes, and support increased protein synthesis. This is especially important when there is limited recovery time between training sessions (e.g., twice per day) or during competition (e.g., multi-game tournament). Food consumed during the first few hours after exercise is crucial for enhancing muscle glycogen replacement. Under normal dietary conditions, complete replacement of muscle glycogen stores may take 24 h after exercise. However, glycogen replacement may be enhanced by manipulating the time and type of foods eaten during the crucial first few hours after exercise. For example, eating high CHO foods immediately and for several hours after exercise hastens glycogen recovery in depleted muscles. When a subsequent exercise session is planned within 6 to 12 h, one recommendation is to consume 1 g of CHO per kg body mass in the first 30 min after the first bout of exercise and again every 2 h up to the subsequent session. Muscle glycogen stores are re-

placed faster by foods with moderate to high GI, such as sports drinks, glucose confectionery, cordials, soft drinks, some fruits, bread and wheat cereals (refer to table 11.2). Fortunately, these foods are generally well tolerated after exercise, and some (e.g., drinks, fruits) also assist with rehydration.

In the **post-exercise recovery period,** injury to skeletal muscle will slightly increase the need for protein (to repair injured tissue) and may also slow the rate of glycogen synthesis (because the muscle's structure is disrupted). There is some evidence that combining protein with high-CHO foods during recovery enhances muscle glycogen replacement compared with high CHO alone (Rankin 1997). Figures 11.1 and 11.2 give some examples of foods containing 50 g CHO and 10 g protein that would be suitable in such instances.

Fluid Loss and Replacement

A well-trained athlete may lose up to 2 to 3 L of water per hour of heavy exercise. Even slight dehydration, equivalent to 2 to 3% of body mass (about 1.5-2.0 L for a 70-kg person), can adversely affect performance in events lasting more than 15 to 20 min. Besides poor performance, dehydration may cause fatigue, muscle cramps, headaches, gastric

---

4 slices bread

1.25 cups cooked pasta

60 g cereal

4 pikelets

2 medium potatoes

2 cups baked beans

1.5 cups lentils or kidney beans

3 apples

2 bananas

50 g jelly beans

1-1.5 sports bars

2.5 muesli bars

750 ml sports drink

600 ml orange juice

Compiled from P. Reaburn and D. Jenkins (eds.), 1996, *Training for speed and endurance.* (St. Leonards, NSW: Allen and Unwin); L. Burke and V. Deakin, 2000, *Clinical sports nutrition,* 2nd ed. (Sydney: McGraw-Hill).

FIGURE 11.1   Examples of foods containing 50 g carbohydrate.

upset and possibly serious heat illness. Thermoregulation occurs primarily through evaporative heat loss (sweating) during exercise, especially in the heat, and fluid replacement is important both during and after exercise. Because absorption of fluid from the gut is limited to about 800 ml per hour during exercise, it is not possible to fully rehydrate during exercise. However, drinking 250 ml every 15 to 20 min reduces fluid loss and corresponding loss of blood volume, aiding thermoregulation and minimising the rise in core temperature. Plain water is sufficient for fluid replacement for exercise up to 60 min duration. For events longer than 60 min, addition of CHO and NaCl (e.g., sports drinks) is generally recommended. Excessive amounts of CHO interfere with water absorption from the gut, but CHO content up to 6% by volume does not impair fluid replacement; most sports drinks contain about 6% CHO by volume.

Thirst is a poor indicator of the need for fluids, and a conscious effort must be made to replace fluids after exercise. A simple guide to the extent of net fluid loss during exercise is the difference between pre-exercise and post-exercise body mass. Whenever possible, this difference should be corrected by adequate fluid replacement before the next exercise session. General recommendations for fluid intake for events lasting longer than 30 min are given in table 11.4. Adding sodium and CHO to fluids (e.g., sports drinks) enhances fluid retention and is often more palatable than plain water. Drinks with caffeine or alcohol should not be used for fluid replacement because these are diuretics (i.e., they increase fluid loss via the kidneys). Adding glycerol to fluids before exercise (hyperhydration) is not any more effective at preventing fluid loss than electrolyte solutions and can produce headache or nausea.

Vegetarian Athletes

Many athletes follow some type of vegetarian diet, either consuming only plant-derived foods (vegan) or consuming plant-derived foods plus only certain animal products, such as dairy products or eggs. As long as their diets are planned and well informed, vegetarian athletes can ensure optimal nutrition. Vegetarian athletes who do not plan their diets are at risk of deficiencies of total energy, protein, calcium, iron, zinc and vitamin B12. Most susceptible are those athletes who avoid animal products without a conscious effort to replace these

---

2 cups cooked pasta

30-35 g lean chicken, beef or lamb

50 g fish

90 g breakfast cereal

220 g (1-1.5 cups) baked beans

50 g nuts

4 slices bread

200 g non-fat fruit yoghurt

Compiled from P. Reaburn and D. Jenkins (eds.), 1996, *Training for speed and endurance.* (St. Leonards, NSW: Allen and Unwin); L. Burke and V. Deakin, 2000, *Clinical sports nutrition*, 2nd ed. (Sydney: McGraw-Hill).

FIGURE 11.2   Examples of foods containing 10 g protein.

TABLE 11.4—Recommended Fluid Intake Before, During and After Competition

Time	Amount
Night before	>500 ml
Upon waking	>500 ml
1 h before	500-1,000 ml
20 min before	250-500 ml
During	250 ml every 15-20 min
After	To replace body mass lost during exercise

Before and during exercise will only be of benefit in events >30 min.

Compiled from H. O'Connor, 1996, "Practical aspects of fluid replacement," *Australian Journal of Nutrition and Dietetics* 53: S27-S34.

essential components from non-animal sources. It is preferable to obtain these nutrients from dietary sources rather than supplements, and consultation with a dietitian may be warranted. Some general guidelines to ensure adequate energy intake and to minimise the risk of nutritional deficiency are to

- include some animal foods such as dairy products or eggs whenever possible;
- consume five to six moderate-sized meals each day to ensure adequate energy intake without discomfort;
- eat energy-dense foods such as nuts, seeds, legumes and dried fruits;
- obtain protein from a variety of foods (e.g., cereals, legumes, nuts, rice);
- eat a variety of fruits and vegetables to ensure adequate vitamin and mineral intake; and
- include calcium-fortified foods (e.g., some breakfast cereals and soy products) if dairy products are not consumed.

In general, the more varied and less restrictive the vegetarian diet, the less likely it is to lead to nutritional deficiencies.

Overtraining

Excessive training may lead to a condition called overtraining syndrome (OTS). OTS is characterised by poor performance in training and competition (despite continued training), persistent fatigue, frequent minor illnesses (such as the common cold and influenza), disturbed sleep and changes in mood state such as depression or loss of motivation. Although OTS occurs in most, if not all, sports, it seems to develop most frequently in endurance athletes training several hours each day (e.g., swimmers, rowers, triathletes, cyclists) and in competitive weightlifters. The exact causes of OTS are not known at present, but contributing factors include

- sudden increases in training volume;
- frequent competition;
- inadequate rest and recovery between training sessions and competitive seasons;
- insufficient nutrition, especially total energy and CHO; and
- high perceived stress levels, whether or not directly related to sport.

Case Study 11.1

As the exercise scientist for a team of cyclists, you are asked to assist the chef/caterer who has been contracted to provide all the team's meals during a 10-day cycle tour. The caterer will need to order and prepare all food to be consumed by the cyclists starting 3 days before the race and continuing for the entire 10 days of racing. This includes food consumed in the mornings and evenings at each day's accommodation, along with food consumed while cyclists are racing during the day.

The chef is creative and enthusiastic about the challenge of working with the team, but she is uncertain as to what particular foods she should prepare to meet the cyclists' dietary needs during the race. Draw up a list of various foods that would be appropriate for the team. Also include menus for 2 "typical" days during the race.

Key Issues

1. What are the cyclists' particular dietary needs during the 10 days of racing? What foods best meet these needs? Why?
2. How can the cyclists balance the need for rehydration and replacement of carbohydrate during and after each day's racing?
3. How will the athletes be able to eat while racing? What foods are recommended and why?
4. How will the chef estimate the quantity of food to be ordered and prepared?
5. Should the cyclists consume any dietary supplements or vitamins throughout the 10 days? Why or why not?

Athletes and coaches are very interested in finding objective indicators or even predictors of OTS that will identify susceptible athletes before symptoms appear. Once performance has begun to deteriorate, it is often too late to adjust training to allow sufficient recovery before important competition. There are myriad purported indicators of OTS, but few have been supported by empirical study. Table 11.5 lists those indicators and predictors of OTS that have been supported by the scientific literature.

Performance deterioration is, by definition, an obvious sign of OTS; decrements of 1 to 20% have been documented in overtrained athletes from a number of sports. A decreased ability to maintain high-intensity exercise, as measured by time to fatigue at 110% of the **individual anaerobic threshold (IAT),** usually on a cycle ergometer, is also a good performance indicator. OTS is associated with decreasing heart rate and blood lactate levels after maximal exercise, most likely due to autonomic dysfunction and decreased production of catecholamines. This is reflected in a decrease in blood noradrenaline levels after maximal exercise and decreased production of the hormone. Because of the expense and inconvenience, hormonal measures are not used as routine markers except in scientific studies of OTS. Changes in mood state occur during OTS, as assessed by the Profile of Mood States (POMS) questionnaire or by the athlete's self-reported analysis of well-being. These include anxiety, depression, apathy, lack of motivation, high perceived stress levels, persistent fatigue not relieved by a rest day and disturbed sleep patterns (e.g., not feeling rested after a long sleep or inability to sleep). Some of these indicators, such as persistent fatigue and high perceived stress levels, may precede the appearance of other symptoms and poor performance; they should be investigated if not resolved with a few days rest.

Other suspected indicators of OTS have not been consistently supported by the research literature. These include blood markers (e.g., serum ferritin or enzyme levels), other hormones (e.g., testosterone, cortisol), early morning heart rate (EMHR) and changes in body mass. Many athletes routinely monitor EMHR as an indicator of OTS, thinking that EMHR rises in advance of OTS. However, most studies of OTS have failed to find any changes in EMHR despite other clear indications of the syndrome. EMHR may be affected by a number of factors including dehydration, temperature and anticipation of the day's events. Measuring maximum

---

TABLE 11.5—Valid and Reliable Markers for Identifying and Predicting Overtraining Syndrome (OTS)

Marker	Expected change during OTS
Performance on standard maximal exercise test (e.g., time trial)	Decreased
Time to exhaustion at 110% IAT	Decreased
Maximal heart rate	Decreased
Maximal blood lactate level	Decreased
Maximal blood noradrenaline level or nocturnal noradrenaline excretion	Decreased
Self-analysis by athlete	Increased fatigue and stress levels, decreased quality of sleep
Profile of Mood States (POMS)	Increased TMD and depression, decreased vigour

Abbreviations: IAT = individual anaerobic threshold as defined by the 4 mmol · L^{-1} method; TMD = total mood disturbance as measured in the POMS.

Compiled from S.L. Hooper and L.T. Mackinnon, 1995, "Monitoring overtraining in athletes: Recommendations," *Sports Medicine* 20: 321-327.

heart rate after training is just as easily performed and is a far better indicator of OTS.

Athletes routinely train intensely, often to the point of overtraining, and it is essential to find a balance between training and recovery. Effective prevention of OTS requires the ability to identify which athletes are showing early signs before actual symptoms occur; the science (and art) of training athletes has not yet reached this point. In the absence of clear indicators and predictors, some general guidelines can be given based on the current state of knowledge about the causes of and contributing factors to OTS. Among these are the following:

► Gradually increase training volume and intensity.

► Progressively introduce new modes of training (e.g., resistance training).

► Periodise training and schedule rest days and recovery sessions.

► Individualise training because there is individual variation in the threshold that induces OTS.

► Identify susceptible athletes based on previous training and performance history.

► Monitor all athletes, and especially susceptible athletes, for early warning signs.

► Ensure athletes rest during the off-season.

Periodisation of Training

Periodisation of training refers to a process of planning the entire season in advance by dividing it into shorter phases, each emphasising one or more particular aspects of training. Training is planned on a daily, weekly, monthly and sometimes yearly basis, often aiming for peak performance at a particular event such as the Olympic Games. Phases are generally divided into preparation (early season), competition and off-season. Each phase is divided into shorter sub-phases, termed *microcycles,* usually lasting 1 week, and *macrocycles,* usually lasting 3 to 5 weeks. Each phase and cycle has a particular focus, for example, to increase endurance capacity during

Case Study 11.2

Sam is 25 and a former State-ranked 10,000-m runner who has recently begun competing in marathons. He has been running about 130 km in eight sessions per week but has recently been forced to reduce this training volume because of extreme fatigue and persistent muscle soreness. Sam works full time as an accountant, and although his employer has been very supportive of his sporting career in the past, she is not pleased with his apparent lethargy and apathy during working hours. He reports that he sleeps poorly and is losing weight because he is often too tired to prepare meals. He has been living on breakfast cereal and take-away food (pizza, fish and chips) for much of the past 3 months.

Sam comes to you for help since you are a well-known exercise physiologist specialising in endurance sports such as marathon running, road cycling and triathlon. He wants to know what is happening to him and how he can resume training in preparation for a major marathon in 6 months. Write a 6-month training program to allow him to compete in this marathon.

Key Issues

1. What is likely the main cause of Sam's fatigue and inability to train? How will you confirm this?

2. What factors have contributed to his current state? What advice will you give to help him address these factors?

3. Are there other possible causes? Would you refer Sam to his doctor or other health professionals? Why or why not?

4. Is it feasible for Sam to compete in a marathon in 6 months? If so, what are the most important factors to incorporate into his training over the next 6 months?

the early season. To avoid overuse injuries and overtraining and to allow rest before starting the next cycle, recovery sessions or days are programmed into the microcycles and macrocycles. The pre-competition taper (reduced training before major competition) should also be programmed into the competition phase.

In planning each microcycle, the coach or athlete must consider its place in the macrocycle and the volume and intensity of training in the previous microcycles. Each microcycle should ensure a balance between different modes of training, for example, dryland (weights) training and pool sessions for the swimmer and weights, sprints and plyometric training for the track sprinter. Adequate recovery is needed between high-intensity sessions, which should be spread evenly across the week. To prevent injury and to allow adequate recovery, it is common for athletes to perform only three high-intensity sessions per week, focusing on other aspects of training in the other sessions. Within each session, the order of activities is also important. Work on speed, power and technique usually precedes general fitness (endurance) exercise since fatigue from prior endurance exercise can interfere with development of power and skill.

Preparation (Early Season) Phase

The main focus of the early season is to develop general fitness (usually some degree of endurance capacity) early in this phase to prepare for high-intensity training both later in the phase and in the competition phase. Enhancing endurance capacity early in the season allows better recovery within and between high-intensity training sessions and during competition involving repeated high-intensity work (e.g., team games). The preparation phase usually lasts for two to three macrocycles (i.e., 6-12 weeks), depending on the sport and length of season. Training begins with high-volume, low-intensity work early in the phase, with volume progressively decreasing while intensity increases later in the phase. Both continuous and interval exercise may be included, depending on the sport. Speed and games athletes often use interval exercise to train at higher intensity and to enhance recovery between repetitions, whereas endurance athletes may include more continuous exercise or longer work intervals with short rest periods.

The preparation phase is also the time to develop muscular strength and hypertrophy as a basis for later speed or power work, especially in contact (e.g., football) or speed (e.g., sprinting) sports. If strength and endurance training are included within the same phase **(concurrent training),** it is possible that the endurance training will interfere with maximal strength development. If development of strength is a priority in the early season, it is preferable that endurance and strength training be emphasised in different macrocycles. Alternating strength and endurance training sessions on different days and avoiding training both within the same session will help maximise strength gains during this phase. During the early season, the focus may also move from general to specific skills.

Competition Phase

After focusing on endurance and strength in the previous phase, the athlete now begins working at intensities as close to race/competition pace as possible ("quality" training). Training thus becomes more specific to the sport and particular event or position (in team games). Training volume is generally lower, but intensity is higher than in the previous phase. For team game athletes, training focuses more on specific skills, strategies and team cohesion. Speed and power athletes shift from a focus on muscular strength to power, plyometric and skill training (e.g., starts and short sprints by the track sprinter). Endurance athletes may add interval work (e.g., track work by the marathon runner). During this phase, the athlete is most susceptible to overuse injuries and overtraining, so programmed recovery sessions and rest days become very important. In sports with weekly competition (e.g., many team game sports), each microcycle may be somewhat similar. In other sports with less frequent competition, and especially in years including international competition (e.g., elite swimming, marathon running, rowing), the program will look very different. Training intensity will build progressively until the taper before the major event(s) (e.g., team selection trials, world championships).

Tapering for Peak Performance

The taper is a period of reduced training, lasting from a few days up to 3 weeks, before major competition. The duration and type of taper are highly variable depending on the sport, the individual athlete and the frequency of competition. Athletes are often trained close to the point of overtraining, and the taper provides sufficient rest to maximise the positive effects of training while minimising the negative effects such as fatigue and muscle soreness. Athletes cannot rest completely during the taper, however, because the effects of detraining begin within a few days of cessation of training. Successful tapering requires a careful balance of sufficient training volume and intensity to maintain fitness while still allowing sufficient rest.

Training volume, intensity and frequency may be manipulated independently in the taper. In the few sports studied (mainly distance running and swimming), it appears that training volume may be reduced by more than 50% over 2 weeks, provided that intensity is maintained. In a study on distance runners, training volume was reduced by 85% while intensity was maintained (at 100% $\dot{V}O_2$max) through interval running over 7 days (Houmard et al. 1994). The taper group improved 5 km time-trial performance by 3% and submaximal running economy (oxygen cost of running at a given pace) by 6%. In contrast, these variables did not improve in a control group of runners who did not taper or in a group of runners who tapered using a similar program except substituting cycling for running. A study on competitive swimmers showed that reducing training volume while maintaining intensity was equally effective using three different methods (reducing training frequency, reducing volume within each session or monitoring subjective responses in swimmers) (Hooper, Mackinnon, and Ginn 1998). In a study on middle-distance runners who performed a 6-day taper of high-intensity interval training, reducing volume by 75% resulted in better 800-m performance compared with a 50% reduction in volume (Mujika et al. 2000).

The requirement of high-intensity training while reducing volume suggests that maintaining adaptations of metabolic pathways and motor recruitment patterns may be important for a successful taper (Houmard et al. 1994). During the taper, other modes of training are usually omitted to reduce fatigue; for example, resistance training is dropped during the taper for swimmers. Changes in levels of stress hormones (e.g., catecholamines; Hooper, Mackinnon, and Howard 1999) and other blood variables (e.g., blood lactate, haemoglobin and red cell concentrations; Mujika et al. 2000) during the taper predict improvement in performance during subsequent competition, suggesting a role for neuroendocrine and biochemical adaptations. The improvement in running economy (Houmard et al. 1994) during the taper suggests that recovery from muscle fatigue or soreness also contributes to a successful taper.

The optimal length of the taper depends on the sport, event or distance, and training history. Short

tapers (less than 1 week) may be effective earlier in the season when accumulated fatigue is lower, but longer tapers (2-3 weeks) may be needed later if the athlete has been training intensely for several months. Tapering appears to lose its effectiveness if done too often (although this has not been thoroughly studied), and the taper must be used judiciously by athletes who compete frequently. It is likely that physical fitness and thus performance will plateau or decline if tapering is the predominant form of training.

Off-Season Phase

The off-season phase is important for rest, recovery and healing of any injuries incurred during the season. High-performance athletes cannot train intensely year-round without appreciable breaks, and omitting the off-season recovery period is likely to lead to poor performance and overtraining in the next season. This phase concentrates on maintaining physical fitness while permitting needed physical and psychological rest. Low- to moderate- intensity endurance and interval training maintain aerobic exercise capacity at a somewhat lower, but acceptable, level than during the season. Speed, power and team game athletes are advised to train once per week using moderately high (60-80% maximal speed) interval training to maintain adaptations in type II skeletal muscle fibres. Athletes who use resistance training during the season also benefit from moderate strength training once per week to maintain muscle mass and strength. Cross-training is useful to maintain fitness, allow recovery from injuries and provide a needed break from a particular sport. The off-season may also provide time to focus on particular deficits, for example, improving flexibility and joint range of motion through a stretching program or correcting an imbalance between muscle groups.

Concurrent Strength and Endurance Training

Many sports require both cardiovascular fitness and muscular strength and power, requiring athletes to undertake both endurance and strength/power training. Including both of these components in the same training microcycle, known as concurrent training, is beneficial for developing all aspects of fitness in recreational and non-elite athletes; however, under some conditions, high-intensity endurance training may interfere with development of muscular strength and power in high-performance athletes. Strength (in high-velocity muscle actions) and power seem to be most affected by concurrent endurance training. In contrast, aerobic power and endurance exercise capacity are not adversely affected by concurrent strength/power training. It is not clear which mechanisms are responsible for this apparent interference in strength and power development by concurrent endurance training.

Strength and endurance training cause very different structural and biochemical changes within skeletal muscle—intense strength training induces hypertrophy and adaptations of the non-oxidative pathways in predominantly type II fibres, whereas endurance training induces metabolic adaptations of the oxidative pathways with less hypertrophy in predominantly type I fibres. It would appear that skeletal muscle cannot maximally adapt to both types of training simultaneously. The negative effect of concurrent training on power and strength at high but not low velocity suggests that neural components may also be involved. In addition, early studies showing interference in strength development may have caused some degree of overtraining by requiring subjects to maintain high-intensity endurance and strength training on a daily basis over several weeks to months. It is thought that daily intense concurrent training does not allow sufficient recovery between sessions, so the athlete begins each subsequent session in a fatigued state and cannot achieve the near maximal strength/power that would be achieved in a more rested condition. A more recent study (McCarthy et al. 1995) showed no interference with strength development during a more reasonable concurrent training program that would be less likely to cause overtraining (3 days per week for each component). Thus, athletes should not be discouraged from training both cardiovascular endurance and muscular strength concurrently, provided that the program is periodised and the coach and athlete are aware of the risk of (and thus seek to avoid) overtraining.

Cross-Training

Cross-training refers to the use of exercise modes that differ from those used in a particular sport. Examples include water running for distance runners and cycling for swimmers or runners. Although cross-training seems to contradict the concept of specificity of training (i.e., benefits are specific to the type of training), there is evidence supporting the use of cross-training for competitive athletes. Introducing cross-training into a training program serves several purposes:

▶ To provide variety and ease boredom
▶ To develop general physical fitness early in the season
▶ To maintain general physical fitness during the off-season or during rehabilitation from injury
▶ To provide recovery training (e.g., the day after competition)
▶ To improve a specific component of physical fitness (e.g., $\dot{V}O_2$max or lactate clearance)
▶ To maintain or intensify training while preventing overtraining or overuse injuries
▶ To promote loss of excess fat

In a study on well-trained distance runners, 5 km running performance was enhanced to a similar extent after 6 weeks of intensified training (increased volume) regardless of mode—interval running or cycling (Flynn et al. 1998). Although the mechanisms responsible for the beneficial effects of cross-training are unclear at present, cross-training appears to maintain or enhance general measures of physical fitness such as $\dot{V}O_2$max. It has been postulated that cross-training may also increase lactate clearance and **lactate threshold,** allowing the athlete to maintain a higher pace (Flynn et al. 1998). This may occur if cross-training recruits skeletal muscle fibres not recruited in the normal mode and induces training adaptations in these fibres, which may then provide additional sites for lactate disposal during exercise. Cross-training does not appear to alter economy of movement (oxygen cost of exercising at a certain pace). However, the topic has not been studied extensively to date, and at present, cross-training is used primarily by athletes to maintain fitness during recovery from injury or in the off-season and to occasionally provide variety during periods of intense training.

Training for Endurance Sports

Although a high $\dot{V}O_2$max is essential for elite performance in endurance sports, it is not the sole determinant of performance. At the elite level, endurance performance is best predicted by the individual athlete's anaerobic threshold (work rate at the inflection point of blood lactate level or minute ventilation) and economy of movement (oxygen cost of working at a given pace). While elite endurance athletes exhibit high $\dot{V}O_2$max values, this does not correlate with performance as highly as anaerobic threshold. One factor that does distinguish top performers from the sub-elite is the ability to perform prolonged exercise at a relatively high percentage, between 80 to 90%, of $\dot{V}O_2$max. In contrast, non-elite or recreational athletes can usually maintain prolonged effort at only 70 to 75% of $\dot{V}O_2$max and the untrained at an even lower relative exercise intensity. Economy of movement is especially important in weight-bearing endurance exercise, such as distance running, or in activities requiring high-level technical skill, such as swimming. Two athletes may have the same $\dot{V}O_2$max, but the athlete with the higher economy of movement will perform better. Elite endurance athletes may be up to 15% more economical than non-elite, suggesting that economy of movement may be trained by improving technique and fitness.

Endurance training often relies on the use of heart rate (HR) or lactate threshold to set exercise intensity. Lactate threshold can be assessed using a staged exercise test of intervals of increasing intensity. Blood is sampled at the end of each stage, and a curve of blood lactate versus work rate plotted. From this lactate curve, a work rate or heart rate at the

point of inflection is then used to set exercise training pace. There are several protocols to determine the lactate threshold, and it is beyond the scope of this chapter to discuss the relative merits of each (Gore 2000).

If assessment of lactate threshold is not possible, a simpler method to set training intensity is using a percentage of maximum HR (HRmax). This requires measurement of actual heart rate during maximal exercise rather than relying on an age-predicted value, which is too imprecise for athletes. HRmax can be measured at the end of 10 1-min intervals of increasing pace, beginning at moderate intensity and ending with an all-out effort. HRmax should be measured immediately after the final interval, preferably with a heart rate monitor. (To prevent injury, it is essential to first complete an extensive cardiovascular and muscular warm-up before the sprints and end with a similar cool-down afterward.) Because HRmax varies by exercise mode and body position, the mode of this test must be specific to the type of training. HRmax will be higher in upright compared with supine exercise, exercise in air compared with in water, and exercise using the entire body compared with isolated body segments. For example, HRmax in running is about 10 beats/min higher than in cycling (less body mass involved) and 10 to 20 beats/min higher than in swimming (supine exercise in water). HRmax is achieved sooner (i.e., at a lower work rate) in a hot compared with a cool environment. Table 11.6 gives general recom-

TABLE 11.6—General Recommendations for Setting Exercise Intensity for Endurance Training Using HRmax

Percentage of HRmax	Purpose and recommendations
65-75%	Recovery between intervals, recovery day after an intense session, after competition
75-85%	30-120 min continuous or interval training to develop or maintain cardiovascular fitness
>85%	Approximates race pace (±5%) 20-60 min continuous or interval training to develop lactate tolerance and fatigue resistance May induce glycogen depletion Generally no more than two sessions per wk

Compiled from P. Reaburn and D. Jenkins (eds.), 1996, *Training for speed and endurance*. (St. Leonards, NSW: Allen and Unwin).

mendations for setting exercise intensity using the HRmax method.

Periodisation of Training for the Endurance Athlete

Periodisation is important for optimising endurance training while avoiding overtraining or overuse injuries (see table 11.7). A solid aerobic base must be set early before quality high-intensity work is undertaken later in the season. A typical microcycle might include one rest day (very important), two recovery sessions (lower-intensity), two moderate-intensity sessions and two high-intensity sessions per week. Macrocycles often include microcycles of varying intensity, for example, a 3-week macrocycle that starts with a hard week, followed by an easy week, then a moderate week, then on to a hard week of the next macrocycle.

The early season (preparation) phase emphasises increasing volume at relatively low to moderate intensities to build cardiovascular fitness and allow the muscles and connective tissue to adapt to high-volume work. Distance rather than intensity is varied, for example, alternating days of long and short runs. Exercise intensity is maintained at less than 85% HRmax or below lactate threshold. To avoid injury, duration of each session and total volume should increase gradually over this phase. As the athlete moves toward the next phase, volume decreases and intensity increases. The mid-season (or pre-competition) phase includes higher intensity quality training

(85-90% HRmax) at slightly reduced volume. Interval training incorporating relatively short rest intervals may be introduced here. During the next phase (speed training), higher intensity interval work (>90% HRmax) is added and volume reduced accordingly so that the athlete can train at near race pace. For both of the latter phases (pre-competition and speed), recovery training or rest days should follow intense sessions or competition. Finally, in the taper over the 7 to 10 days before competition, intensity and frequency are maintained but volume is reduced, perhaps by 30 to 50%. A shorter taper (2-3 days) may be used for competition early in the season when there is less accumulated fatigue.

Training for Muscular Strength, Power and Endurance

Muscular strength, power and **endurance** are important components of physical fitness required by many, if not most, sports—from sports requiring grace and skill, such as gymnastics and diving, to those requiring pure speed, such as sprinting, or sheer strength, such as power weightlifting. Strength and power training are now integral parts of training for many sports, even those considered mainly endurance activities such as cycling, rowing or swimming.

TABLE 11.7—Periodisation of Training for the Endurance Athlete

Phase	Length	Intensity	Volume
Early season	12-16 wk	<85% HRmax	Moderate to start, increasing to high
Mid-season (pre-competition preparation)	6-8 wk	Increase to include 85-90% HRmax twice per wk	Decrease volume from previous phase
Speed training	4-6 wk	Increase to include >90% HRmax or at race pace	Decrease volume from previous phase
Taper	7-10 d	Maintain intensity	Greatly reduce volume

Compiled from P. Reaburn and D. Jenkins (eds.), 1996, *Training for speed and endurance*. (St. Leonards, NSW: Allen and Unwin).

Muscular strength, power and endurance are separate components of muscular fitness, and each requires specific training to obtain optimal results. Muscular strength is defined as the maximum force or torque exerted by a muscle group in a single movement. Muscular power is the product of strength and speed (force × velocity or force per unit time). Muscular endurance reflects the ability of a muscle group to generate force repeatedly in multiple contractions. Different activities require different relative contributions of each. For example, rowing requires high levels of muscular power and endurance, whereas Olympic weightlifting requires high levels of muscular power and strength.

There is generally a direct relationship between these three components of muscular fitness, but improving one component does not necessarily cause increases in the others. For example, sprinting requires maximum power to be developed against low resistance, and strength training alone will do little to improve sprint speed. At the other extreme, pure strength sports such as weightlifting require training at near maximum strength. Thus, the desired outcome dictates the specific type of training. In addition, many sports, such as team games, require optimising all three components of muscular fitness using periodised training. The mode of training, along with other important variables such as speed of movement, movement pattern (e.g., in one or more planes) and relative degree of force to be generated, must also be considered when developing a program to train muscular fitness. The following sections discuss general training principles to increase muscular strength and power; specific guidelines for muscular training in children are discussed in chapter 9.

Training for Muscular Strength

Training to maximise muscular strength requires the muscles to work at near maximum capacity; this is generally in the range of 4 to 8 repetitions per set at 80 to 90% of maximum strength (1 RM). The optimum may be 5 to 6 RM, but a variety of intensities is recommended to avoid monotony. Unless the objective is to isolate a particular part of a movement, lifts should encompass the full range of motion of a muscle group. In general, gains in strength are related to training volume (sets × repetitions), but there is no single combination of sets and rep-

etitions that is most effective. Large strength gains may be achieved in the less experienced with only 1 set of high-intensity work. In contrast, the experienced weightlifter needs multiple sets (3-8 for each muscle group) to induce further neural and structural changes. Maximal strength development appears to require maximal voluntary muscle actions, but that does not necessarily require working at 1 RM (maximal strength). Rather, at least some of the workout must include exercise to temporary "failure" of the muscle group. For example, by definition a set at 6 RM (a resistance that can be lifted six but not seven times) should induce temporary failure after the sixth lift. Muscular strength can increase without an increase in muscle mass, especially at the onset of a program when neural adaptations account for most of the improvements in strength.

Training should be periodised to induce progressive overload without overtraining. The experienced weightlifter usually aims to achieve muscular hypertrophy through high-volume work early in the season, progressing to more high-quality, intense strength work. Between 48 and 72 h is needed for full recovery of strength after an intense workout, and a split routine may be necessary to accommodate a complete training program (discussed later in the chapter). As mentioned earlier, endurance training may interfere with development of muscular strength. Athletes performing concurrent training (both strength and endurance) should ensure that endurance training is performed on alternate days to allow sufficient recovery. Alternatively, strength and endurance work can be emphasised in different microcycles.

Training for Muscle Hypertrophy

Skeletal muscle will hypertrophy (increase in size) after high-intensity resistance training. In human skeletal muscle, hypertrophy occurs primarily through an increase in size of individual muscle fibres and connective tissue. Although data from both human and animal studies suggest that hyperplasia (increase in fibre number) may occur in response to heavy strength training, any contribution to increased contractile protein and increased strength is likely to be minimal. Skeletal muscle hypertrophy depends on the type, intensity and volume of training. Hypertrophy requires a large volume of training over time (i.e., weeks to months) and is specific to the motor unit recruitment pattern. According to the size principle of muscle fibre recruitment, hypertrophy in the larger, more forceful type II fibres requires high-intensity work at near maximum strength. For example, muscle biopsies of endurance athletes show hypertrophy of type I (slow twitch) fibres with normal-sized type II (fast twitch) fibres. Strength and power athletes who perform high-intensity strength training exhibit hypertrophy of type I and II fibres.

Athletes seek to increase muscle size for several reasons. In the sport of bodybuilding, muscle size and definition are major determinants of performance. Strength and power athletes seek to increase muscle size in light of the general relationship between muscle cross-sectional area and strength; that is, increasing size should also lead to increased strength. Athletes in contact and collision sports require muscle bulk to guard against injury and to effectively perform many skills (e.g., tackling). In the periodised training program, most athletes focus on hypertrophy during the pre-season, in preparation for later strength, power and skill training. Hypertrophy is accomplished through high-volume, lower resistance training, usually involving 3 to 5 sets of 8 to 20 RM, two to three times per week. While this may be appropriate for strength and power athletes such as sprinters, games athletes and powerlifters, more extensive hypertrophy may be required in some sports (e.g., power weightlifting, bodybuilding). These athletes use higher volume training, usually 3 to 6 sets of 8 to 12 RM but sometimes up to 10 to 15 sets. In addition, several exercises are performed for each muscle or muscle group.

Training for Muscular Power

Since muscular power involves both strength (force) and speed (velocity), both components must be trained. There is some debate as to the optimal training resistance and velocity to maximise power development. Research generally shows that changes in power are related to the velocity of movement in both testing and training; that is, the largest increases in velocity are observed when testing is at the same velocity as training. The principle of specificity implies that the training velocity and movement pattern should closely simulate that required of the sport. Thus, the choice of training velocity depends on the desired outcome. Sprinting (pure speed) requires a different training pro-

gram than Olympic weightlifting (power and strength). Athletes using power training often periodise their training to first focus on muscular strength and hypertrophy during the pre-season, followed by more specific power training during the competition phase. It is important to continue strength training even when the primary focus shifts to muscular power.

The shape of the force-velocity curve indicates that, in a concentric movement, a muscle group's maximal force is exerted at zero velocity, and force declines as velocity increases. Maximal power development occurs in the mid-range of this curve, at 30 to 50% of maximal force; training for power therefore requires relatively light loads to be lifted rapidly. However, in most traditional methods of resistance training, a large proportion of the movement includes deceleration rather than acceleration of the weight. For example, the squat requires rapid and forceful acceleration at the start of the movement, but most of the remaining movement involves deceleration to control the bar. Thus, high force and power are achieved only for a short time and within a narrow range of movement. To optimise power development, it has been suggested that training requires near maximum power and acceleration throughout the entire range of movement to minimise the deceleration phase (Wilson 1994). So-called ballistic lifts such as the squat jump allow the weight to be projected into space using specialised safety equipment. These movements may incorporate both resistance and plyometric training to maximise power output.

Plyometric Training

Plyometric training is another type of power training used by many speed and power athletes, especially sprinters and jumpers. **Plyometrics** makes use of the stretch-shortening cycle in which skeletal muscle generates more force when a concentric contraction is immediately preceded by stretch of that muscle. Pre-stretch of the muscle augments subsequent force by two mechanisms: (1) activation of the stretch reflex and (2) elastic recoil generated within elastic components of the contractile filaments and connective tissue. The stretch-shortening cycle is a natural part of many movements, such as the backswing (e.g., in golf, tennis or cricket) or countermovement before a jump (e.g., bending the knees before jumping, as in the rebound in basketball or spike in volleyball).

Examples of commonly used plyometric training include the following:

> ▶ Simpler examples for beginners or children—skipping and hopping
> ▶ For the more experienced athlete—depth-jumping (e.g., dropping from a bench and then immediately jumping), medicine ball catching and throwing, and bounding

Although it is clear that plyometric training enhances explosive power (the vertical jump, for example), the responsible mechanisms have not yet been identified. They likely involve a combination of neural and structural adaptations.

The major benefit of plyometric training is that movements are sport specific (e.g., jumps for basketball or volleyball athletes) and are performed at the high velocity and acceleration needed for sport. Weightlifting, whether using free weights or weight machines, cannot simulate sport-specific movements at the high velocities encountered in many sports. The disadvantages of plyometric training include the potential for injury from high-impact force (e.g., depth jumping), the need for prior strength training experience and the often difficult task of determining optimal training loads.

The optimal number of repetitions and sets for plyometric training is not yet known, and research to date shows improvements with many different combinations of variables. There are, however, a number of recognised precautions for the use of plyometric training. Because repetitive impact movements increase risk of injury, intense plyometric training is recommended for mature athletes (i.e., not children or adolescents) and only after considerable strength-training experience. One year of intense strength training and the ability to perform a back squat of at least 1.5 times body mass are accepted as prerequisites before beginning intense plyometric training; strength training should be continued during the phase incorporating plyometrics. Obviously, an injured athlete should avoid plyometrics until muscular strength and endurance are regained and the injury completely healed. In a periodised program, plyometrics is usually introduced in the competition phase, after strength and hypertrophy development in the preparation phase. Training should be progressive, starting with few repetitions and sets and progressing gradually. Plyometrics should be performed no more than two to three times per week and only after an extensive muscular warm-up that includes stretching. The muscles should be rested for at least 48 h between sessions. Because injury is most likely to occur when the muscles are fatigued, plyometric exercises should be performed at the start of a session before any strength or endurance work. Long rest intervals (5 min) are needed between sets of plyometrics.

Training Mode

There is a wide variety of training modes to enhance muscular strength, power and endurance. The choice of mode depends on access to equipment, desired outcomes, the athlete's experience and particular components of muscular fitness to be targeted. Several terms are used to describe modes of muscular strength training:

> ▶ Isometric training refers to a muscle movement in which force is generated but muscle length remains constant.
> ▶ Dynamic resistance exercise refers to a movement in which force is generated while the muscle changes length, either shortening (concentric movement) or lengthening (eccentric movement).
> ▶ Isotonic exercise is one type of dynamic movement against a constant resistance (e.g., a barbell). This term is really a misnomer because it implies that the muscle tension remains constant (iso = same, tonic = tension), whereas in reality the external resistance remains unchanged while muscle tension varies with joint angle. The term isotonic training has been replaced by terms such as isoinertial or dynamic constant external resistance training.
> ▶ Variable resistance exercise is another type of dynamic training that uses a weight machine to vary the external resistance through levers, pulleys or cams. The intention is to alter the resistance at different joint angles to maximally tax the muscle throughout its range of motion.
> ▶ Isokinetic exercise (constant velocity) is a movement in which the speed or angular velocity of movement is controlled by the machine, and force is measured throughout the range of motion.
> ▶ Concentric movement refers to a muscle action in which the muscle shortens while generating force.
> ▶ Eccentric movement refers to a muscle action in which the muscle lengthens in a controlled manner while generating force. Eccentric motion is a natural part of many movements, such as landing

after a jump or walking downhill. Eccentric muscle actions are essential for stabilising the body or particular muscle groups, for example, to maintain balance when landing after a spike in volleyball or to decelerate the arm at the end of a throw. Many movements combine concentric and eccentric actions in sequence, for example, raising (concentric action) and lowering (eccentric action) the bar in a biceps curl.

Each training mode has advantages and disadvantages. For example, although isometric movements are used extensively for injury rehabilitation or for individuals with joint disorders such as arthritis in which there is restricted range of motion around a particular joint, they are of limited benefit for the healthy athlete because improvement in strength is specific to the joint angle used in training. Isokinetic movements may allow maximal torque to be exerted throughout the range of motion, but speed is controlled so the athlete cannot vary rate of force development and may not be able to train at near maximal velocity. Isoinertial and variable resistance machines permit both eccentric and concentric movements, but these are not often sport specific. Optimal training for muscular strength and power requires creative combinations of different modes and training techniques to accommodate these advantages and disadvantages. To use the sprinter as an example, pre-season training might focus on muscle hypertrophy and pure strength early in the season using isoinertial (e.g., free weights) or variable resistance training. As the season progresses, training would then switch to incorporate power training with weights and plyometrics.

Eccentric Training

As mentioned previously, eccentric or "negative" training refers to movements in which the muscle lengthens while generating tension. Eccentric muscle actions are integral to many movements (e.g., maintaining balance during footstrike in running, decelerating the arm when throwing). Most resistance training movements have both eccentric and concentric components; for example, pushing or raising the bar is often a concentric action, while returning the bar to the starting point often requires an eccentric movement (think of a biceps curl or leg press). For any given muscle group, development of maximal muscular strength appears to require both concentric and eccentric muscle actions. Compared with concentric training alone, combined eccentric and concentric training results in greater improvements in the ability to generate force in both eccentric and concentric movements. Thus, effective resistance training must incorporate some means of working muscles both eccentrically and concentrically. Free weights and isoinertial and dynamic resistance machines can easily accommodate eccentric training simply because returning the weight to its starting position usually requires an eccentric movement. Some, but not all, isokinetic machines permit eccentric movements.

The optimal resistance for eccentric training is still a matter of debate. As indicated by the force-velocity curve, force output is greater in eccentric compared with concentric movements of the same muscle group. Thus, eccentric training with a resistance that can be lifted concentrically requires only sub-maximum force in the eccentric movement. To use the biceps curl as an example, the maximum resistance (weight) is limited to that which can be lifted in the concentric phase (flexion at the elbow). To perform the eccentric movement (lowering the weight via extension at the elbow) requires less than the maximal force that can be exerted eccentrically by the biceps. For each muscle group, it is thought that the optimal eccentric training intensity is 100 to 130% of maximal force exerted in the concentric movement. There are several ways to train at intensities above 100% of 1 RM force. Using weight machines, the concentric movement (lift or push) can be performed with both arms (or legs), with only one limb used for the eccentric (lowering) phase. Using free weights, a spotter can help in the concentric movement, and the athlete alone lowers the weight. Some isokinetic machines allow controlled eccentric movements using resistance in excess of 1 RM. When performing eccentric movements, it is important to ensure that the movement can be controlled and that resistance is not excessively high. Since eccentric training induces more muscle damage (and thus soreness) than concentric training, it must be used judiciously and with appropriate recovery between sessions, especially for the novice or when returning from injury.

Training Frequency

The optimal training frequency for development of muscular strength and power is not clear at present. The optimal frequency requires a careful balance of other training components (e.g., endurance, skill), the athlete's experience (elite and more experienced can generally tolerate more frequent training), phase of the season (i.e., early season or competition) and risk of overtraining or injury. At least 48 and possibly 72 h appear to be needed for recovery of strength between high-intensity sessions training the same muscle groups. Novice or less experienced athletes show great improvements in muscular strength with only two high-intensity resistance training sessions per week. For experienced resistance athletes, at least three sessions per week may be required for maximal strength gains. It is not uncommon for elite weightlifters to train twice per day for short periods (i.e., a few days). However, changes in technique and muscular power occur within a few days, raising questions of safety and training effectiveness with continued twice-daily training. If twice-daily sessions are needed, split routines are recommended. Split routines are used if a session would be too long to fit within a single session. Split sessions may involve repeating multiple sets of the same exercises at different times during a single day or, more often, grouping exercises of closely related muscles together in the same session and alternating these with exercises of different muscle groups in a different session. For example, the upper body may be worked in one session and the lower body the next. Split routines allow high-volume training to be performed while still providing needed recovery.

Training for Team Games

Training for team games usually requires a combination of endurance, sprint speed, skill and muscular strength or power. The relative mix of these components will vary by sport, position within the sport, age, training history and specific skills to be developed. It is essential to first understand the event requirements, that is, the relative importance of endurance, sprint speed, strength/power and skill to performance for each sport and sometimes each position. This may include time motion analysis, in which a match is filmed and analysed for different levels of activity for different positions. For example, analysis might include the amount of game time spent in sprints, jogging or other movements and the intervals between. This information is then used to develop a specific training program. Heart rate monitoring in a game may also be used to determine appropriate training intensities.

Periodisation of Training for the Team Game Athlete

The serious team game athlete likely would have maintained some level of aerobic fitness during the off-season via low-intensity endurance exercise. Table 11.8 briefly summarises periodisation of training for the team game athlete. In the early season,

TABLE 11.8—Periodisation of Training for the Team Game Athlete

Phase	Endurance training	Speed training	Resistance training
Early season	Long duration, low-moderate intensity Not on days of resistance training	Short sprints (3-10 s) with long rests (60 s)	Hypertrophy: 8-15 reps Strength: 2-6 reps 2-3 sets, 2-3 d/wk
Mid-season (pre-competition preparation)	Decrease frequency and volume Add interval work	Specific to sport Increase intensity to competition pace Add acceleration and agility work	Sport-specific power 30-50% 1 RM in fast movement 2-3 d/wk
Competition	Once per wk to maintain fitness	Once per wk to maintain fitness	One strength + one power session per wk

Compiled from P. Reaburn and D. Jenkins (eds.), 1996, *Training for speed and endurance*. (St. Leonards, NSW: Allen and Unwin).

non-specific endurance exercise (e.g., cross-training) is used to establish an endurance base. Good endurance fitness assists recovery between intervals during intense training and in matches. Training volume gradually increases while exercise intensity remains low to moderate (70-85% HRmax). The preseason also includes some brief speed work, resistance training and skill development. Speed training focuses on good form in short sprints (3-10 s), with long rest intervals (60 s) to avoid injury. Speed training should be performed when the athlete is not fatigued (e.g., early in a training session). Resistance training focuses on enhancing strength and, when needed for contact sports, size (hypertrophy). The relative importance of resistance training depends on the sport, position, age and experience. Developing strength requires high-intensity work at close to maximum strength using high resistance and low repetitions (e.g., 2-6 reps per set, 2-3 sets). Hypertrophy training involves higher repetitions (8-15) and higher volume (2-4 sets). At this stage, no more than two to three strength sessions should be performed each week because 36 to 72 h recovery is needed to maximise strength gains. To prevent injury and maximise training effort, a proper cardiovascular and muscular warm-up is essential before speed and resistance training sessions. As mentioned earlier in the chapter, endurance training can interfere with maximum strength development, so endurance and resistance training should be performed on alternate days if included in the same macrocycle.

During the mid-season before regular competition begins, training focuses on maintaining endurance and strength while developing sport-specific fitness, speed and power. Endurance training volume decreases as intensity increases, and sport-specific interval training is introduced. Intensity of speed work gradually increases to approximate (or even exceed) competition pace. Training is added to improve acceleration from different starting positions (e.g., standing, crouching, jogging) and sport-specific agility (e.g., ability to change direction, stop and start quickly). Resistance training now focuses on developing sport-specific power, using lower resistance but with fast, explosive movements. Rather than working against heavy resistance as in pure strength training (e.g., 80% 1 RM), power training is best performed as fast movements against moderate resistance (e.g., 30-50% 1 RM). These actions

Case Study 11.3

Greg is 21 years old and plays Rugby Union (back-row position). He sustained a hamstring muscle strain early in the off-season during a friendly game of touch. The injury has healed after successful physiotherapy and flexibility work, but he is now in relatively poor physical condition after 2 months with little exercise. He has 4 months to prepare for the upcoming season.

After a recent fitness test, Greg's coach identified that he needs to significantly improve cardiovascular endurance, muscular strength and power, and speed. Provide an overview of the 16 weeks of training available to the athlete that includes specific work on the fitness components needing improvement. (You may find it easiest to draw a graph showing the relative importance of each component over the 16 weeks.) Include within the 16 weeks repeat testing of his physical fitness. Also provide a "typical" 7-day training block within the 16 weeks.

Key Issues

1. When and how will you re-assess physical fitness during the 16 weeks? How will you establish the effectiveness of the 16-week program?

2. How often should Greg train during the 16 weeks? Indicate frequency (on a weekly basis) for each of the types/modes of training.

3. What potential scheduling problems might arise in trying to improve the various aspects of fitness identified by the coach? How will these be addressed when developing the training program?

4. Which fitness component (endurance, strength, speed, power) should be developed first, second, and so on, over the 16-week period? How will improvements in each area be maintained once the focus has shifted to another component?

should mimic, as much as possible, movements used in the particular sport.

During the competition phase, recovery after matches and between sessions becomes essential for preventing overtraining and overuse injuries. The day after the match is devoted to recovery, perhaps as a rest day or incorporating stretching, cross-training (e.g., water running) and other regeneration techniques such as massage. Each weekly or more frequent match may be considered equivalent to one high-intensity endurance training session. Maintenance of endurance ability may require only up to two additional sessions—a brief (10-15 min) session at near competition pace and a lower intensity longer session that may incorporate skill or agility drills. During the competition phase, speed may be maintained using brief sprints or drills (e.g., bounding) emphasising proper technique. These should be performed early in the session, after a good warm-up but before endurance or skill training. Resistance training aims to maintain muscular strength and power developed in earlier phases. One or two sessions per week is usually sufficient, with one session devoted to maintaining strength (low reps, high resistance, low volume) and the second session devoted to sport-specific power. During the off-season, the team game athlete should perform moderate-intensity endurance exercise to maintain aerobic capacity. One session per week of interval training at higher intensity will help maintain speed and muscular power. It is important to recognise that cardiovascular fitness and muscular strength will decline to some extent during the off-season. This is necessary to allow the athlete time to recover between seasons and to begin the next season fresh.

Training for Speed

Speed requires the body to be moved over a defined distance as quickly as possible. To optimally plan a speed-training program, it is first important to analyse the type of speed needed. Factors to consider include the duration of the sprint (from a few seconds to perhaps 2 min), whether there is a single sprint or multiple sprints, the duration of the rest intervals between sprints, and whether the sprint is in a straight line or requires other movement patterns. Understanding the nature of the speed requirements then dictates the type of speed-training program. For example, a 100-m track sprinter needs to develop speed in a straight line, whereas a football or soccer player needs to develop the ability to move quickly in different directions. To give another

example, a basketball player must be able to sprint repeatedly while fatigued, whereas a track runner runs only a single sprint at a time during competition.

To effectively train sprinting ability, the sprint is broken down into specific components that can be trained individually. These include

- reaction to a signal (e.g., the gun start in swimming, movement by an opposing player in a team game);
- acceleration, or the ability to achieve maximal speed quickly (e.g., the first 20 m of a sprint, the run-up in long jump);
- the ability to maintain and readjust balance (e.g., running with the ball around or through the defence in football, passing the ball downcourt in netball or basketball); and
- the ability to maintain speed and form while fatigued (e.g., at the end of a long sprint, as in the 200-m butterfly or throughout the 400-m hurdles).

Timing specific stages of a sprint can help identify weaknesses to be targeted for improvement. For example, in track sprinting (or any game sport requiring straight running), timing lights can be used to time each 20 m of a 120-m run. These times can be used to determine if there are weaknesses in the start (reaction to a signal, acceleration), middle or end (ability to maintain speed while fatiguing).

Acceleration is important for short sprint events, team game sports and some explosive movements such as jumping events in track. Acceleration may be required from a complete stop (at the start of a track or swim race) or from slow movement (in many team games), and the athlete may need the ability to accelerate and decelerate repeatedly (as in a team game). As such, acceleration is trained over short distances (10-20 m), from a complete stop or moving start, and using single or repeated efforts. Shorter distances and more complex movement patterns may be appropriate for some sports such as tennis or squash.

Maintaining speed while fatigued is essential for longer sprints (30 s to 2 min) or for repeated shorter sprints, when muscle creatine phosphate has been depleted and lactate levels are high. This type of sprinting is said to require **lactate tolerance,** the ability to continue high-intensity work despite high lactate levels (and thus reduced pH) in skeletal muscle. It is especially important to train lactate tolerance for events requiring the athlete to maintain technique during fatigue, as in a 200- or 400-m swim or the 400-m hurdles, or to sprint repeatedly over time, as in many team games. Training generally includes multiple repeats with relatively short rest intervals (see table 11.9). The body adapts to this type of training by increasing lactate clearance and oxidation by other tissues and increasing the buffering capacity of skeletal muscle and blood.

High-intensity sprint training is recommended no more than three times per week. It is likely that such training induces microscopic damage to skeletal muscles requiring more than 24 h to repair. Moreover, there is a belief among speed athletes and coaches that the nervous system also requires recovery between sessions, although this has not been thoroughly studied in the scientific literature. It is recommended that speed athletes allow at least 1 day between each high-intensity sprint session; this time can be devoted to developing muscle flexibility and strength. Periodisation of training is also important because continued high-intensity speed training over several months is likely to lead to stagnation in performance, overuse injury or OTS.

Many speed athletes also use resistance training to develop muscular strength and power. As described earlier in the chapter, speed athletes should use a periodised training program to first develop muscular strength and hypertrophy in the early season and then focus on power in the competition phase. Muscular strength and endurance are important for maintaining proper form during speed events. For example, sprinting and jumping require good core strength (strong postural and abdominal muscles).

Stretching and Muscle Flexibility

Stretching is an essential but often overlooked part of the athlete's training. Poor muscle flexibility and joint range of motion not only increase risk of muscle-tendon and joint injury but may also compromise performance in many, if not most, sports. For example, in sprinting and the long jump, stride length, power and technique may be compromised by poor flexibility in the ankle and hip. Agility in game sports such as soccer, football and basketball may also suffer because of poor flexibility. Even strength athletes such as Olympic weightlifters require good flexibility of the hips, knees and shoulders. Muscle-tendon length often declines as a result of resistance training without attention to muscle flexibility; shortened tendons and muscles limit range of motion and may predispose the athlete to injury. Thus, stretching should be an integral part of an athlete's training. In some sports such as sprinting or gymnastics, an entire training session may be devoted to flexibility work.

Regular flexibility training induces structural changes in skeletal muscle and associated tendons, resulting in increased resting length of the muscle-tendon group. Four types of stretching are used in sports training: static, dynamic (or ballistic), slow movement and proprioceptive neuromuscular facilitation (PNF). Static stretching is most commonly used because it is simplest and least likely to cause injury. In static stretching, the muscle is relaxed and

TABLE 11.9—Exercise and Rest Intervals for Interval Training

Exercise duration	Rest duration	Intensity[a]	Fitness component	Example of event relevant to training
2-5 min	2-8 min	85-90%	Endurance	Middle distance, long distance
30-120 s	2-6 min	90-95%	Lactate tolerance	Long sprint, middle distance
20-45 s	3-5 min	>95%	Sustained speed, technique	Sprint, team games
5-30 s	15-150 s	>95%	Speed, power, acceleration, technique	Sprint, team games
6-15 s	1-2 min	100%	Speed, power, acceleration, technique	Short sprint, team games
3-6 s	30-45 s	100%+	Acceleration, technique	Short sprint, team games

[a]Intensity as a percentage of maximum pace over the specified distance.

Compiled from B.S. Rushall and F.S. Pyke, 1990, *Training for sports and fitness*. (Melbourne: Macmillan Australia).

lengthened to the point of tension (slight discomfort but not pain), and this position is held for 10 to 60 s. This type of stretching is recommended for general warm-up and cool-down for all athletes and for injury rehabilitation. Dynamic, or ballistic, stretching is more active, involving bouncing into the stretched position. It has fallen out of favour recently because it is associated with increased risk of injury and delayed-onset muscle soreness. However, many sports involve movements requiring ballistic stretching (e.g., gymnastics, wrestling, diving, ballet), and ballistic stretching is of value for the competitive athlete provided that certain precautions are taken. Ballistic stretching should be undertaken by athletes with good flexibility and a long history of flexibility training; however, a warm-up of extensive static and slow movement stretching should always be performed first. As its name implies, slow movement stretching involves stretching through a slow movement. Examples include neck, trunk or arm rotations. Slow movement stretching is of value as part of the warm-up, placed between static and ballistic stretching.

PNF stretching is an advanced technique requiring competent instruction to be effective and to avoid injury. There are several methods of performing PNF stretching, all based on the observation that voluntary contraction of muscle before stretching causes reciprocal inhibition of its antagonist, permitting greater range of motion and stretch of the agonist. The muscle to be stretched is first contracted concentrically, followed by relaxation and stretching. PNF stretching often requires a partner, which may limit its convenience and require additional time. Although PNF stretching may be of value for rehabilitation of an injury and for athletes requiring extensive flexibility (e.g., ballet dancers, gymnasts, wrestlers), it may not necessarily be superior to a combination of the other types of stretching for many athletes. The choice of stretching technique depends on the athlete's experience, sport requirements, available time and injury history. Regardless of which techniques are used, it is essential to plan flexibility training to the same extent as other training components.

Summary

High-performance athletes have specific needs in terms of their training and preparation for competition. Whereas any number of physical activity programs may suit the average person desiring to improve health and general physical fitness, athletes need individualised training to enhance specific components of their physical performance. Training is strategically planned in advance (periodisation), often for months or even years, leading up to key competitions. Optimal nutrition is central to continued quality training, recovery and competitive performance. Adequate hydration during and after exercise is also critical for an athlete. In planning the training season, athletes, coaches and sport scientists must carefully balance the need for daily high-intensity, high-volume training against the risk of overuse injury or overtraining. Cross-training may give athletes the opportunity to continue intense training while preventing overuse injury or overtraining. Tapering (reducing training volume while maintaining intensity for 1-3 weeks before major competition) is associated with improved performance in sports requiring high-volume training such as swimming and distance running. Muscular training to improve strength, power and muscular endurance is now integral to training for most athletes, even those in endurance sports, but it must be specific to the desired outcomes. Success at team games requires a combination of many components of physical fitness, and each component must be strategically targeted in training programs. Finally, although often overlooked, muscle flexibility is also a critical part of training for all athletes; lack of muscle flexibility may impair performance and increase the risk of injury.

Selected Glossary Terms

anaerobic threshold—During exercise of increasing intensity, a point at which the metabolic demands of exercise must be met by increasing contribution by the anaerobic glycolytic system, producing excess lactic acid.

carbohydrate (or **glycogen**) **loading**—The dietary practice by athletes of increasing carbohydrate intake to very high levels and reducing training volume, thereby enhancing muscle glycogen synthesis and storage.

concurrent training—Training for both muscular strength and cardiorespiratory endurance within the same training cycle.

cross-training—Maintaining fitness by training using another mode of exercise different from the specific sport; alternatively, using a variety of different types of activities to achieve physical fitness.

glycaemic index (GI)—A measure of the magnitude of rise in blood glucose 2 h after ingestion of 50 g of a particular food relative to pure glucose.

glycogen—Polymer of multiple glucose molecules; the main storage form of glucose in the body, primarily in muscle and liver; provides a major substrate for high intensity exercise.

individual anaerobic threshold (IAT)—During exercise of increasing intensity, a point at which the metabolic demands of exercise must be met by increasing contribution by the anaerobic glycolytic system, producing excess lactic acid.

iron-deficiency anaemia—Iron deficiency, characterised by clinically low concentrations of red blood cells, haemoglobin and serum ferritin (the body's storage form of iron).

lactate threshold—A point during exercise of increasing intensity at which blood lactic acid levels begin to rise exponentially above resting levels.

lactate tolerance—The ability to continue exercising at a high intensity despite high muscle and blood lactic acid levels.

muscular endurance—The ability of a muscle or muscle group to generate force repeatedly or continuously over time; an important component of sports requiring repetitive application of force, such as swimming, rowing or cycling.

muscular power—The rate at which a muscle or muscle group can develop force, defined as force per unit time; an important component of explosive movements such as sprinting, jumping and throwing.

muscular strength—The maximum force a muscle or muscle group can generate in a single maximal contraction or movement.

overtraining syndrome (OTS)—In athletes, a state of persistent fatigue, poor sport performance, mood state alterations and other symptoms resulting from prolonged periods of excessive training with inadequate rest and recovery.

periodisation of training—A process of dividing an athlete's season into phases and planning a varied training program to optimise performance at certain times and to avoid overtraining.

plyometrics—A type of power training used by speed and power athletes that includes exercises to pre-stretch the muscle group before each movement to enhance muscle force and power.

post-exercise recovery period—The period after intense exercise (training or competition) when the body returns to a resting state. During recovery, the body restores resting levels of substrates (e.g., glycogen) and fluids (e.g., blood volume), and repairs injured tissue.

tapering—Practice by athletes of reducing training volume and possibly intensity for up to 3 weeks before a major competition.

Student Activities and Study Questions

1. What is considered the best way to train muscular power using resistance training? Is it better to train for pure strength and hypertrophy using high loads, or are lower loads better? What does the recent research literature say about this?

2. What factors enhance glycogen replacement after depletion by prolonged exercise? What factors interfere with glycogen replacement? What foods would you recommend athletes eat, and avoid, if wishing to maximise glycogen replacement after endurance exercise?

3. Arrange a visit to a State Academy or Institute of Sport or other venue where high-performance or professional athletes are training. What roles do exercise scientists play in optimising training of these athletes?

4. Find out from different athletes (e.g., swimmers, runners, rowers, cyclists) the methods they use for tapering before major competition. Are there differences between sports? Between different athletes within a sport? Can you identify reasons for these differences? How have these athletes developed their tapering strategies (trial-and-error, reading the scientific literature, word-of-mouth, tradition within a sport)?

5. What is the difference between bodybuilding, powerlifting and Olympic lifting? Which of these sports requires the most strength? Power? How do training programs differ for these different sports? Why? If possible, attend training sessions for each and observe similarities and differences between training techniques.

Section 4

LEADERSHIP AND MANAGEMENT FOR THE EXERCISE MANAGER

The previous sections have established the expertise and technical skills of exercise managers to facilitate participation in physical activity across the wider community. They discussed the processes of health risk screening, physical fitness assessment, physical activity prescription and programming, evaluation and promotion of physical activity across the population from healthy individuals to those with disease or impairment to high performance athletes. Building on these processes, we now add, in section 4, the leadership and management skills so necessary to succeed in the business world. Whether working for yourself, or for others, exercise management is conducted in a professional environment involving other people. The concepts of leadership and business management discussed in section 4 will assist you in providing your technical skills more effectively and more efficiently, resulting in more enjoyment and satisfaction in your work. The two chapters have a practical emphasis and include the associated theory to help you gain an understanding of what makes leaders, managers and employees successful in a wide variety of physical activity settings.

Effective leadership and management skills are essential for every organization with aspirations of long term sustainability. These skills can be learned and it is hoped that this section will be a resource for ongoing reference during your career, whether in the physical activity setting or elsewhere, since the suggestions in each chapter have application across other fields of endeavour.

Skills developed through the study and practice of leadership and management will enhance your job prospects and give you confidence for tackling the problems you are sure to meet in your work, whether your role is leader, manager or employee. There is a specific focus on effective business planning, conduct, and evaluation as these skills are the basis of business management. Communication is also covered in detail because effective communication is vital to an organisation's internal efficiency and to good relations with clients, investors and other organisations.

The aim of this section is to show the broad scope of management issues related to physical activity settings. By necessity it is not comprehensive or exhaustive on any topic but provides a good basis for further study. Further study is particularly recommended as you move to higher managerial positions. Recommended readings have been selected to provide not only further knowledge in the area but also sound practical advice.

CHAPTER 12

Leadership and Human Resource Management

Quality service to clients is an essential component of exercise management. However, quality service can only be provided if exercise managers are competent in a variety of professional, technical and business skills. Success also depends on interpersonal skills, such as being able to effectively interact with clients, staff, colleagues, superiors and people from other organisations. This chapter presents concepts and strategies for the successful **management** of human resources. These form the basis of essential skills for effective **leadership,** which is the foundation of good human resource management.

Role of Leadership in Management

Successful organisations need both good leadership and good management. Although their tasks overlap, leaders and managers achieve their goals differently. Managers organise, control and review systems, whereas leaders provide visions for change in the systems and inspire people to work within them. Management and leadership skills complement each other—the most effective manager is also a good leader.

What Is Leadership?

Leaders are individuals who guide a group of people to accomplish goals that will benefit others. These goals provide a valuable purpose: they are the basis for the group's commitment to the leader's authority and to each other. By working together to achieve common goals, employees are committed not only to the leader but also to the leader's purpose. Staff appreciate leaders who understand the desired results and know what needs to be done to achieve them. While maintaining this focus on results, leaders must also display leadership attributes including appropriate values, motives, skills and behaviours. A wide array of attributes is observed in successful leaders, although outstanding leaders sometimes lack one or more of these common traits. For example, charisma is considered a common leadership trait, but it is not always observed in leaders. What *is* observed in all leaders is the ability to bond a group of people together to work toward a particular purpose.

Good Leadership in Exercise Management

Good leaders are guided by a set of ideals that shape the goals of a business so that profitability is an outcome and a measure of success but not an end to itself. In exercise management, the core ideology of excellent service to the client will never change over time, although practices and strategies to provide this will need continual evolution to stay in tune with technical, cultural and client changes. This never-ending quest for excellence, progress and innovation is part of the inner ideology of a good leader in exercise management. Although charismatic qualities are not needed for successful exercise management leadership, dissatisfaction with the status quo is a requirement in our field. Thus, a core goal is the search for continual improvement in the quality and value of services through progress and growth in specific policies, procedures and practices.

A specific skill of leaders in the exercise setting is the development of a team to build and maintain a business. Being a leader means spending time helping team members successfully complete their work. The more time leaders invest in their team, the more loyalty and productivity result. Leaders must guide a group of people to achieve a common task, to work as a team, and to respect and develop its individual members. This is particularly important in the physical activity environment where teams are often multidisciplinary and their members' skills and knowledge overlap to some degree (e.g., members from fields of health, science, medicine and physiotherapy). The better the working relationships among such a team, the more effective the outcomes it will achieve; it is the team leader who is responsible for establishing and enhancing these relationships.

Many people have innate leadership skills, but there is general agreement that a person can be trained to be a leader if a real desire to help others exists. For example, personal skills that can be learned include effective **planning,** chairing meetings, and methods of persuasion and explanation. The specific functions of leadership vary in different environments but in an exercise setting include those listed in figure 12.1.

Context and Leadership

Leaders do not work in a vacuum. They are always part of a given social, cultural, political, technical and economic environment that is constantly changing. Environmental factors that affect leadership may be internal or external to the workplace, but they all have a direct influence (both positive and negative) on how leaders function. The constraints of a particular working environment that may influence the way leaders operate include the culture of the profession and organisation, available resources and expectations of others. Good leaders have a clear picture of the structure of their organisation, their position in it and the constraints within which they work. These constraints are posed by the health of the economic system in which the organisation operates, the technology influencing the organisation's processes, the political and legal systems regulating the organisation and the sociocultural environment where customs, values and demographics determine how people will interact with an organisation. The latter is particularly important in the exercise setting because many people are always involved (e.g., clients, other health professionals, accountants and equipment suppliers).

In considering all these constraints, leaders understand the need for clearly identified management

---

Ensure work meets organisation's vision and goals.

Plan work, set tasks to achieve it and set a time line for completion.

Delegate tasks to staff and instruct them on the processes involved.

Set standards and outcomes required.

Hire, appraise, develop and dismiss staff.

Control, monitor, motivate and reward staff.

Set an example of behaviour expected of staff.

Provide conflict resolution and stress management when required.

FIGURE 12.1 Functions of leadership in an exercise setting.

procedures, including those for allocating responsibilities and monitoring the successful completion of tasks. Although the modern workplace may require staff to work with minimal direct supervision, employees often do not have the self-management skills required to work effectively and efficiently without some level of management and overall guidance. With flexible, adaptive and strategic approaches to management, leaders help their staff learn to work well with growing autonomy and thus avoid the following scenario (author unknown):

> A work place had staff called Everybody, Somebody, Anybody and Nobody. An important job needed to be done. Everybody was certain that Somebody would do it. Anybody could have done it but Nobody did it and Somebody got angry because it was Everybody's job. Everybody thought Anybody could do it but Nobody realised that Everybody wouldn't do it. In the end, Everybody blamed Somebody when Nobody did what Anybody could have done.

It is indisputable that exercise managers must have specific technical skills; this forms the basis of trust between the exercise manager and the client. While this is a priority, other essential skills are also required. The exercise manager must develop a philosophy of good leadership if values and goals are to be set that foster a productive business with ethical standards. The need for a code of **ethics** in the

workplace signifies the importance of social competence for the exercise manager when dealing with clients, staff and colleagues. Modern exercise managers should be competent in making decisions, allocating responsibilities and recruiting specialists to support them if required. This is only possible if exercise managers have well-developed leadership skills for working in a social environment.

Common Characteristics of Good Leaders

Many studies of management have assessed the attributes that describe successful leaders; some of these are presented in figure 12.2. While leaders are nearly always perfectionists with good interpersonal skills, they also have the ability to inspire their followers to worthwhile purposes. In the exercise setting, great leadership is not provided by those who look for outcomes of money, status or promotion but by those who aim to benefit others, whether through health improvement or performance enhancement. This important requirement involves demonstration of the leader's values, motives and competence, and it revolves around the leader showing (not simply saying) that he or she is committed to helping workers and clients achieve their goals. Some examples of how leaders show their commitment to the staff's success are included in figure 12.3.

By setting an example of what is required from staff, a leader can create an atmosphere that promotes

Commitment

Confidence

Consistency

Courage

Empathy

Honesty

Humour

Industry

Initiative

Integrity

Intellectual capability

Justice

Perseverance

Reliability

Responsibility

Tact

FIGURE 12.2   Characteristics of effective leaders.

Keep staff informed.

Consult staff and involve them in decision making.

Provide staff with challenges.

Delegate responsibility.

Promote teamwork by recognising the whole team.

Acknowledge work done well.

Assist staff to improve their skills.

Motivate staff by providing purpose for their work.

Demand high standards.

FIGURE 12.3   How leaders demonstrate commitment to their staff.

efficiency and effectiveness. If the leader can prove that he or she is positive, calm, confident, encouraging and hardworking, it provides employees with a role model for their own actions because the leader's disposition is nearly always contagious. Indeed, the skills that make exercise managers good leaders are the same skills that make their personnel effective with their peers, subordinates and clients. Listening empathetically, cooperating with others to achieve joint goals and eliciting the assistance of others when needed are all examples of good leadership skills.

Leadership skills are more readily developed when exercise managers regularly assess strengths and weaknesses that affect their own performance. In setting goals for improvement, leaders should consider

- ▶ their own appropriate health and exercise practices ("practising what they preach"),
- ▶ keeping abreast of innovation in practice and technology,
- ▶ developing new skills and knowledge,
- ▶ current attitudes and beliefs related to health and exercise,
- ▶ opportunities at work for testing alternate approaches, and
- ▶ taking time out for reflection.

A combination of minor changes to daily routines and major time allocations for continuing professional development, participating in professional organisations, attending and presenting at conferences, seminars and short courses, and contributing to professional publications will help exercise managers achieve their goal of continual professional development.

Importance of Planning

Planning is the ability to identify relevant issues, develop courses of action and effectively allocate resources to ensure achievement of objectives. It revolves around identifying tasks, personnel and support to achieve a specific result. The following steps provide a logical approach to planning for the exercise manager:

1. Identify the main tasks.
2. Obtain relevant information.
3. Write a realistic outline for action.
4. Consider the possible alternatives.
5. List the pros and cons of the main options.
6. Write a program and time line to achieve the result.
7. Evaluate success/failure/shortcomings.

Good leaders involve their staff in the planning process so that they will be more committed to making the plan work. For example, employees may be included in **brainstorming** sessions, asked to provide feedback or involved in discussions as the plan is developed. Other strategies of good leaders include contingency plans, maintaining some flexibility in the plan and searching for creative solutions with staff. In its simplest form, planning requires a leader to answer the questions of *how, who, when, what, where* and *why*.

How Is Leadership Measured?

Leaders are generally selected from the most technically competent workers in an organisation. However, the skills needed for technical excellence and those needed for success in leadership are rarely the same, although not mutually exclusive. With technical work the emphasis is on individual ability and performance, whereas with leadership the focus is on team effort, processes and outcomes. Success in leading a team is measured by the team's performance, not the leader's performance.

Outstanding leadership is demonstrated by constant inspiration of others, promotion of high employee morale and team spirit, and achievement of group goals through delegation, training and development of staff. These qualities are not easily measured. When people are asked to describe their "good bosses", they often use the phrase *tough but fair*. These characteristics reflect a leader's standards and it is therefore useful to study the systems the leader has in place in the organisation, rather than considering the leader's individual qualities, because a leader usually strives to maintain his or her own standards in the work produced by the staff. Effective leadership requires that employees have faith in the leader's judgement on the required standards; they must trust the leader to direct them correctly in achieving the organisation's goals. Simple rating scales (for example, from *completely trust the leader* to *do not trust the leader at all*) are useful for evaluating such factors.

Examples of Good Leadership

Three examples of good leadership that show how managers can constructively affect the people with whom they work are provided in this section. These examples describe managers motivating and developing individual staff and managing a team.

Example One (Leader: Claire)

Claire begins a meeting: "I've called this meeting so that we can go over our new client group. You will already have read the outline of the job, including background information on the organisation, a description of the client group—our first opportunity to work with people with mental illness—their requirements, tasks for each of you, the time line for achieving component tasks, the outcomes expected and the performance criteria".

At the top of a white board, Claire writes the importance and relevance of the job and summarises it by saying, "Our mission is to prove that we can provide exceptional care for this new type of client. We have been working toward this opportunity for over a year. A successful outcome will lead to more interesting work for all of us in the future".

Claire then outlines the tasks for each person and encourages discussion, listening carefully to each person's comments and concerns and summarising the decisions on the white board. She allows plenty of time for staff members to discuss ways of making the tasks more efficient, for example, sharing of repetitive tasks to make the work more satisfying for each member. Claire uses brainstorming to generate creative ideas for handling some problems. At this point, she insists on ideas being presented with no assessment of the suggestions until after employees have exhausted their contributions.

During the meeting, items requiring action are tabulated and a specific person allocated to undertake each item. The meeting is closed with agreement on the time of the next formal discussion for the staff and the date on which each member will receive minutes of the meeting.

The first example shows how an exercise manager outlined a new job so that the workers clearly understood its importance, their individual roles and the outcome required. This manager (Claire) understood the need to provide her staff with information that gained their commitment to a worthwhile mission, for this is what makes individuals want to work together as a team. Notice also how Claire used specific tools (written instructions, face-to-face meeting, white board, mission statement, open discussion, brainstorming, minutes of the meeting) to provide clear guidance and expectations of her staff.

Example Two (Leader: John)

JOHN TO ANGELA:

"Angela, I really appreciate that you have been making an effort to use some lateral thinking in solving some of our concerns with this corporate fitness program. I know you like to work independently, but make sure you discuss these good ideas with the team before acting on them. We all need to work together if we're to keep this program on budget and also maintain interest for those who have been with us for a long time".

JOHN TO MARK:

"Mark, you're working well with this corporate fitness program, but you don't seem very happy. Are you worried about making decisions on the new equipment layout on your own? Would you like to run some ideas past me now?"

JOHN TO ZOE:

"Zoe, you're really flying with the new exercise routines. Let me have the final draft as soon as it's ready".

The second example of good leadership shows how a manager (John) considers the differences in his staff when helping them learn to cope better with more autonomy in their work. This manager avoided the mistake of thinking that all his personnel are alike. By trying to understand how each is different and providing appropriate encouragement based on individual needs, John recognised and used the differences positively to allow his staff (Angela, Mark and Zoe) to improve. Notice how John dealt differently with the three staff members: Angela was provided with feedback and asked to work more with the rest of the team. Mark was assisted personally on a one-to-one basis, but Zoe was given only brief feedback and a reminder to give him the work when it was finished.

Example Three (Leader: Alex)

ALEX TO SAM:

"Sam, I'm glad Grant promised you time off today to go to that conference on new exercise science technology. It will put you behind in your program development work, but I hear that you have asked Judy to cover your personal training clients while you're away and she has agreed. When you return, will you send a report on the conference to the other staff?"

ALEX TO DIANE:

"Diane, I understand that you feel you should skip the computer skills course tomorrow because the monthly client reports are not finished. I don't think they'll have a problem with giving us an extra day so that you can go. I'll phone the manager and see if he agrees".

ALEX TO YVONNE:

"Yvonne, you're the only person we have who can handle elite pentathletes. Have you arranged to take Judy with you next time so she can learn the ropes? We need to have someone to backstop you if you're away".

The last example shows how a manager can ensure that workers are properly trained and encouraged to develop skills, allowing them to do their current work more efficiently. It is better to prepare staff for more demanding work than to get into the vicious cycle of not developing staff because everyone is too busy. There are several reasons why employees may be "too busy"; two of these are lack of training and shortage of personnel (perhaps because other staff have left because of lack of opportunities to advance through appropriate training). No matter how busy a work group is, this vicious cycle can be avoided by good leadership.

Continual training is a necessity in the rapidly changing field of exercise management. Alex avoided the mistake of forgoing staff training and development because of a busy work environment by prioritising training in individual development plans, setting aside time for development, ensuring that employees used their training in their work as soon as possible and providing opportunities for cross-training during work (this is essentially staff teaching other staff on the job).

Human Resource Management

The proper management of human resources, an important function in any business, assists in achieving the goals and objectives of an organisation by considering the most effective use of staff resources. The exercise manager must perform several functions to ensure good human resource management. These include the following categories, which will be covered in the remainder of the chapter:

- ► Team building
- ► Communications
- ► Staff selection, appraisal and development
- ► Conflict and stress management

Team Building

A group of individuals working together can be more effective if they function as a team. This requires the group members to commit themselves to the team and its mission. Because most workers are used to being supervised and evaluated on an individual

---

Case Study 12.1

Cathy has just been appointed the manager of a group of five health professionals to implement a new health and wellness program for a large organisation. She is preparing for the first meeting of the group. Only Cathy and one other person have worked together before. Cathy knows she needs several strategies over the next few months to bring the group together to work effectively as a team. Her planning will consider administration tasks such as drawing up a project plan with tasks, delegations and time lines; support mechanisms such as regular individual and team meetings; reporting processes including written documentation and progress reports; and opportunities to link the group together as a team. Draw up Cathy's ideas for the first meeting and indicate those items that Cathy will use for team building.

Key Issues

1. What will Cathy's goals be for the first meeting?
2. What factors does she need to consider when planning the work ahead?
3. What strategies will she use to commence building strong working relationships among the group?
4. Will it be necessary for Cathy to monitor the group? How will she do this? Will she include this in the discussion at the first meeting?

basis, exercise managers need to encourage employees to keep their primary focus on team performance rather than on individual performance.

Exercise managers create positive attitudes in their staff by considering group dynamics and what motivates their employees to work hard. This is largely achieved by providing common goals and values, for these are what define a team. By providing opportunities for positive group experiences with shared goals, individual staff members will become a functional unit. Creating this teamwork approach is an important function of a leader. It includes focusing on team performance rather than individual performance, letting the team have responsibility for correcting and improving the performance of individuals, rewarding the team not individuals and making team performance an important component of each individual's performance appraisal.

In building effective teams, exercise managers are required to set administrative and interpersonal standards, delegate tasks and then support the team in executing these tasks. Standards by which the team must work are needed so that all individuals know what is expected of them. Administrative standards include expectations of operational skills such as who will liaise with clients, how meetings will be conducted and how reports will be handled. Interpersonal standards describe how individuals will treat one another. An important example is insisting that

ideas may be criticised but not the individual who presented them. This is crucial for maintaining a team because criticising a person rather than an idea leads to arguments or other emotional responses and takes the focus from the idea to the person.

Delegation is another important skill required of a team leader. The leader or exercise manager chooses what to delegate, to whom, and when. In delegating, the exercise manager retains the accountability for the task, but the responsibility and authority for carrying it out is given to staff members. There are several reasons for delegating tasks, including giving the exercise manager time for team management tasks such as planning and development of staff skills, confidence and satisfaction. The most common tasks to be delegated include those that are routine (e.g., payment of accounts and personnel, sorting of mail, personal client interactions, tracking of client programs), although planning, organising and coordinating tasks may also be delegated. Managers are most effective when they prioritise management tasks and delegate operational tasks. For example, managers do not normally delegate tasks such as setting objectives, developing and monitoring teams, or improving organisational processes. Effective delegation also requires good briefing skills; these are described in the next section. Strategies to consider for helping minimise mistakes when tasks are delegated to staff are included in table 12.1.

TABLE 12.1—Considerations When Delegating Tasks to Staff

Process	Consideration
Level of delegation expected	Full responsibility: act on own initiative; no referral
	Partial responsibility: some initiative expected; refer periodically
	No responsibility: no initiative required; fully briefed
Preparation of staff	No preparation: staff are competent to handle task
	General instructions: requirements and outcome expected
	Explanation: detailed instructions and briefing
	Demonstration: presentation, practice and correction provided
	Training: course or instruction and assistance
Level of support	No special consideration
	Only outcome reviewed
	Assistance available on request
	Periodic check on progress
	Close and continuous assistance

Case Study 12.2

Matthew and Sally are business partners about to provide new exercise classes at their corporate health centre in the city. A new staff member, Jacqui, has been employed part time (15 h/wk to be allocated as follows: 7 h of classes, 3 h of class preparation, 5 h of administration). Matthew and Sally have just had an argument over what tasks Jacqui will actually be allowed to do. The issue is that Matthew wants Jacqui to do tasks that Sally thinks she should not be given until they have had time to assess her capabilities. Matthew asks you, as Jacqui's supervisor, to prepare guidelines for her tasks for the first 3 months of her employment so that Sally will give her the opportunity to show that she can appropriately handle them. You use the considerations in table 12.1 and select five tasks: preparation of class content, delivery of classes, marketing of new classes, maintenance of special equipment for her classes and conducting a survey to gather clients' feedback on the new classes.

Key Issues

1. Using table 12.1, what level of delegation, preparation and support do you consider appropriate for each of the five tasks for Jacqui?

2. Did Sally's concern influence your decisions?

3. What changes would you hope to be making to the guidelines after the first 3 months?

One of the important benefits of delegating work to the most appropriate employee is optimisation of the profitability of the work. It has been suggested that as much as 40 to 50% of work is done by staff more highly qualified than needed (Maister 1993). This results in lower profitability, and it also means that development of staff skills, morale and motivation are lower than they could be. A common reason given for reluctance to delegate is the time required to supervise junior workers. However, staff training is an important long-term business approach that results in development of the organisation as well as the employees.

Another important task of a team leader is staff support. This includes encouraging participation in group activities, encouraging workers to expand their skills or try new activities, welcoming staff suggestions, actively promoting employees inside and outside the organisation, encouraging team spirit and fully informing staff about details related to their work. With support, staff are able to function at their optimal levels.

Communications

Good **communication** skills underpin many of the management skills described elsewhere in this chapter. For example, good communication between managers and personnel requires that managers listen to staff feedback. Indeed, one of the most important communication skills of an effective manager is the skill of listening. But listening itself is not enough; what the manager does with this feedback is just as important. Moreover, being a successful exercise manager may be more about the way things are done than about what is done. If a decision is made against the advice of staff, a good manager will offer explanations for the decision during face-to-face discussion and not hide behind e-mail, paper or voice mail communication. Newsletters, magazines and other forms of communication also have their place but are more effective if used as a supplement to face-to-face communication. When choosing a communication medium, the situation, information to be relayed and the skill, sensitivity and experience of the communicator should be considered. For example, a manager altering staff work hours will meet less resistance if a formal meeting is held to discuss the changes than if they are communicated via e-mail with no opportunity for employee input before a decision is made.

Communication takes up a large proportion of most managers' time. Personal contact between employees and managers has been identified as a significant factor influencing staff attitudes to communication in organisations and the concept of *walking the talk* is therefore a popular management strategy. However, it has been suggested that, on average, 75% of oral communication is ignored, misunderstood or quickly forgotten (Bolton 1996), requiring managers to back up face-to-face discussions with written summaries of the meeting.

Of the many communication skills, there are three specific areas in which exercise managers should be proficient: **briefing** staff, leading meetings and **controlling** staff.

Briefing Staff

The main purpose of briefing is to allocate tasks, distribute resources and set performance measures. Skills needed include

- ▶ preparation (thinking ahead and planning the brief so it is complete and logical),
- ▶ clarification (providing detail so there is no confusion),
- ▶ simplification (providing details that are readily understandable), and
- ▶ conviction (enthusiasm for the work and clear identification of its purpose).

The exercise manager should explain the task (objectives, aims, purposes), give reasons why decisions have been made, allocate tasks to staff members and set the outcomes required. In keeping a balance between order and freedom, the exercise manager should answer the question "What is my role?" for each staff member. For example, a team of exercise managers responsible for a national football team may include a biomechanist, exercise physiologist, masseur, physiotherapist and sports physician, among others. It is important for optimal performance of the athletes that all members of the exercise management team have clearly defined roles, an ordered structure and processes within which to work, along with the freedom to fulfill their roles within set guidelines without continual interference.

Leading Productive Meetings

Meetings must be interactive in order to be productive. It is generally agreed by researchers that we can only listen effectively for 30 to 60% of the time, and effective listening is greatly reduced the longer we listen without talking or responding in some way. Therefore, discussion is an important tool for making meetings work well. All employees can take a leadership role at some time during meetings by contributing to the discussion. This is usually most effective if staff have read background material, thought about issues in advance and prepared in other ways such as researching relevant additional materials and remembering to take diaries to the meeting. Documentation is another method to achieve an effective meeting. For example, an agenda distributed in advance is an important tool for ensuring a meeting is productive. Additionally, meetings should be followed up with written communication (usually in the form of minutes, meeting notes or action summaries) confirming what was covered and the decisions made.

Controlling Staff

It is the manager's role to persuade personnel to carry out tasks as the organisation expects. This requires effective controlling skills. Most effective managers provide a balance between **nurturing** staff and being demanding; the ability to nurture staff is the hallmark of a good leader. Genuine concern for their welfare is intuitively detected by employees, and this helps the manager maintain an appropriate level of control. A manager who is too strict will not only send the message that he doesn't trust his staff, thereby demotivating them, but also restrict his staff's ability to make decisions on their own and thus stagnate their development. For example, compare the controlling demonstrated by two different managers (Laura and Michael) who have been listening in on the beginning of a conversation between their staff member (Rachel, a gym receptionist) and an irate customer:

> Laura immediately comes over to Rachel and dismisses her with:
> "I'll deal with this! You check the tennis booking".
> Michael, however, listens to the conversation for a few minutes then comes over to Rachel and continues to listen without interrupting while Rachel attempts to sort out how the misunderstanding occurred. When the conversation appears to be concluding he says to the customer:
> "I'm the manager and I add my apology to Rachel's. We're sorry the misunderstanding occurred and we'll do our best to see that it doesn't happen again".

Notice the use of Michael's *"we're"* and *"we'll"* and his support of Rachel by allowing her to continue the discussion with the customer; in contrast, Laura shows both Rachel and the customer that she has no trust in Rachel's ability to bring the conversation to an appropriate conclusion. Michael is likely to provide Rachel with constructive feedback on her handling of the situation, pointing out both good and poor components so that the scenario is both a learning and a motivating one, whereas Laura is likely to criticise Rachel afterward, continuing to be unsupportive and demotivating.

By nurturing staff so that they feel valued for their contributions, they are more likely to perform at their best. While good performance requires praising so that employees know that they should not settle for less in the future, poor performance also needs to be recognised and controlled. Controlling skills are needed in situations that require reconciliation of differences among workers, relieving of group tension with humour and disciplining of staff for failing to maintain agreed standards. It is also the manager's role to identify sources of current or potential problems and develop strategies for overcoming them.

To avoid the need for controlling skills, the exercise manager should be aware of the circumstances that cause problems and try to sense when a possible problem is imminent. Asking questions at this time may prevent the problem from occurring. Listening is also an important managerial skill in such situations because staff are more likely to listen to managers who listen to them. Other ways of avoiding the need for controlling skills are to consult staff on matters that affect them and to fully explain all decisions; employees are more likely to support procedures if they are consulted before decisions are made.

Negotiation is another important component of controlling staff. Both managers and employees are more likely to achieve satisfactory personal outcomes in negotiating if they first consider their objectives and what concessions they are prepared to make. Then during the discussion, negotiation involves an assessment of the conflict and the common ground before any agreement is reached on the course of action.

Disciplining staff is a controlling skill required when staff make mistakes or fail to maintain agreed standards. Getting all the facts before taking action allows the manager time to decide how best to approach the situation. Firm correction is needed whenever the consequences of such behaviour are serious, for example, if the staff member has been untruthful, has been rude to a client or has publicly refused to follow agreed policies. However, the majority of mistakes made by employees are usually done with the best intentions. In this case, criticism combined with a compliment may be a good reaction from the manager. By showing workers that their efforts are still appreciated even though a specific action may not have been appropriate, managers can avoid staff becoming resentful and losing their motivation to work. For example, if a poor decision is made that will not have serious consequences, the manager may acknowledge what was done correctly before indicating where action was unsatisfactory and then finish positively by showing how the incident may have been handled appro-

priately. This technique is used in sports coaching and is called "sandwiching" because the negative reaction (criticism) is sandwiched between two positives (a compliment and the behaviour required in future). For example, a manager, John, might discipline a staff member, Mark in the following way:

> "Mark, you've been coming up with some good ideas for the new clinic's equipment, but you shouldn't have told the rep from that company that we didn't want any of their new models. It would have been better if you had said we hadn't made a final decision. That way we keep our options open in case the funding comes through for the more expensive models".

Whatever way staff are criticised, it is important that the manager provides an opportunity for learning more appropriate behaviour. The discussion should therefore include

▶ what behaviour should not have happened,

▶ what should have happened that did not happen,

▶ what behaviour should be continued, and

▶ how the behaviour could be corrected.

Knowing when to criticise and when not to criticise is a skill that managers learn mostly through experience. Empowering staff to make their own decisions, try new ideas and take calculated risks for improvement is an important role of human resource management. Acting as a coach and mentor and leading employees so that they don't need controlling are the aims of a good manager.

Staff Recruitment, Appraisal, Development and Rewards

One of the roles of a manager is to plan and monitor staffing, which may be considered one of the most critical activities of management—an organisation is often said to be "only as good as its people". In the exercise environment, staffing represents the major component of the budget. Staffing includes hiring of staff, setting of individual performance requirements, provision of training and resources, monitoring performance, providing feedback and opportunities for development, and taking action if performance is unsatisfactory.

Staff Recruitment

Staff recruitment is an important component of human resource management for the leader in an exercise environment. Hiring the right personnel requires ongoing human resource planning and allows organisational strategies and goals to be met. Consideration of the job requirements and the necessary qualifications and qualities remains integral to staff selection and training.

Many organisations today prefer to use overtime, volunteers, or contract or temporary workers to overcome short-term staffing needs. However, equitable, competitive and timely staff selection enhances the organisation's image as an attractive exercise site and avoids the disruption often seen with long temporary appointments or unfilled vacancies.

Although the staff selection process has subjective elements, objectivity is enhanced by establishing selection guidelines and an informed committee. A **job description** is prepared or updated for the position to reflect the tasks and responsibilities required. This also forms a framework for the selection criteria, including knowledge and skills, qualifications, experience and relevant personal qualities. Techniques for choosing the selection committee, advertising, short-listing applicants, conducting interviews, making selection decisions, advising applicants and providing feedback are useful skills for every exercise manager.

Monitoring Staff

Staff need to be monitored to check that standards are maintained and that employees remain correctly focused in line with management expectations. Through observation, support, direction, regulation and restraint, the exercise manager helps staff consider their time management in performing daily tasks. The aim is to work toward a self-control situation where management has to intervene as little as possible. Clear expectations, frequent communications and accountability in an environment of trust and mutual respect will reduce concerns and result in better creativity and more productive work than will a multitude of rules, restrictions and controls.

In the previous example when John disciplined Mark for prematurely advising a supplier that new equipment would not be required, it would be appropriate for Mark to ask John for a review of the guidelines of his role so that he is able to consider these as he completes the new clinic layout. This would reduce the likelihood of the possibly demotivating experience of having his work performance again criticised.

Performance at work is influenced not only by ability but also by the level of understanding of the job required. If employees clearly understand their individual roles in the organisation, they are more likely to perform better than if their roles are ambiguous. Performing well is accompanied by intrinsic and extrinsic rewards that lead to job satisfaction and, ultimately, to increased effort and better performance. Monitoring this sense of fulfilment among staff is one of the human resource roles of the exercise manager.

Staff Appraisal

Performance appraisal techniques are used to evaluate staff. The exercise manager must keep performance data in order to continually assess each individual's contribution and to provide feedback on work completed. Regular appraisal interviews, where positive practices and outcomes are considered followed by suggestions for improvement, help employees evaluate their own performance and that of the group.

The purpose of evaluation is to determine whether staff are working efficiently and effectively to achieve the organisation's goals and objectives. Appraisals aim to improve staff performance through the review of performance measures, the provision of constructive feedback and the suggestion of opportunities for career development. They do not take the place of recognising good performance, or dealing with poor performance, when it occurs. However, appraisal interviews benefit employees by providing recognition, feedback, career planning and catering for work needs. When feedback is provided, the exercise manager should encourage staff to consider the suggestions in figure 12.4.

Listen carefully.

Ask questions for clarity.

Paraphrase the feedback in your own words.

Acknowledge the point of view and agree with what is true.

Before responding, consider taking time to think it through.

Decide whether you will change your behaviour and, if so, the process to achieve this.

FIGURE 12.4   Considerations for staff being provided with feedback.

A time consuming but important role for the exercise manager is determining what and when performance measures should be taken and then maintaining these data. Constant monitoring is essential so that interventions can occur quickly when expectations are not met, thus reducing the need for conflict resolution and stress management. Performance indicators are often based on specified outcomes, actions and timetables, areas in which assessment can be objective and meaningful for staff. In addition, data on performance indicators must be interpreted within the context of the work environment. Another important aspect of the appraisal process is feedback that provides constructive and non-judgemental critical analysis. Feedback should always be based on performance and effectiveness criteria and not on a person's character. Conducted successfully, the process should act as a motivational tool for the staff and is most effective if employees are involved in developing strategies for making changes. Feedback is commonly focused in an annual performance appraisal that considers

- past performance,
- future work (targets, priorities, standards, strategies),
- matching of perceptions of what can be achieved, and
- improvement of skills, knowledge and behaviour.

A clear record of the discussion and its results is an important outcome of the performance appraisal. This may include a specific performance rating and statement for each job responsibility, comments on overall performance with emphasis on strengths and areas for improvement, and plans to improve performance with a focus on development. Before the interview, a list of duties and responsibilities should be made for review. Other areas to be discussed might include quality and quantity of work; knowledge of job, policy and objectives; cooperation and dependability; attendance and punctuality; initiative; and supervisory or technical potential. The exercise manager may also consider a "360° appraisal" where an individual is rated by his or her immediate superior, peers and subordinates.

Staff Development

New staff or staff who are new to a role require an orientation program in which duties are explained and expectations defined. An action plan then outlines the tasks required (in priority order) and where

to find assistance and resources. If monitoring indicates that performance is below expectations, the manager should work with the staff member to determine the source of the problem and develop strategies for improvement. If performance is satisfactory, the manager may take the role of a coach when the employee takes the initiative to request assistance to improve. Through coaching, the manager may provide opportunities for similar work in another environment, more challenging work or different work to further develop the staff member's abilities. Encouraging employees to critically evaluate their own performance, to suggest improvements or alternatives in the way they perform, and to invite constructive criticism will establish an environment for honesty and thus maximise opportunities for staff development. Figure 12.5 offers considerations for managers giving feedback.

Inviting criticism from personnel presents an excellent learning opportunity for managers. Providing regular opportunities for staff to contribute feedback to their manager will not only improve the manager's performance and that of the organisation but also the manager's positive relationship with the staff. In addition to the considerations in figure 12.5 for providing employees with feedback, the manager should listen carefully without reacting defensively to criticisms, consider ideas seriously, acknowledge useful ideas and implement these wherever possible. Reciprocal supportive communication in which positive outcomes as well as problems are discussed openly and honestly between a manager and staff is the ultimate in a working relationship.

Give positive feedback before negative and finish with positive feedback.

Be exact, descriptive, clear and unambiguous.

Give specific examples.

Do not be judgemental.

Speak for yourself, not others.

Use "I" not "you" (e.g., "I feel annoyed when you are late" not "You are always late").

Do not use questions (e.g., "When will you be early for a change?") but "I" phrases that indicate a problem to be resolved (e.g., "I notice that you are often late").

FIGURE 12.5   Considerations for managers providing feedback.

Setting up procedures in such a way that employees work in an environment that encourages them to improve their skills is good human resource management. This should be very much like training an athlete. Managers are most effective when they think and perform as a coach rather than a supervisor. A coach does not tell an athlete to keep trying different things until a new skill is learned and then the reward will be a day off. Rather, the coach leads the athlete through a set of gradually more difficult drills, rewarding the athlete after each one is mastered until the skill is learned. Coaching points for staff development are included in figure 12.6.

Managers should also consider assisting employees to look for opportunities to develop their skills. Today's jobs are often so intense that opportunities to concentrate on improving skills and developing new ones can be easily missed. To keep up with new developments in the exercise management field, staff must continually seek opportunities and then diligently take action so that learning and improvements occur. For example, yearly attendance at AAESS workshops and seminars and SMA conferences would significantly assist in staying abreast of developments. Figure 12.7 provides some considerations to help staff maximise their skill development.

Awareness of staff strengths and weaknesses and their impact on others is also an important management skill, as is the identification and promotion of original thinking, ingenuity, innovation and readiness to accept challenges. Since development of the human personality is shaped not only by genetic predisposition but also by education and training, staff management requires consideration of suitable opportunities for assisting employees with these qualities. Some strategies for enhancing staff creativity are given in figure 12.8.

In the exercise management profession, managers can motivate their staff to creatively look after clients by making it clear to employees that they are responsible for their clients' satisfaction and at the same time making it clear to clients that the staff are responsible for looking after them. Directing concerns and complaints back to staff to deal with, but being available to discuss problems without taking over, leads to staff empowerment, creativity and learning. If employees perceive an open and trusting environment for discussion, they will be more likely to keep the manager informed about their work. This is a fundamental organisational requirement for good management because it makes managers aware of information that may be important for the organisation's direction or impending problems that may be prevented.

Be aware of your weaknesses.

Ask managers to provide opportunities to develop skills.

Ask colleagues to provide feedback on your work.

Seek out a mentor outside your immediate worksite.

Organise professional development at annual staff appraisal.

Attend professional organisations' meetings, courses and workshops.

FIGURE 12.7   Considerations for staff seeking to develop their skills.

Monitor performance and reward and recognise good performance.

Communicate progress to increase awareness and show all staff why they are important.

Consider awarding productivity bonuses.

Consider the drawback of raising expectations that cannot be met.

Use motivators such as recognition and advancement.

FIGURE 12.6   Coaching points for staff development.

Facilitate thought-provoking discussions.

Discuss individuals' ideas in team meetings.

Develop ideas and investigate their implementation.

Bring different ideas together into team processes.

If ideas cannot be implemented immediately, target them for future consideration.

FIGURE 12.8   Strategies that promote staff creativity.

Staff Rewards

For effective motivation in the workplace, it is important to reward staff who excel. This not only shows that the manager values their hard work, it will also influence other employees to excel and increase their drive to achieve organisational goals. Ignoring high achievement is a mistake; managers should be quick to notice and reward good work. Strategies for providing rewards in the workplace (see figure 12.9) fall within four categories: recognition, advancement, better work and better working conditions. The most important type of reward in the workplace is recognition. Employees understand that managers cannot always provide monetary rewards or even formally recognise their achievements, but for many people working in exercise management, great satisfaction is gained from being told that they have fulfilled or exceeded expectations.

Giving frequent rewards, usually in the form of praise, is an effective way of creating a happy workplace and promoting teamwork. When staff work as a team, it is particularly vital that each member continually acknowledges the contributions and successes of the others to ensure that no one feels taken for granted or unneeded. Further, group rewards usually result in everyone in the group helping each other perform well and improve because each member has a vested interest in others doing well.

Conflict and Stress Management

Conflicts arise in even the best-managed organisations as a result of misunderstandings, incorrect or insufficient information, and mismatches of personal goals and organisational goals. Not all conflict is bad or requires managerial response; conflict of ideas can be useful as long as the focus remains on the ideas and not on the people involved. However, when conflict becomes disruptive or personal, or threatens work output, it needs resolution by the team with assistance or at least support from the manager. Steering the team between complete avoidance of conflict, which reduces the team's effectiveness and growth, and continuing conflict, which eventually destroys the team, is the manager's responsibility. Several methods of dealing with conflict have been identified. They include avoiding, accommodating, compromising, competing and collaborating as outlined in figure 12.10. However, work is sometimes more demanding than staff can accommodate, and conflict and stress are the outcome. Conflict resolution and stress management are nearly always very time consuming for the exercise manager.

Workplace stress is a global phenomenon. In the United States, stress claims represent more than 15%

Recognition: acknowledgement and praise through written or verbal media, including face-to-face communication, certificates, plaques, newsletters, e-mail or staff meeting announcements

Advancement: promotion in status, salary, responsibility or job security

Better work: more interesting or appealing work or more variety

Better working conditions: improved physical environment, more freedom, "perks" (e.g., car)

FIGURE 12.9   Staff rewards.

Avoiding: Deliberately ignoring problems and avoiding confrontation is useful when problems are trivial or may go away on their own, priorities are elsewhere, others are better at handling the situation or time is needed for staff to cool down.

Accommodating: Giving in is useful when the leader is wrong, the issue is not as important for the leader as for the staff or an atmosphere of harmony is more important.

Compromising: Coming to some agreement is useful when an interim measure is needed, there is pressure to make a decision or mutually exclusive goals are involved.

Competing: Win-or-lose decisions are useful when a quick decision is vital, the issue is vitally important or the leader is certain the decision is correct.

Collaborating: Problem solving to find a solution that everyone is content with is useful when the issue is too important for compromise, commitment to the outcome is needed, different interests need to be merged or learning the process is part of the objective.

FIGURE 12.10   Strategies for resolving conflict.

of all occupational claims, and approximately 10% of workers' compensation claims in Australia are related to stress. Stress at work is caused by many factors including working long hours, instability of working conditions, poor communication, poorly defined job descriptions, organisational change (mergers, takeovers, downsizing and structural change), high demand for productivity, demanding clients and superiors, dependence on technology and close scrutiny of individual performance. These can often leave a worker swinging between loyalty, hope and commitment and anxiety, anger and depression. In the past, stress was hidden by sick leave and holiday leave, and although this often remains the case, stress claims within workers' compensation are now commonplace.

Because exercise itself is recognised as a management strategy for stress, the exercise manager is ideally suited to help staff with stress management. Some approaches to stress management include monitoring workloads, involving staff in decision making, resolving conflict quickly and developing a culture in which staff are supportive of one another.

Effective communication is particularly essential for diffusing stress because it is needed to create an environment in which conflicts of interest, personal problems and staff shortcomings can be constructively handled. However, stress has a negative influence on communication. In situations of stress or conflict, staff are particularly resistant to information with which they do not agree and tend to hear what they want to hear (selective listening). This is another reason why good communication skills are a required characteristic of exercise managers.

Summary

Leadership and human resource management in the exercise setting require refined skills across a broad range of areas such as planning, building teams and recruiting, appraising, developing and rewarding staff. Leadership and human resource management are most effective when managers make extensive use of their best interpersonal skills. These include all forms of communication (written and oral), especially when briefing and controlling staff or resolving conflict and stress. Central to all these skills is the core ideology of never settling for the status quo. The search for improvement in every aspect of human resources is central to effective relations with staff, clients, peers and superiors.

Case Study 12.3

Damien is the manager of a personal training business with three employees, Katie, Nick and Reece. Generally, the group gets on well together, but in the last week Nick and Reece have not talked to one another. Damien thinks it is because Nick has become so tired he has lost his sense of humour and is sharp with everyone. Nick's client base has grown recently, and he is looking unwell and concerned about an old injury that is causing him pain again. Katie's client load is also at a maximum, and Reece has declined to take on some of Nick's clients until after his final-year university exams next month. Damien knows he has to better manage the situation, but his youngest son is in hospital and he is reluctant to take on any of Nick's clients himself. Furthermore, he has previously tried to solve a similar scenario by putting on more staff, but the clients complained because they want to have the trainers they know. Considering figures 12.9 and 12.10 and other information provided in the text, how would you approach the group if you were Damien?

Key Issues

1. How will Damien open the group's discussion?
2. What outcomes are needed in this scenario?
3. Are any of the strategies for resolving conflict (figure 12.10) useful here?
4. How could Damien use rewards?
5. What would you put in place for the future considering that this has happened before?

Selected Glossary Terms

brainstorming—A group's generation of ideas through non-critical discussion.

briefing—Allocating tasks and resources and setting performance measures.

communication—Exchange of information and ideas between individuals.

controlling—Monitoring and correcting an organisation's activities to achieve goals.

delegation—Process of entrusting staff with tasks for which the leader is responsible.

ethics—Moral principles that provide guidelines for behaviour.

job description—A summary of what an employee does in his or her work.

leadership—Influencing others' behaviour to accomplish group goals.

management—Administration (includes planning, organising, controlling) of resources (human, physical, financial, information) to achieve organisational goals.

negotiation—A process of resolving conflict by searching for a solution to a problem that is satisfactory for all parties involved.

nurturing—Genuine support, encouragement and development of another.

planning—The process of deciding how to achieve an organisation's goals.

Student Activities and Study Questions

1. Choose three different leaders from your past (e.g., family, school, sport, hobbies, work), and list their positive and negative qualities. What were the three most significant positive qualities and the three most significant negative qualities that made these leaders memorable for you? Now choose a leadership role you have undertaken and list the positive and negative qualities you feel you displayed in that role. Use your lists to consider how leaders you have been involved with in the past have influenced your leadership style. Have you emulated the good qualities of the leaders who made a positive impact on you and refrained from displaying the negative qualities that you remember of poor leaders? What qualities could you benefit from strengthening for your future leadership as an exercise manager?

2. Attend and observe a group meeting of an organisation (sport, business, hobby). What functions did the leader of the group perform during the meeting? What characteristics from figure 12.2 did the leader display? Did these functions and characteristics assist in making the meeting efficient? Did they help bring about the outcomes for which the meeting was called?

3. Prepare your ideal but realistic job description as an exercise manager in a corporate environment with 300 staff and its own health and wellness centre. In developing this job description, consider job descriptions you have acquired for at least two managers in settings other than health and wellness. What leadership tasks have you omitted and why have you omitted these? How will this affect your success as a leader in this corporate organisation? What human resource management tasks have you omitted and why? How will you ensure these tasks are appropriately maintained for the successful management of this health and wellness centre?

4. Discuss with three people the concerns they have at work. Select a concern you have not yet experienced and one of your own concerns. What similarities and differences are there between the two concerns? What strategies might you use to avoid the two concerns in the future?

5. As the leader of a group of three staff, you are aware that the group is finding the worksite excessively stressful. As a result, work practices, particularly communication, are much less effective than usual. What would you do to address this issue? After you outline the process required to overcome this issue, make a list of the possible strategies you may consider for implementation. What leadership qualities and skills do you draw on in forming this plan? Are there other qualities and skills that will be helpful in implementing the plan?

CHAPTER 13

Business Management

Every **organisation** needs effective management to be successful, and businesses in the exercise industry are no different. Managing is the process of getting things done through others. It involves planning, organising, motivating and controlling, and these functions are never ending. Whenever one issue is dealt with another needs attention. However, many managers find their role very rewarding, perhaps because of their involvement and responsibility in so many aspects of the organisation. Together with an understanding of the exercise inductry, exercise managers need an understanding of business processes in order to create and maintain a successful business. This chapter covers these processes including business planning, marketing, financial management, management of programs, facilities and equipment and risk management. It also addresses legal issues including workplace health and safety and business writing.

Organisational Structures

Understanding and defining the structure of the organisation allows the exercise manager to be clear about the responsibilities and tasks of all management and staff. This provides a basis for fulfilling the objectives of the organisation. With new or very small organisations, the structure is usually simple and clear: who is doing what, when and why is understood by all involved. However, in large organisations, assumptions about these functions can result in less than optimal working conditions. Along with the organisation's culture, its structure may promote or restrict ideal communication networks and impinge significantly on the working environment.

The way a business is structured can have a profound impact on its development and success. A large business develops diagrammatic charts of its **organisational structure** to illustrate the lines of communication and how functions are divided among the staff. Consider figure 13.1, which shows two possible structures for the same staff of a commercial fitness centre. Each clearly indicates the chain of command and accountability of staff, while also reflecting the different levels of responsibility. For example, if a junior employee wants to introduce a new service, knowing the organisational structure of the business will be important for determining which other staff members might be involved in discussions and decision making. Some organisational structures may require discussion with several employees; others may require discussion with only one superior. In this example, according to the model presented in figure 13.1a, the customer service officer would initially discuss offering a new service with the aerobics instructor and the equipment coordinator before taking the idea to the front desk manager. In contrast, in the model presented in figure 13.1b, the customer service officer would discuss the idea with the front desk manager who would discuss the idea with the aerobics instructor and the equipment coordinator. The organisational struc-

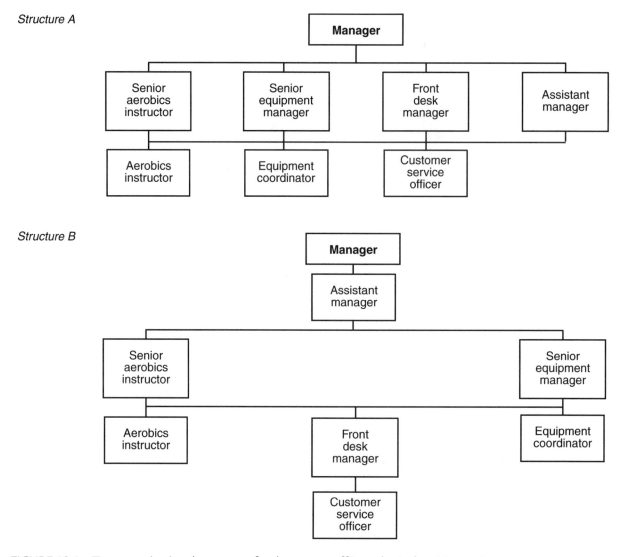

FIGURE 13.1   Two organisational structures for the same staff in a physical activity setting.

ture of a business, therefore, has an effect on the types of communication networks established and the group dynamics of the staff. Further, if a business is to develop optimally, some flexibility may be required in its organisational structure as it diversifies and grows.

Exercise management is a service industry that provides assistance to clients based on the use of its main asset: its staff. The staff's knowledge, judgement, creativity and problem solving are what the business sells. Businesses are most effective when they provide services to a niche market. For example, a business that offers services ranging from personal training for elite sports teams to exercise programs for the overweight and unfit general public will need to work very hard at a consistent organisational image that does not confuse clients and the public.

This image may be compromised if the business attempts to be too diverse. A business should therefore clearly define its service range, and this should be reflected in its organisational structure.

Business Plans

A **business plan** summarises the goals, objectives, structure and strategies of a business. This document is developed before starting or expanding a business and is reviewed at least every 3 or 4 years. An important function of a business plan is to provide a record of assessment of both the viability of the business idea and the ability to provide a product or service. In reporting the results of the feasibility study, the business plan provides clear evidence of the business opportunity, why it exists, and how the business will operate. Factors critical to the success of the business (as shown in figure 13.2) are

identified in the feasibility study. This process of thoroughly investigating a commercial idea before starting a business is particularly important if financial assistance is required.

Provides direction and focus

Shows financial institutions that the idea is viable

Shows profitability on paper before investment

Reduces ad hoc decisions

Indicates operating procedures

Requires consideration of competitors

FIGURE 13.2   Reasons for writing a business plan.

Scope and Purpose of a Business Plan

To prepare for the success of a business, a business plan should encompass management, **market research,** marketing strategies, operations, financial planning and an **action plan** as detailed in figure 13.3. A short summary at the beginning of the business plan, called an executive summary, provides an overview of the essential information. The executive summary is a crucial part of the business plan because it must convince the reader that the business idea is viable and entice the reader to read further. The business plan answers the following questions:

EXECUTIVE SUMMARY

- management team
- business opportunity
- establishment costs
- financial projection

MANAGEMENT

- business concept
- mission statement
- manager's qualifications and skills
- regulatory issues
- trading name
- legal structure
- business premises
- product/service(s)

MARKET RESEARCH

- current state of industry
- market size and trends
- potential clients
- test market results
- competition and competitive advantage
- "SWOT" analysis

MARKETING STRATEGY

- product
- price
- place
- promotion
- people

OPERATIONS

- development status
- facility
- equipment
- layout
- staffing
- procedures

FINANCIAL PLAN

- establishment costs
- source of funds
- projected income
- projected costs
- cash flow forecast

ACTION PLAN

- tasks
- dates
- person responsible

FIGURE 13.3   The scope of a business plan.

► Is there sufficient demand for the product or service?

► Can demand be covered by the resources available?

► Can the business make a profit?

► Will the profit be sufficient to justify the investment?

Management

The management section of a business plan includes an outline of the business concept, the **mission statement,** goals, values, manager's qualifications and skills, regulatory issues relevant to the business, its trading name, legal structure, business premises and the product/service(s) to be offered.

The mission statement clearly describes what the business expects to achieve. It answers the question "Why do we exist?" and provides staff, clients, investors and others with a clear statement of the purpose of the business. Mission statements often include references to clients, the product/service(s), professional and financial satisfaction for managers and staff, and growth of the business. It may also state the beliefs and philosophy of the organisation, as in some of the following mission statements:

> American College of Sports Medicine: The American College of Sports Medicine promotes and integrates scientific research, education, and practical application of sports medicine and exercise science to maintain and enhance physical performance, fitness, health, and quality of life.

> Australian Association for Exercise and Sports Science (AAESS): AAESS is a professional organisation which is committed to establishing, promoting and defending the career paths of tertiary trained exercise and sports science practitioners, who are in turn committed to best practice and client well-being.

> Brisbane fitness centre: To provide the community with safe, scientifically based exercise programs conducted ethically and with excellent standards of facilities and services for members.

Setting goals helps to identify what the business expects to accomplish. The acronym SMART indicates important aspects of goal setting:
Specific: clear and precise in their expectations
Measurable: performance indicators included so achievement/success can be measured
Achievable: realistic for the organisation to achieve
Relevant: clearly related to the organisation's work

Time frame: a specific time assigned for accomplishment

The identification of core values is also recommended for new businesses and for businesses as they change and re-evaluate. If several values (e.g., trust, respect, teamwork, commitment, open communication, creativity/innovation) are maintained as a central, essential guide for all work, then the business is more likely to stay true to its mission and original reason for being established.

Market Research

Market research is the systematic gathering, recording and analysis of data related to **marketing,** an essential function of any business. Marketing is the process of enticing clients to purchase the products or services that the business offers. Good market research skills enable employees to develop effective marketing strategies. For example, market research provides essential information on the current state of the industry, market size and trends, potential clients, the competition and any competitive advantage the business might have. It also offers the means of assessing strengths, weaknesses, opportunities and even threats and how these can be implemented to the advantage of the business. Typical methods for gathering this information include

► surveying through questionnaires and interviews;

► acquiring data from media and journal articles, government and commercial publications, company records and the like; and

► conducting experimental research to assess how changes in manipulated variables affect other variables.

Market research is the first step in establishing the feasibility of a business idea. It allows planning of how the service will be priced, promoted and delivered to meet the goals of the business. It identifies prospective clients' needs and wants and how these might be satisfied with consideration to the expertise of the business and its competition. In deciding if a business idea is feasible, the service to be provided has to be analysed in terms of its demand. The following questions must be asked:

► What services are needed/wanted?

► What fee is attractive?

► Who are the competitors?

► How do competitors market their services?

▶ What are competitors' strengths and weaknesses?

▶ What opportunities exist for establishing the services?

▶ Are there any threats to establishing the services?

▶ What strategies can be identified to benefit from the strengths and opportunities and deal with the weaknesses and threats?

▶ How can clients be enticed to use the services of the new business?

A critical part of market feasibility research is identifying similar businesses in the vicinity of the proposed business. If there is competition, then features that make the business distinct should be clearly identified. Differences might include fees, accessibility, quality of services or facilities, and special needs for which the business will cater. These advantages also help identify a profile of the potential clients of a business so that they can be targeted in marketing strategies.

A **SWOT analysis** (**S**trengths, **W**eaknesses, **O**pportunities and **T**hreats) is a helpful tool for examining internal strengths and weaknesses of a business and identifying the external opportunities and threats that may affect how the business functions. A SWOT analysis is usually recorded in a matrix

table (see figure 13.4). This matrix can be expanded as in figure 13.5 to help managers develop strategies from the SWOT analysis to benefit business operations. To show how weaknesses and threats will be overcome or covered and how strengths and opportunities will be maximised, the matrix allows development of strategies as follows:

▶ SO: strategies utilising strengths and external industry/market opportunities of the business

▶ ST: strategies using strengths of the business to reduce the impact of external threats

▶ WO: strategies attempting to reduce internal weaknesses by utilising external opportunities

▶ WT: strategies attempting to minimise the impact of internal weaknesses and external threats

The aim is to generate as many strategies as possible to address issues raised in the SWOT analysis. After each strategy, a reference can be included to indicate the source of the reasoning (e.g., O1, W3, as depicted in figure 13.5).

Marketing Strategy

Establishing clear marketing goals will keep the business focused and help maintain effective marketing

---

INTERNAL FORCES

Strengths	Weaknesses
▶ New equipment	▶ Limited staff numbers
▶ Excellent location of facility	▶ No staff for new aerobic program
▶ Surplus from last year's budget	▶ Unattractive exterior of facility
▶ 5% increase in membership last year	

Opportunities	Threats
▶ Housing estate opening within 2 km	▶ New gym opening in nearby suburb
▶ New Government funding programs	▶ Low membership fees offered by opposition
▶ Development of new aerobic program	▶ High inflation

EXTERNAL FORCES

FIGURE 13.4   SWOT analysis for a business in a physical activity setting.

	Strengths	**Weaknesses**
	1. New equipment	1. Limited staff numbers
	2. Excellent location of facility	2. No staff for new aerobic pro gram
	3. Surplus from last year's budget	3. Unattractive exterior of facility
	4. 5% membership increase	
Opportunities	**SO**	**WO**
1. Housing estate new opening within 2 blocks	1. Distribute flyers in new housing estate (O1, S3)	1. Paint exterior and order signage (O1, W3)
2. New government funding programs	2. Develop a proposal for Active Australia funding (O2, S1, S2)	2. Hire more staff (O2, O3, W1, W2)
3. Development of new aerobic program	3. Develop new marketing materials (O1, S1, S2, S3)	
Threats	**ST**	**WT**
1. New gym opening in nearby suburb	1. Restructure membership fees to match competition (T1, T2, S3, S4)	1. Refurbish facility's exterior (T1, W3)
2. Low membership fees offered by opposition	2. Develop a special seasonal membership (T1, T2, T3, S4)	2. Hire casual staff to cover busy periods (T1, W1)
3. High inflation		

FIGURE 13.5   Matrix of strategies developed from SWOT analysis in figure 13.4.

strategies. The marketing strategy places the consumer at the focal point and assumes the business will provide what people want to purchase and not what the business wants to sell. The business must therefore find out what people want or need so that it can offer the right marketing mix (the right product at the right price, available through the right channels and presented in the right way). This requires assessment of the five Ps: people, product, price, place and **promotion.**

In order to keep the first P (people, i.e., customers) as the focus of marketing, exercise managers think not about producing products or services but about satisfying clients. An accurate profile of potential customers is therefore important for establishment of appropriate marketing strategies. This prevents selling (a focus on the needs of the seller to convert products into cash) and encourages marketing (a focus on satisfying the needs of the buyer). In the case of exercise management, the second P (product) is a service such as physiological assessment and advice, sports training or rehabilitative care. New businesses usually prosper most successfully if they do not attempt to offer a wide range of services initially but instead concentrate on a portion of the market (what is called a market niche or segment). Services that competitors have ignored, will ignore or are unable to provide make ideal market segments. The third P (price) is what is paid for the service or product. Price is often decided by market forces outside control of the business, and because the business must be financially viable, costs must be thoroughly analysed (refer to section on financial planning). The fourth P (place) describes the geographical area in which the service will be provided; it should be appropriate to the other Ps. For example, an exclusive gym for high-fee-paying clients would be appropriate in an inner city area close to this type of clients' worksites but not for an industrial area where workers may have low incomes. Promotion, the fifth P, is the communication between the business and the client to inform, educate or persuade. The decisions that make communication techniques the most effective are based on

- the promotion objectives (e.g., to affect behaviour, knowledge or attitude),
- resources available (especially human and financial),
- the type of organisation,
- the type of product,
- target markets (e.g., size, demographics, geographical location),
- the competition, and
- legal issues.

More than one promotional method is usually used in a **promotional mix** of the following four categories:

1. **Advertising** (non-personal, paid communication usually presented through newspapers, magazines, television, radio, signs, direct mail, billboards, brochures and so on)
2. Personal selling (face-to-face promotion between seller and potential consumer; also includes telephone, video conferences and interactive computer links)
3. Sales promotions (includes telemarketing, point-of-purchase displays, newsletters, giveaways, special events, open house days, exhibitions, sponsorships, free "come and try" sessions and seminars)
4. Publicity (unpaid promotion such as being the subject of a newspaper, magazine, television or radio feature)

In the exercise environment, marketing techniques are used to promote a professional service primarily to attract new clients. Printed articles, brochures, direct mailings, electronic advertising, and free "come and try" sessions and seminars all work well in enticing clients to try a new business in the exercise setting. Advertising aims to broadly generate new business, while specific targeting of new clients is achieved through referrals, newsletters, personal letters and phone calls. Whatever promotional technique is used, some consideration should be given to the focus of attention; the more diverse the focus of attention, generally the weaker the impact. This is often referred to as the "raspberry jam" theory because the further an amount of jam is spread on bread, the weaker the taste).

Using a number of simultaneous methods is best for marketing a new business. In addition to deciding what marketing techniques to use, decisions must also be made concerning the allocation of time and finances and how the effectiveness of the techniques chosen will be assessed. If clients are not resulting in referrals for an existing business, a high priority should be to provide better service and foster existing client relations rather than broad marketing for new clients. In the exercise setting it is easier and cheaper to keep an existing customer than it is to gain a new one. A commonly used technique is to offer incentives to existing clients who introduce new clients to the business.

Operations

The operations section of the business plan considers how the business will operate: its procedures and processes, staffing structure, program management, and facility and equipment needs and management. These are covered in detail in later sections of this chapter because their effective planning and control are essential to a successful business in the exercise setting.

Financial Plan

The financial feasibility analysis requires projections of income and expenses. The foundation of these projections is based on the market analysis and, for an existing business, on past financial records. Potential sources of data for a new business include similar businesses in other locations and published industry averages or standards. Initial or pre-opening expenses including capital expenses, equipment and supplies should be considered as well as ongoing operating expenses as outlined in figure 13.6. In the planning process, pricing and quantity are important decisions. A common pricing strategy in the exercise setting is to use psychological pricing by which clients are charged fees they would expect to pay. Setting break-even goals is an important task determined through a **break-even analysis.** It considers expenses (variable and fixed) and what income needs to be generated to reach a break-even point (where income equals expenses). A loss occurs below the break-even point and a profit above it. A simple example is shown in figure 13.7.

INITIAL OR PRE-OPENING EXPENSES

Capital (purchase of land, building, refurbishment, signage)

Equipment (computers, furniture, telephone/fax, photocopier, exercise equipment)

Supplies (office supplies, tools and other items renewable every year, security, first aid supplies, uniforms)

OPERATING EXPENSES

Fixed (rent, interest charges, insurance, equipment leases)

Variable (wages [approximately 70% of expenses for businesses providing services in the exercise environment], advertising, electricity, taxes, depreciation, equipment maintenance and repairs)

FIGURE 13.6   Initial and operating expenses for a business in the exercise setting.

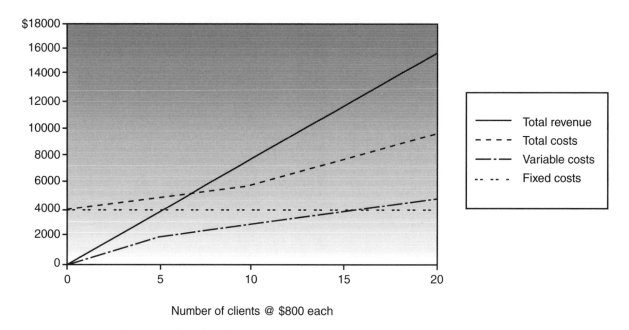

Number of clients @ $800 each

FIGURE 13.7   Break-even analysis for a business in a physical activity setting.

New businesses usually require financial support from investors or financial institutions. The rate of return on the investment must first be calculated to determine whether the investment will be profitable. The investor must obtain a minimum of 10 to 15% on the return of the investment, otherwise it would be better to invest in other areas that have less risk. Repayment of the principal amount borrowed as well as the interest must be considered in the operating costs. Overestimation of income and underestimation of expenses are common for new business owners, who may not fully appreciate the complexities of the business. A thorough financial feasibility study is the best insurance against poor investment, and a good accountant is usually of significant assistance in this task. An accountant is also helpful for locating potential investors and maintaining a focus to ensure the financial obligations to these investors are met. For a small business, a bank is often the source of short-term cash needs and for long-term financing, other options may include finding a business partner or merging with another small business.

Action Plan

Action plans show how the business will achieve its goals by documenting (usually in a simple table format) what and when action will be taken and who will be responsible. By reminding management and staff what has to be done, this tool supports the business planning. It lists specific strategies to be implemented by specific people by specific dates, thus providing an easy checking device to maintain focus and assess progress. An example of an action plan is provided in table 13.1.

Facility and Equipment Management

An important issue for managers in the exercise setting is the selection and maintenance of facilities and exercise equipment. The expense is usually considerable and includes costs associated with purchases or leasing, maintenance, insurance, repairs, storage, and training and monitoring of staff in correct maintenance procedures. Facilities are usually leased, at least on an initial basis while the profitability of the business is established. Equipment is either bought or leased. There are advantages and disadvantages of both purchasing and leasing equipment, some of which are shown in table 13.2. To assist in deciding the best approach, the advice of a qualified accountant is usually recommended.

Once the decision is made whether to purchase or lease equipment, it is then necessary to decide the type of equipment and the best supplier. To help exercise managers address equipment decisions, the following information is required for developing a purchase plan:

▶ Clients' service needs (the most important consideration for gaining and maintaining clients)

▶ Suppliers' reputation (assists in ensuring quality purchases)

▶ Suppliers' buying power (affects price and suppliers' sustained sales)

▶ Warranty conditions (affects possible maintenance costs and value for money)

▶ Servicing support (essential for ongoing availability of equipment for use)

TABLE 13.1—Action Plan

Action required	Personnel	Completion
GENERAL		
Review all programs' objectives	Matthew	15 June
Prepare draft strategic plan for next year	Steve	30 June
Prepare retreat	Sue	Completed
Prepare budget projections for strategic planning group	Judy	30 June
Develop stretching poster for gym	Sally	Completed
Organise subsidy for staff development seminar	Sam	12 August
MARKETING		
Investigate competition's programs and report to strategic planning group	Sally	30 June
Prepare promotional kit for new program	Sue	15 July
Send promotional material to high schools	Sue	Completed
Follow up with Wendy on opportunities for testing new program for schools	Sally	Completed
Finalise proposal for conducting survey of all clients	Judy	30 August
Investigate electronic advertising	Sam	30 August

TABLE 13.2—Advantages and Disadvantages of Purchasing and Leasing Equipment

Advantages	Disadvantages
PURCHASING	
Capital investment	Loss of capital which could be used in other ways
Resale value	Repair costs when warranty expires
Purchase is a tax deduction	Loss on resale
Depreciation is a tax deduction	Less likely to keep equipment current
Freedom to sell or update	
LEASING	
Tax deduction	Stranded with equipment until lease expires
Repairs may be covered by supplier	No capital investment
Regular turnover so stays current	Tax deduction of depreciation not used
Cheaper than buying	No resale value

▶ Price (value for money)

▶ Suitability of equipment (consider in relation to client expectations, other equipment and the facility's characteristics such as space and layout)

▶ Meeting of Australian safety standards (provides confidence in purchase and important for fulfilling care requirements)

▶ Maintenance requirements (affects ongoing costs and staff who ensure requirements are met)

▶ Storage size and ease (equipment that is stored between sessions needs to be easily packed and moved and must fit in available space)

▶ Durability of equipment (affects maintenance and life of items)

▶ Aesthetic appeal of equipment (consider items in regard to others for consistent and appropriate style of facility)

To ensure full value is obtained from the equipment, regular maintenance is required. Maintenance procedures should be developed so that the following are considered:

▶ Staff are assigned specific responsibilities.

▶ Staff are trained in proper care and use of equipment.

▶ Clients are supervised in the proper use of equipment.

▶ Manufacturer's instructions are followed to ensure warranty and legal requirements are met.

▶ A maintenance schedule is developed.

▶ Specified maintenance procedures are followed.

▶ Maintenance service records are kept for all equipment.

▶ Accountability for maintenance is assured by requiring staff to sign and date service records.

▶ Equipment is stored appropriately.

Program Management

Management of successful programs in the exercise setting requires effective planning, **budgeting, client-centred service, program evaluation** and business writing. These are covered in the following sections.

Planning

Planning is vital to the success of a program. Programs that are thoroughly planned generally oper-

Case Study 13.1

Emily is assisting a client with rehabilitation exercises in a hospital clinic when the room is filled with a piercing yell. All eyes turn toward the sound. It is immediately clear that a client has fallen from an exercise bike and is in great pain on the floor beside it. Emily rushes over to the elderly, obese woman on the floor. As she tries to concentrate on the process she should follow to deal with the situation, she can't help but notice that the bike seat is tipped and bent. Emily is intensely angry; the injured client cannot move because of the pain in her back, and Emily knows that this could have been easily avoided. She recently told the facility manager several times that the bike seat was near failure and needed urgent replacing. She decides to write a plan for the facility's future equipment management since the current procedure is ad hoc and not documented in their procedures manual. What would you include in this plan?

Key Issues

1. What is the main goal of Emily's plan?
2. Consider questions about who, what, when, where, why and how?
3. What information will Emily seek before she begins writing her plan?
4. How important will it be to include her superiors in the process of writing her plan?

---

ate in a smooth manner, meet client expectations, achieve desired outcomes and are innovative. Lack of planning leads to disgruntled clients and staff and eventually to unsustainable businesses. Three phases need to be examined when planning a program:

1. Client anticipation
2. Client participation
3. Client reflection

When planning a program, many managers focus too heavily on the phase of client participation and fail to adequately cover the other important elements. For example, the manner in which phone enquiries are handled (anticipation) or the design of the exit route from the facility (reflection) can influence a client's overall perception of a program.

Budgeting

As the tool for evaluating financial performance, budgeting is an important ongoing task for business management. It is used for planning, monitoring and controlling the work of the business and forecasting future business outcomes. There are several different types of budgets, each with a different purpose, including capital, operating, cash and profitability budgets. Only two specific budgets will be discussed here—the budget to forecast cash flow and the budget to show profitability as these two are essential for the effective short- and long-term management of a business.

Cash Flow Budgets

Cash flow budgets are financial records showing when and how much cash will move into and out of a business; they are kept so the business can make sure it will be able to meet expenses such as wages, suppliers' invoices and taxation payments. Market research or previous years' budgets provide the information used to set up the budget. Incoming funds from sales or services and outgoing money to cover expenses are the basis of a cash flow budget. Seasonal trends due to factors such as holidays and weather patterns are important considerations for averting difficult financial times in the exercise setting. The example shown in table 13.3 indicates an opening cash balance at the start of the year of $1,000. After total receipts of $4,000 and expenses of $2,000, the net increase ($2,000) results in a cash balance at the end of January (and for the commencement of February) of $3,000. This process allows the exercise manager to be continually aware of the finances available for use in the business and reduces the likelihood of being caught unable to pay expenses.

Profitability Budgets

Profitability budgets are financial records showing which work is profitable and which is not; they are essential for keeping a business viable. Unlike the cash flow budget, this type of budget does not reflect cash resources at any particular time because it considers non-cash items such as depreciation of

TABLE 13.3—Example of a Cash Flow Budget

Item	January	February	March	April
INCOME				
Cash sales	$2,000	$2,500	$3,000	$3,000
Credit card sales	2,000	3,500	4,500	4,000
Total income	4,000	6,000	7,500	7,000
EXPENSES				
Wages	$1,500	$1,500	$1,500	$1,500
Other	500	600	900	1,000
Total expenses	2,000	2,100	2,400	2,500
Net increase/decrease	2,000	3,900	5,100	4,500
CASH BALANCE				
Start	$1,000	$3,000	$6,900	$12,000
End	$3,000	$6,900	$12,000	$16,500

equipment and invoices not yet paid. A profitability budget monitors expenditure and income related to different types of work, allowing a business to discern where it should focus its work in order to be most financially successful. An example is provided in figure 13.8.

Client-Centred Service

Because exercise management is a service industry in which services are "experienced", the attitude, confidence and manner of the staff are very important. A client-centred approach places the client at the focus of all work considerations and conduct. The goal is a caring image presented by cooperative, responsive and adaptable staff who always explain services to clients without being asked, anticipate clients' needs and consult clients regarding important decisions.

This philosophy of providing special care to all individuals at all times is central to client-centred service. Because clients have dealt with organisations providing other services (e.g., medical and accounting practices), they can easily define the quality of service experienced and patronise a business with certain expectations. A client-centred approach gives clients new to the exercise setting (e.g., an individual

employing a personal trainer for the first time) the best chance to overcome their concerns and uncertainties. For example, at their first meeting with an exercise manager, new clients are likely to be feeling

RECEIPTS

Memberships	$550,000
Product sales	12,000
	$562,000

EXPENSES

Operational costs	$150,000
Equipment purchases	100,000
Loan repayments	60,000
	$310,000
Surplus for year	$252,000
Surplus at beginning of year	$100,000
Surplus at end of year	$352,000

FIGURE 13.8   Example of a profitability budget.

Case Study 13.2

Alison and her manager, Ian, were discussing the first meeting Alison had just had with her new client, Louise. Alison could tell that Ian was not entirely happy with the way she had conducted the meeting. Ian told her that most staff have a natural tendency to judge, evaluate and correct inaccurate statements made by clients. He then said: "This is what you did in your meeting with Louise. Her body language was telling me that she was feeling like many clients do on their first meeting with our staff—uncomfortable about sharing their personal details with you, worrying about showing you that they don't know as much about exercise as they should, and wondering whether you know what you're doing and whether you'll look after them as they're hoping you will. Louise looked uncomfortable during your whole meeting, so I'd like you to come up with some strategies to help her overcome these feelings at your next meeting."

Alison had several ideas. At the next meeting with Louise, she first greeted Louise with a smile and a bright hello and asked Louise about her week, making a mental note to follow up on two things she said this time at their next meeting together. Alison was careful to find something positive to say in response to Louise's comments about her exercise during the week and to sandwich any negative comments between positive ones while also avoiding judgemental responses. Alison also made an effort to reassure Louise that her actions were a good first step and to encourage her to do more. Finally, Alison monitored her voice and behaviour, checking that she was not being patronising but listening with empathy. Can you think of other ideas for Alison?

Key Issues

1. What are Alison's goals for her next meeting with Louise?
2. How might Alison check whether she achieved these?
3. What process could be implemented to ensure Alison becomes proficient at using these strategies?

insecure, exposed, skeptical, suspicious and perhaps worried.

Attaining Client Satisfaction

Client satisfaction is crucial to the success of a business and dependent on the exercise manager clearly understanding what the client wants from the service. Exercise managers who make assumptions about clients' needs without asking them may never be able to provide client satisfaction; satisfaction will only be gained by asking probing but not intrusive questions to find out what clients really want. Often, clients will tell exercise managers that they are happy with the services provided when in fact they are not. Only a small number of clients readily provide detailed information to help exercise managers completely satisfy them. Figure 13.9 gives some steps that will assist the exercise manager to attain client satisfaction. For example, in a personal training business, the trainer must consider a client's fitness, health, medical history and goals to develop an attractive and effective program for the client. Further, the client should be allowed to play a significant role in the decision-making process because clients who

Listen and reflect back the client's needs.

Provide more than one program that satisfies the client's needs.

Provide details of costs, advantages and disadvantages of each program.

Recommend a preferred program.

Listen while the client comments on the programs, answer questions and clarify where required.

Allow the client to decide on the program to be implemented.

FIGURE 13.9 Attaining client satisfaction.

feel left out of the decision-making process are likely to be dissatisfied with the service provided by the trainer.

An important factor for attaining client satisfaction is **service quality.** This should not be taken for granted but should be approached in a systematic way by implementing procedures for enhancing the client's exercise experience. Some strategies are included in figure 13.10. In addition to the implementation of strategies to assist staff in providing quality service, exercise managers can provide feedback to staff on their implementation of the strategies, particularly by recognising and rewarding achievement; this might be considered the best method of ensuring that employees focus attention on enhancing client service.

Sustaining Client Satisfaction

To sustain client satisfaction, exercise managers must strive to provide services that consistently meet or exceed clients' expectations on an ongoing basis. If this is achieved, clients will be inclined to remain with the business and recommend it to other potential clients. Exercise managers must consistently monitor employees and demand that they meet set standards if client satisfaction is to be sustained. This requires an ongoing staff training program. Other strategies include the constant attempt to improve the delivery of services and to maintain or increase the amount of client contact, giving the business a competitive advantage over its competitors. Competitive advantage is further enhanced if staff skills (technical, interpersonal and business) are improved beyond those of other organisations.

Another strategy for sustaining high-quality customer service is the assessment of clients' satisfaction with current work and the implementation of improvements they suggest. Client feedback, especially through written questionnaires, provides a measure of accountability for keeping staff aware of client satisfaction with service. While written questionnaires are an important tool for gathering information, they also have limitations (e.g., biased sampling because of dissatisfied clients who just take their business elsewhere and are not prepared to provide any feedback). The benefit of probing discussions between staff and clients, particularly with those who have not continued with the business, cannot be overestimated. However, it is essential that client feedback is not just collected but also acted on. When clients take the time to provide feedback, they usually watch to see the result. For example, if a client using rehabilitation equipment tells staff that access to a particular piece of equipment is a problem because others are using it for extensive periods, the client will be waiting for staff to do something so that access is easier. If no action is taken, the client is likely to be dissatisfied with the response. Further, if staff make access easier only for this one client and not for all clients, then an opportunity to improve the service has been lost. Whatever strategies are employed, there must be dedication to continual improvement if client satisfaction is to be maintained.

Program Evaluation

A business must be flexible, continually adapting to maintain a match between the organisation's capabilities and responsibilities and the wants and needs of clients. Doing so ensures that satisfaction is gained from both sides. Important considerations are the organisation's competition, and political, economic, cultural, environmental, technological and legal trends. If the business is to remain current or innovative, these factors must be constantly monitored. An important component of this process is program evaluation.

Businesses conduct program evaluations to establish the value of programs and to review their operations. This allows informed decisions for improving practices, modifying procedures, meeting the ever-changing needs of clients, establishing accountability and developing new programs. It is unlikely that a business will have a single evaluation procedure that can meet all its needs for evaluating its different programs. Therefore, managers usually adopt different procedures based on the following questions:

► What is the purpose of the evaluation?
► Who will assess the findings of the evaluation?
► How will the findings be used?
► What are the issues to be addressed?
► What process will be used to address these issues?

Keep high standards of appearance and cleanliness of facilities and staff.

Ensure staff are prompt, happy, and reliable.

Employ staff with caring philosophies and excellent interpersonal skills.

Assist staff in keeping their knowledge and skills up to date.

Continually provide interesting and relevant information and explanations for clients.

FIGURE 13.10   Enhancing client service.

► What resources are available?

► What data must be collected?

► How will the data be collected?

► How will the data be analysed?

► How will the findings be presented?

Program evaluation permits informed decision making when altering program delivery, staffing, budgeting and promotion or determining whether objectives have been met. It also provides evidence of how clients see the offered services, how well the services are meeting their needs and how successful innovations have been. Record-keeping systems track growth and attrition and, as such, are an important source of this information for a business. When collecting data during evaluations, important issues include consideration of clients (e.g., not expecting clients to repeatedly complete long questionnaires) and keeping staff performance as a separate appraisal.

In the physical activity setting, the program manager is usually responsible for the program evaluation. However, in some cases, external consultants may conduct specific evaluations. The findings are most often provided in written reports to stakeholders and discussed in meetings, where an oral presentation may be provided. The focus of an evaluation is the effectiveness of programs in terms of client satisfaction and other outcomes such as improved fitness and well-being and also the program's efficiency in terms of cost versus benefit. Evaluation is particularly important when there is a need to justify continued or additional financial support of a program. However, the ultimate aim of program evaluation is to allow the implementation of improvements to better satisfy clients.

Business Writing

Businesses depend heavily on well-composed written communication because it conveys information, ideas and requests for action while providing a reflection of the organisation's style and professionalism. Communicating effectively through written material is a skill like any other technical skill. It requires a foundation of good writing principles and ongoing practice. When writing business documents, consideration should be given to the use of

► the same language as for verbal presentation,

► a level of formality appropriate to the reader,

► active rather than passive voice,

► visual appeal and up-to-date presentation,

► coherent structure and

► relevant details.

Poorly written business documents are ineffective and counterproductive. A well-written document is

► clear, specific and unambiguous;

► inviting in appearance;

► free of jargon, clichés and stiff or boring language;

► correctly addressed;

► based on short paragraphs;

► free of grammatical errors; and

► not worded flippantly or in condescending tones.

Before writing a document, several steps should be followed to plan an outline (see figure 13.11). Preparation starts by first defining the target audience, the reason for writing and what the reader should think, do or feel when he or she reads the document. The next step is to list the information to be included. Answering the questions posed by who, what, when, where, why and how is an important part of the business writing process. It is helpful to set out a structure for the document and an order of presentation of the information before the document is drafted, edited and proofread.

In editing, the draft can be improved by

► using shorter words, sentences and paragraphs;

► explaining needed technical terms;

1. *Prepare:* define purpose and what reader should think/do/feel
2. *Organise:* determine information needed (ask who, what, when, where, why, how) and structure of document
3. *Draft:* write first draft starting with easiest section
4. *Edit:* consider structure, content, style, presentation
5. *Proof:* ask someone to check the document for you

FIGURE 13.11   The steps in planning business writing.

► eliminating jargon and other industry-specific language;

► using lists with bullets to highlight items visually;

► simplifying explanations;

► eliminating repetition and unnecessary words; and

► taking advantage of having someone else check it for clarity.

The goal should be a document that meets the four Cs (clear, concise, correct and complete), written to express not impress. A well-written document conveys to readers (who may be potential clients or investors) that a business is well managed and that the staff are competent and skilled. A poorly written document conveys the opposite: staff may be careless or lack technical skills.

Risk Management

All businesses, especially those in the exercise setting, set the stage for a wide variety of possible accidents, injuries and incidents. Managers must be aware of their legal responsibilities and roles in minimising risks for clients, staff and other individuals such as contractors and visitors. Given current **legislation,** there is an expectation that managers will be proactive in their responsibility for the welfare of their staff, clients and others by identifying possible sources of risk, assessing the extent and severity of these risks and planning for their minimisation. This process is called **risk management** and is outlined in figure 13.12.

Managers are said to be negligent if they breach their legal duty of risk management and this carelessness results in unintentional harm to others. In addition to possible harm to staff, clients and other individuals, **negligence** results in loss of clients, legal expenses, medical costs, increased insurance costs and other expenses such as the replacement of staff or diverted staff time to deal with the repercussions of incidents. A comprehensive risk management strategy is an essential part of long-term strategic planning as well as day-to-day management. It has many benefits including fewer accidents and illnesses, lower staff absenteeism, lower workers' compensation premiums and improved work efficiency.

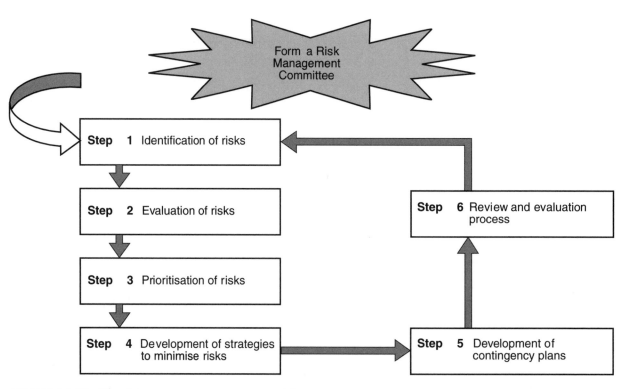

FIGURE 13.12   The risk management process model.

Risk management is the responsibility not only of the manager but of every staff member. For a business to successfully implement a risk management plan, employees must be familiar with the organisation's procedures and regulations. The establishment of day-to-day procedures and regulations is the key to ensuring risk management plans are followed and staff are safety-conscious. This includes safety inspections and investigations, regular maintenance schedules, accident reports and staff training. An important initial procedure is the establishment of risk management plans that include the identification of risks, the assessment of these risks and the development, implementation and monitoring of strategies to reduce risks, along with emergency procedures to minimise the impact of incidents when they do occur.

Identification of Risks

Understanding how specific activities affect clients, staff and other individuals is important for identifying hazards inherent to the activities and environment of the exercise setting. Examples include movement, use of equipment, noise and manual handling. This process requires managers to walk around the workplace and carefully assess with their staff where possible hazards may occur, providing an excellent opportunity for management to involve employees in decision making; staff are likely to be well aware of day-to-day processes that generate risks. Potential sources of risk in different exercise settings are included in table 13.4.

Risk Assessment

After identifying possible sources of risk, the extent or severity of the effects of each risk should be considered. The potential for serious injury or illness and the probability of the risk's occurrence are determined by first giving a score to the frequency of occurrence (ranked on a scale of 1 [highly unlikely] to 5 [will occur]) and to the severity of occurrence (ranked on a scale of 1 [negligible impact] to 5 [devastating consequence]). The frequency score and the severity score are subsequently multiplied to give a ranking between 1 and 25. The risks are then ranked to give an order of risk priority from very severe to minor. An example is included in table 13.5.

Developing, Implementing and Monitoring Strategies to Reduce Risks

Controlling, eliminating and reducing hazards is the expected outcome of risk management. Managers must show that they are continually identifying and managing exposure to risks and taking reasonable precautions and exercising proper diligence to reduce risks. Best practice in the exercise setting requires that professionals adhere to stringent processes. For example, health risk screening before exercise assessment using the American College of Sports Medicine's current guidelines is an internationally recognised standard for best practice in risk management for exercise managers.

Identifying strategies to reduce risks is the first step, which must be followed by setting in place procedures for implementing the strategies and then monitoring that they are being correctly followed. Some ideas for strategies for the exercise setting are provided in figure 13.13. Tracking this process is an essential component of risk management. Records of incidents, procedural changes and monitoring methods provide important documentation of the organisation's control measures. Furthermore, all staff are responsible for seeing that these processes are implemented, and a workplace health and safety

TABLE 13.4—Potential Sources of Risk in Different Exercise Settings

Clinical setting	Fitness centre	Sports club
Client's condition is exacerbated	Client drops free weight on foot	Player slips on wet concrete
Employee injures back when supporting heavy client	Client's valuables stolen from locker room	Spectator suffers food poisoning from canteen food
Employee injures hand trying to repair equipment	Employee steals stock	Spectator falls from grandstand
Client trips over mat left in walkway	Client gets burned in hot shower	Referee hit by spectators' drink cans

officer is an essential appointment in every business. This officer's responsibilities include ensuring that staff follow risk management procedures such as completion of accident reports, submission of reports to management and implementation of new procedures introduced after incidents occur.

Emergency Procedures

Emergency procedures are needed to deal with incidents caused by both human influences and natural forces (e.g., storms, floods). The design of emergency procedures for an organisation is an essential component of risk management, and the inclusion of professional advice is highly recommended. The procedures should detail step-by-step instructions of what should be done in an emergency and should be generic so that they can be adapted to all emergency situations. Management has a responsibility to ensure that procedures are in place and that staff are familiar with them; this requires regular practices, such as evacuation in case of fire, and regular updating of responsive actions, such as would be taught in a first aid course.

TABLE 13.5—Example of Risk Assessment

Risk	Frequency	Severity	Score	Rank
Fall on wet change room floor	4	4	16	1
Injury on treadmill	3	4	12	2
Electrical shock from faulty fan	2	5	10	3

Know the relevant workplace health and safety laws, regulations and guidelines.

Immediately replace or substitute worn or damaged equipment.

Redesign workplace and exercise layouts for safety.

Timetable activities that have a risk component when staff and clients are fresh.

Develop new procedures when old ones are shown to be unsafe.

Train staff in new practices.

Provide protective equipment when advantageous.

Provide instructions and warnings about possible risks.

Screen clients to identify those particularly at risk due to poor health, injuries, disabilities, etc.

Provide adequate supervision of activities.

Limit number of clients so facility is not overcrowded.

Carefully consider how activities expose clients to risks.

Select and maintain equipment for safety.

Have readily accessible medical assistance.

Regularly review all aspects of operations for safety.

Keep staff first aid qualifications up to date.

Consider access and layout to reduce exposure to risks.

FIGURE 13.13   Strategies for reducing risks.

Case Study 13.3

Mark and James were on their way to the local football field for training. It was James' birthday and they were early, so they stopped at the pub for a few drinks. An hour later after several beers each, Mark and James became very agitated by the trainer's demands to complete set drills. In a fury, Mark decided he'd had enough training and jumped a fence dividing the field from the change rooms. Unfortunately, Mark did not clear the fence and spiked himself badly in the leg. An ambulance was called to take Mark to hospital where he required surgery. Mark later filed a suit against the trainer for negligence by not preventing him from training when intoxicated. The football club immediately updated its risk management plan. However, James thought that this was insufficient and wrote to the club to suggest several other considerations for follow up to ensure the incident was not repeated. What would you include if you were James?

Key Issues

1. The strategies listed in figure 13.13 are not exhaustive for reducing risks in physical activity settings but give some ideas of the strategies that James might include. What would you add to this list?

2. Do the requirements for workplace health and safety in the exercise environment shown in figure 13.14 assist in developing more strategies for this particular incident?

Legal Responsibilities

The community expects to be protected against negligence or careless conduct by all professionals including exercise managers; the only response to this expectation is to operate in an arena of meticulous care. There is great uncertainty at present concerning **litigation** over negligence and the degree of protection the community expects. With this in mind, only the highest priority can be given to considerations of legal issues in the exercise environment.

A **duty of care** exists between an organisation and its clients because of the nature of the business relationship between the two parties. Managers who fail to identify risks could be seen as breaching their duty of care to their clients. For example, if an instructor notices a client performing a squat technique incorrectly but decides to say nothing, the instructor could be held liable for a breach of duty of care because of negligent **omission.** Solicitors, lawyers, Legal Aid and insurance companies are all sources of legal assistance; businesses in the exercise setting are recommended to develop professional relationships with these groups to ensure professional indemnity and other types of insurance such as public liability and workers' compensation are appropriately covered.

Further, there are many issues relating to appropriate workplace conduct for staff. These include staying up to date with relevant legislation, including equal employment opportunity (EEO) acts that prohibit discrimination based on a person's sex, religion, race, colour, ethnic origin, birthplace, descent, political affiliation, disability, marital status or pregnancy.

In Australia, approximately 250,000 people suffer from work-related health problems every year. Keeping workplaces safe requires systematic and ongoing management. Employers have an obligation to take reasonable precautions and exercise diligence to ensure that the workplace is free from disease or danger of injury. To achieve this, management must first identify hazards with the potential to cause injury or disease and then take action to reduce the risk of exposure. For some workplace risks, there are compliance and advisory standards; where there is no standard about a particular risk, managers may choose how they will meet their obligation to manage exposure to the risk. Proactive behaviour is required to anticipate risks rather than merely reacting after an incident has occurred. Not identifying an obvious risk puts a business in a position to be liable for failure to identify and deal with the risk. Figure 13.14 provides an outline of procedures required for managing exposure to risk in the exercise environment.

In Australia, the highest percentage of work-related health problems involves the back (approximately 25%). Back injuries cost an estimated $1 billion in medical payments and workdays lost

Write a policy outlining commitment to WHS and include procedures manuals.

Allocate to staff roles of responsibility and accountability for WHS.

Develop a system for consultation with staff so that WHS issues are discussed.

Regularly evaluate hazards and their control measures.

Regularly contact governing body for up-to-date information and provide this to staff.

Provide training for new staff and in-service training for ongoing staff.

Ensure equipment is regularly inspected and maintained appropriately.

Develop an accident and incident reporting system.

Provide emergency planning (e.g., evacuation signs).

FIGURE 13.14   Workplace health and safety (WHS) requirements for the exercise environment.

every year. Other problems include open wounds, noise pollution, occupational overuse syndrome and occupational stress. Occupational overuse syndrome (once termed *repetitive strain injury*) has been shown to occur more often if detrimental psychosocial issues are not addressed in the workplace. These issues are closely related to occupational stress, one of the fastest growing work-related health problems in Australia today. Management practices are considered to be an important underlying cause, and thus prevention of work-related health problems has become a focus for managers. If managers, staff and WHS professionals all work together in a coordinated manner to identify potential problems and their solutions, fewer workdays will be lost, workers' compensation claims will be reduced and relationships between management and staff will be improved.

Summary

You cannot have a business without a business manager. Managers will always be needed to perform the endless functions of planning, organising, evaluating and improving businesses. In the exercise setting, business managers have a dynamic and challenging role. The industry is becoming profoundly profit driven, requiring managers to administer highly effective and efficient programs and facilities. To do this, good management skills are vital. Managers must strive to ensure that changing needs of clients are being met and business practices are streamlined to continually meet or exceed client expectations. This is the start of good business practice in the exercise setting; it should be supported by best practice in risk management and other business skills such as marketing and budgeting.

Selected Glossary Terms

action plan—Specific tasks and those responsible for executing them to ensure strategies are implemented.

advertising—Paid form of presentation of goods or services by an identified organisation.

break-even analysis—Procedure to identify the point when an organisation stops taking a loss and starts making a profit on sales of goods or services.

budgeting—The preparation of a plan or forecast of future financial operations.

business plan—A document outlining the business strategy, structure and operation.

client-centred service—Work focused on the customer.

client satisfaction—The effectiveness an organisation achieves in meeting its customers' requirements.

duty of care—Responsibility to act in a required manner of care.

legislation—A statute or act derived by Parliament.

litigation—Conduct of legal proceedings by parties before a court.

marketing—Determining the needs and wants of potential clients and how to deliver the desired satisfaction.

market research—The process of gathering information for management to decide on a course of action.

mission statement—The primary purpose of an organisation.

negligence—Duty of care breached through a careless act or omission that results in damage.

omission—Failure to act that may constitute an offence where duty of care exists.

organisation—A group of people working in a structured and coordinated way to achieve their goals.

organisational structure—The pattern of formal grouping of people and their tasks.

program evaluation—Systematic collection and reporting of information on the delivery of a client service.

promotion—Communication to inform, persuade and influence potential clients.

promotional mix—Group of promotional tools including advertising, personal selling, sales promotions and publicity.

risk management—The process of identifying, evaluating and minimising risks that may lead to harm, together with the development of contingency plans and ongoing review of procedures.

service quality—The customer's perceived level of the provided service.

SWOT analysis—A component of the marketing plan that identifies an organisation's strengths, weaknesses, opportunities and threats.

Student Activities and Study Questions

1. Compare the equipment and layout of two gyms of comparable size. What are the similarities? What are the differences? Are there reasons for the differences? What benefits are there in the gyms' selections? Try to talk with staff and/or clients to ask them what they like and dislike about the equipment and layout. Do they have reasons for their likes and dislikes?

2. A new gym is targeting business people on their way to and from work. Dimensions of the equipment room are 15 × 20 m with a height of 2.2 m. As the gym manager, you have $400,000 to spend on equipment, but this must also cover maintenance for 3 years. What equipment would you buy assuming there will be no further funding for equipment for 3 years? List the brand names and prices of all items. How much did you allow for maintenance? On what did you base this?

continued

continued

3. The management of a small private hospital where you are working decides to investigate the feasibility of introducing an exercise rehabilitation clinic. You are asked to take on this investigation. What will be your mission statement for the clinic? What headings will you use to guide the feasibility study?

4. Choose a business with which you are familiar and perform a SWOT analysis. Extend this to a matrix of strategies (an example is shown in figure 13.5) to show the marketing strategies you would use to assist this business.

5. Outline a schedule to evaluate one physical activity program provided by your university or school. Use the questions provided in the section on program evaluation to guide you.

APPENDIX

Åstrand-Rhyming Submaximal Cycle Ergometer Test[1,2]

A single-stage, 6-min submaximal bicycle ergometer test designed to estimate maximal oxygen consumption. A steady-state heart rate between 125 and 170 beats per minute (bpm) is required.

1. Adjust seat height of the bicycle.

2. Record resting heart rate and blood pressure.

3. Determine the client's initial workrate based on gender and fitness status:

   ► males, unconditioned: 50 W or 100 W

   ► males, conditioned: 100 W or 150 W

   ► females, unconditioned: 50 W or 75 W

   ► females, conditioned: 75 W or 100 W

4. Start the client cycling at the determined workrate. Monitor heart rate (HR) and rating of perceived exertion (RPE) each minute and blood pressure every 2 min.

5. Following 2 min, the workrate may need to be adjusted if the initial workrate is not generating a heart rate response between 125 and 170 bpm.

   ► For clients >40 years, if the HR is <120 bpm then increase the workrate by 25 W to 50 W. The client will need to cycle at this second workrate for 6 consecutive min.

   ► For clients >40 years, if the HR is >120 bpm then continue at the same workrate for 4 min (6 min total).

   ► For clients <40 years, if the HR is <130 bpm then increase the workrate by 50 W. The client will need to cycle at this second workrate for 6 consecutive min.

   ► For clients <40 years, if the HR is >130 bpm then continue for 4 min (6 min total).

6. If the heart rate measured in the sixth minute is within 5 bpm of the heart rate measured in the fifth minute, then reduce the workload for a cooldown. If the difference in heart rate between the fifth and sixth minute is greater than 5 bpm, then have the client continue for another minute until two consecutive heart rates are within 5 bpm (to a maximum of 10 min total exercise time). The test should be stopped if the heart rate >170 bpm or >90% APMHR or RPE >17.

7. Cooldown: have the subject pedal with little or no resistance for 4 min, monitoring heart rate every minute and blood pressure every 2 min. Following 4 min, have the client remain seated until HR <100 bpm.

8. Offer the client a drink of water and unhook any equipment (e.g., sphygmonomometer, heart rate monitor).

9. Calculate the results:

    a. Using the tables provided for males (table A.1) and females (table A.2), locate the final heart rate and workload and the corresponding prediction of maximal oxygen consumption in $L \cdot min^{-1}$.

    b. Multiply this score by the age-correction factor (table A.3).

    c. To convert the absolute score ($L \cdot min^{-1}$) to a relative score ($ml \cdot kg^{-1} \cdot min^{-1}$), multiply by 1000 and divide by the client's body weight.

TABLE A.1—Prediction of Absolute Maximum Oxygen Consumption ($L \cdot min^{-1}$) From Heart Rate and Workload on a Bicycle Ergometer (Males)

Heart rate	50 W	100 W	150 W	200 W	250 W
120	2.2	3.5	4.8		
121	2.2	3.4	4.7		
122	2.2	3.4	4.6		
123	2.1	3.4	4.6		
124	2.1	3.3	4.5	6.0	
125	2.0	3.2	4.4	5.9	
126	2.0	3.2	4.4	5.8	
127	2.0	3.1	4.3	5.7	
128	2.0	3.1	4.2	5.6	
129	1.9	3.0	4.2	5.6	
130	1.9	3.0	4.1	5.5	
131	1.9	2.9	4.0	5.4	
132	1.8	2.9	4.0	5.3	
133	1.8	2.8	3.9	5.3	
134	1.8	2.8	3.9	5.2	
135	1.7	2.8	3.8	5.1	
136	1.7	2.7	3.8	5.0	
137	1.7	2.7	3.7	5.0	
138	1.6	2.7	3.7	4.9	
139	1.6	2.6	3.6	4.8	
140	1.6	2.6	3.6	4.8	6.0
141		2.6	3.5	4.7	5.9
142		2.5	3.5	4.6	5.8
143		2.5	3.4	4.6	5.7
144		2.5	3.4	4.5	5.7
145		2.4	3.4	4.5	5.6
146		2.4	3.3	4.4	5.6
147		2.4	3.3	4.4	5.5
148		2.3	3.2	4.3	5.4
149		2.3	3.2	4.3	5.4
150		2.3	3.2	4.2	5.3
151		2.3	3.1	4.2	5.2
152		2.3	3.1	4.1	5.2
153		2.2	3.0	4.1	5.1
154		2.2	3.0	4.0	5.1
155		2.2	3.0	4.0	5.0
156		2.2	2.9	4.0	5.0

Heart rate	50 W	100 W	150 W	200 W	250 W
157		2.1	2.9	3.9	4.9
158		2.1	2.9	3.9	4.9
159		2.1	2.8	3.8	4.8
160		2.1	2.8	3.8	4.8
161		2.0	2.8	3.7	4.7
162		2.0	2.8	3.7	4.6
163		2.0	2.9	3.7	4.6
164		2.0	2.7	3.6	4.5
165		2.0	2.7	3.6	4.5
166		1.9	2.7	3.6	4.5
167		1.9	2.6	3.5	4.4
168		1.9	2.6	3.5	4.4
169		1.9	2.6	3.5	4.3
170		1.8	2.6	3.4	4.3

TABLE A.2—Prediction of Absolute Maximum Oxygen Consumption (L · min^{-1}) From Heart Rate and Workload on a Bicycle Ergometer (Females)

Heart rate	50 W	75 W	100 W	125 W	150 W
120	2.6	3.4	4.1	4.8	
121	2.5	3.3	4.0	4.8	
122	2.5	3.2	3.9	4.7	
123	2.4	3.1	3.9	4.6	
124	2.4	3.1	3.8	4.5	
125	2.3	3.0	3.7	4.4	
126	2.3	3.0	3.6	4.3	
127	2.2	2.9	3.5	4.2	
128	2.2	2.8	3.5	4.2	4.8
129	2.2	2.8	3.4	4.1	4.8
130	2.1	2.7	3.4	4.0	4.7
131	2.1	2.7	3.4	4.0	4.6
132	2.0	2.7	3.3	3.9	4.5
133	2.0	2.6	3.2	3.8	4.4
134	2.0	2.6	3.2	3.8	4.4
135	2.0	2.6	3.1	3.7	4.3
136	1.9	2.5	3.1	3.6	4.2
137	1.9	2.5	3.0	3.6	4.2
138	1.8	2.4	3.0	3.5	4.1
139	1.8	2.4	2.9	3.5	4.0
140	1.8	2.4	2.8	3.4	4.0
141	1.8	2.3	2.8	3.4	3.9
142	1.7	2.3	2.8	3.3	3.9
143	1.7	2.2	2.7	3.3	3.8
144	1.7	2.2	2.7	3.2	3.8
145	1.6	2.2	2.7	3.2	3.7
146	1.6	2.2	2.6	3.2	3.7
147	1.6	2.1	2.6	3.1	3.6
148	1.6	2.1	2.6	3.1	3.6
149		2.1	2.6	3.0	3.5
150		2.0	2.5	3.0	3.5
151		2.0	2.5	3.0	3.4

(continued)

Heart rate	50 W	75 W	100 W	125 W	150 W
152		2.0	2.5	2.9	3.4
153		2.0	2.4	2.9	3.3
154		2.0	2.4	2.8	3.3
155		1.9	2.4	2.8	3.2
156		1.9	2.3	2.8	3.2
157		1.9	2.3	2.7	3.2
158		1.8	2.3	2.7	3.1
159		1.8	2.2	2.7	3.1
160		1.8	2.2	2.6	3.0
161		1.8	2.2	2.6	3.0
162		1.8	2.2	2.6	3.0
163		1.7	2.2	2.6	2.9
164		1.7	2.1	2.5	2.9
165		1.7	2.1	2.5	2.9
166		1.7	2.1	2.5	2.8
167		1.6	2.1	2.4	2.8
168		1.6	2.0	2.4	2.8
169		1.6	2.0	2.4	2.8
170		1.6	2.0	2.4	2.7

TABLE A.3—Age Correction Factor

Age	Factor	Age	Factor
15	1.10	32	0.909
16	1.09	33	0.896
17	1.08	34	0.883
18	1.07	35	0.870
19	1.06	36	0.862
20	1.05	37	0.854
21	1.04	38	0.846
22	1.03	39	0.838
23	1.02	40	0.830
24	1.01	41	0.820
25	1.00	42	0.810
26	0.987	43	0.800
27	0.974	44	0.790
28	0.961	45	0.780
29	0.948	50	0.750
30	0.935	55	0.710
31	0.922	60	0.680

[1]Adapted, by permission, from J. Schell and B. Leelarthaepin, 1994, *Physical fitness assessment in exercise and sport science,* 2nd ed. (New South Wales: Leelar Biomediscience Services): 162-167.

[2]From Åstrand and Rodahl (1986).

YMCA Submaximal Aerobic Fitness Test[3]

A multiple-stage submaximal bicycle ergometer test to estimate maximal oxygen uptake. Two to four, progressive 3-min stages are performed in an attempt to attain two consecutive steady-state heart rates between 100 bpm and 85% APMHR.

1. Adjust the seat height.
2. Record resting heart rate and blood pressure.
3. Start the client cycling at 25 W (stage 1). Monitor heart rate (HR) and RPE every minute and blood pressure once in stage 1.
4. Determine the HR in the third and follow the flow chart in table A.4 to determine the workrate for stage 2.
   a. if the HR is <80 bpm, then increase the workrate to 125 W,
   b. if the HR is between 80 and 89 bpm, then increase the workrate to 100 W,
   c. if the HR is between 90 and 100 bpm, then increase the workrate to 75 W, or
   d. if the HR is >100 bpm, then increase the workrate to 50 W.
5. Monitor HR and RPE every minute and blood pressure once in stage 2.
6. Following 3 min at stage 2, set the third workrate according to stage 3 in table A.4 and monitor HR, RPE and blood pressure as in the previous stages.
7. If two consecutive HRs between 100 and 85% APMHR have not been achieved, then have the client complete stage 4 (table A.4).
8. If two consecutive HRs between 100 and 85% APMHR have been achieved, then reduce the workrate and have the client cool down.
9. Cooldown: have the subject pedal with little or no resistance for 3 min monitoring heart rate every minute and blood pressure after 2 min. Following 3 min, have the client remain seated until HR <100 bpm.
10. Offer the client a drink of water and unhook any equipment (e.g., sphygmonomometer, heart rate monitor).
11. Calculate the results:
    a. Plot the two final HRs versus workrate on the graph shown in figure A.1.
    b. Draw a line through the two points to the APMHR.
    c. From this point, draw a vertical line through the horizontal axis.
    d. Record the absolute $\dot{V}O_2$max (L · min^{-1}) predicted from the intersecting line.
    e. To convert the absolute score (L · min^{-1}) to a relative score (ml · kg^{-1} · min^{-1}), multiply by 1000 and divide by the client's body weight.

TABLE A.4—Protocol for the YMCA Submaximal Bicycle Ergometer Test

Stage 1		25 W		
	HR <80 bpm	HR 80-89	HR 90-100	HR >100
Stage 2	125 W	100 W	75 W	50 W
Stage 3	150 W	125 W	100 W	75 W
Stage 4	175 W	150 W	125 W	100 W

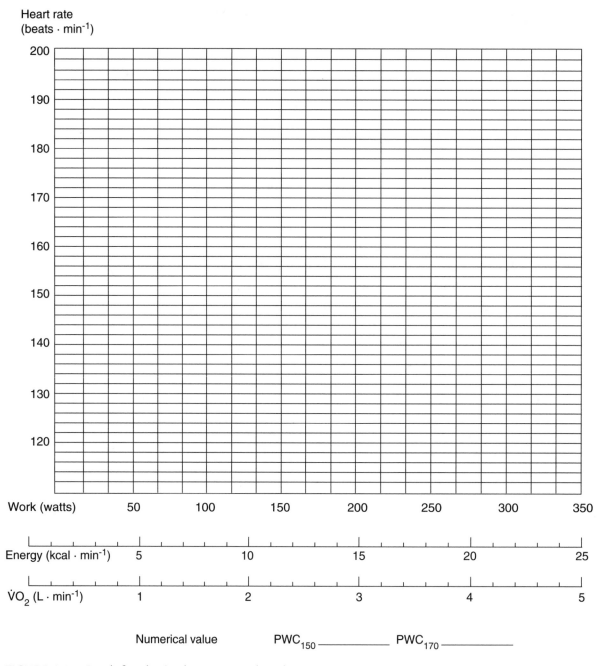

FIGURE A.1   Graph for plotting heart rate and workrate.

Adapted, by permission, from L. Golding, C. Myers, and W. Sinning, 1898, *Y's way to physical fitness*, 3rd ed. (Champaign, IL: Human Kinetics).

GLOSSARY

acquired brain injury (ABI)—Traumatic brain injury resulting in permanent damage to the affected area of the brain, which may involve cognitive or physical impairment.

action plan—Specific tasks and those responsible for executing them to ensure strategies are implemented.

Active Australia—An Australian public health initiative to promote and improve participation in sport and physical activity across the population; founded in 1996.

activities of daily living (ADLs)—Physical tasks required of independent living, such as dressing and feeding oneself, walking, transferring into and out of bed or a chair, housework and stair climbing.

adherence—Maintenance of a treatment or protocol.

adoption—Beginning a recommended treatment or protocol.

advertising—Paid form of presentation of goods or services by an identified organisation.

age-predicted maximum heart rate (APMHR)—Estimated maximum heart rate, calculated as 220 minus age; used to determine recommended exercise intensity (e.g., exercising at a pace that elicits a heart rate equivalent to 60% of APMHR).

agility—The ability to change direction while maintaining balance.

American College of Sports Medicine (ACSM)—The largest sports medicine and exercise science professional organisation in the world, dedicated to promoting and integrating scientific research, education and practice in sports medicine and exercise science; founded in 1954.

anaerobic capacity—Average work output over 30 to 60 s in an all-out exercise test, often using cycle ergometry.

anaerobic glycolysis—The capacity of muscle cells to produce energy (ATP) and the body to perform exercise using the anaerobic glycolytic metabolic pathway.

anaerobic power (or peak power)—The highest power output generated during the first 3 to 5 s of an all-out exercise test, often using cycle ergometry.

anaerobic threshold (AT)—During exercise of increasing intensity, a point at which the metabolic demands of exercise must be met by increasing contribution by the anaerobic glycolytic system, producing excess lactic acid.

angina—Discomfort or pain in the chest, often radiating to the shoulders, arms, neck or jaw, resulting from myocardial ischaemia.

antagonist muscle—A muscle or muscle group that opposes the movement of another muscle group.

anthropometry—The scientific measurement of the human body and its skeleton, including measures of circumferences, body diameters, skinfold fat thickness and body mass.

atherosclerosis—A pathological process resulting in potentially obstructive lesions in the major arteries, in particular the aorta, and coronary, carotid, iliac and femoral arteries.

Australian Association for Exercise and Sports Science (AAESS)—The professional body representing exercise and sport science professionals in Australia; founded in 1991.

balance—The ability to control physical movement of the body and maintain stability.

ballistic stretch—A type of stretching exercise that requires the participant to continuously move, or bounce, throughout the movement; this type of exercise may mimic movements to be performed, such as kicking a football.

barriers—Real or perceived reasons affecting an individual's ablity to engage in an activity or belief (e.g., lack of time can be a real or perceived barrier to participation in physical activity.)

basal metabolic rate (BMR)—The lowest rate of energy expenditure to maintain the body in its basal state, measured in the morning in a fasting state under controlled laboratory conditions.

behavior change—A complex process of altering an observable activity, usually a lifestyle habit, influenced by both external and internal stimuli.

best practice—The use of advanced methods and technology, usually backed by research and recommendations by professional organisations, to provide the highest quality of professional service or care.

blood gas analysis—Measurement of arterial P_aO_2 and P_aCO_2.

blood glucose—The amount of the simple sugar glucose measured in the blood; normal postprandial blood glucose is <10.0 mmol $\cdot$ L^{-1}

body mass index (BMI)—The ratio of body mass (in kg) to height (in metres squared), expressed as kg $\cdot$ m^{-2}; a simple method to determine an optimal body weight range.

bone mineral density—Amount of bone tissue (bone mass) per unit volume, reflecting the mineralisation of bone.

brainstorming—A group's generation of ideas through non-critical discussion.

break-even analysis—Procedure to identify the point when an organisation stops taking a loss and starts making a profit on sales of goods or services.

briefing—Allocating tasks and resources and setting performance measures.

budgeting—The preparation of a plan or forecast of future financial operations.

business plan—A document outlining the business strategy, structure and operation.

cable tensiometer—A device used to measure isometric strength at a specific angle.

caloric threshold—Used in exercise prescription to estimate the minimal or optimal amount of energy to be expended in a specified period of time.

carbohydrate (or **glycogen**) **loading**—The dietary practice by athletes of increasing carbohydrate intake to very high levels and reducing training volume, thereby enhancing muscle glycogen synthesis and storage.

cardiac rehabilitation—A multifaceted secondary prevention program to help patients return to an active and satisfying life after some type of cardiac event; includes interventions to facilitate weight loss, smoking cessation, blood lipid and blood pressure management, effective use of prescribed medication and physical activity.

cardiorespiratory fitness (CRF)—The ability to perform prolonged exercise, quantified in a test of maximum oxygen consumption ($\dot{V}O_2max$) or time to fatigue at a certain work rate.

cerebral palsy (CP)—A non-progressive neurological disorder of movement or posture caused by lesions in the upper motor neurons of the brain occurring before, at or soon after birth; the main impairment involves loss of control of muscle tone and spinal reflexes, specifically the ability to move, balance and maintain postural control.

chronic fatigue syndrome (CFS)—A debilitating condition characterised by excessive fatigue persisting for more than 6 months for which there is no other identifiable clinical cause. Symptoms include cognitive and sleep disturbances, generalised muscle weakness and soreness, fever, and swollen or painful lymph nodes.

chronic obstructive pulmonary disorder (COPD)—A group of conditions characterised by airway obstruction; the most common forms are asthma, emphysema and chronic bronchitis.

circuit resistance training—Resistance training in which the subject moves quickly between exercise stations, with little rest (<1 min) between different exercises; a good way to combine muscular and aerobic conditioning.

client satisfaction—The effectiveness an organisation achieves in meeting its customers' requirements.

client-centred service—Work focused on the customer.

communication—Exchange of information and ideas between individuals.

compound exercise—An exercise movement using multiple muscles and joints, for example, a squat.

concurrent training—Training for both muscular strength and cardiorespiratory endurance within the same training cycle.

confidentiality—Maintaining privacy regarding all personal and health information obtained from a client during, for example, health risk screening, physical fitness testing and exercise programming.

contraindication—A condition, system or impairment that suggests that the desired treatment (e.g., physical activity) is inadvisable.

controlling—Monitoring and correcting an organisation's activities to achieve goals.

core stability—Muscular endurance and strength of the abdominal and trunk muscles needed for spine stability and postural control.

coronary angiography—An invasive technique used to fluoroscopically outline the coronary arteries; coronary angiography is used to diagnose coronary artery disease and help plan revascularisation if necessary.

coronary artery or heart disease (CAD or CHD) risk factor—A health, behaviour or lifestyle factor that, based on epidemiological evidence, is known to be associated with the development of coronary artery disease (or narrowing of the coronary arteries).

cross-training—Maintaining fitness by training using another mode of exercise different from the specific sport; alternatively, using a variety of different types of activities to achieve physical fitness.

cystic fibrosis (CF)—A genetic disease affecting primarily the lungs in which altered cellular transport of chloride ions affects hydration of cells, resulting in excessively salty sweat and thick mucus. Accumulation of thick mucus in the lungs causes frequent infection, which may lead to scarring and permanent damage.

delegation—Process of entrusting staff with tasks for which the leader is responsible.

disability-adjusted life year (DALY)—An estimate of potential life years lost because of premature death, disability and poor health.

duty of care—Responsibility to act in a required manner of care.

dynamic balance—Maintaining postural control during movement, as in reaching while standing or regaining balance after a sudden disturbance.

dynamometer—A device used to measure isometric strength.

dyslipidaemia—Blood lipid levels outside the recommended levels; in particular, concentrations of total cholesterol, high-density lipoprotein cholesterol, low-density lipoprotein cholesterol and triglycerides.

dyspnoea—Shortness of breath or difficult or laboured breathing, especially during physical activity, associated with pulmonary and some types of cardiovascular disorders.

echocardiography—Evaluation and interpretation of images of the heart, heart chambers, heart valves and myocardial blood flow using non-invasive ultrasound technology.

electrocardiogram (ECG)—A graphic recording of the electrical activity of the heart.

ergometer—A device used to measure muscular work performance and able to be calibrated, for example, the Monark bicycle ergometer.

ethics—Moral principles that provide guidelines for behaviour.

evaluation—A process to collect and analyse important information to guide decision making; in the exercise context can be applied to development of programs for individuals, groups, communities or organisations.

exercise—A subcategory of physical activity that is planned and structured with the intention of improving or maintaining physical fitness.

exercise-induced asthma (EIA) or bronchospasm (EIB)—Acute narrowing of the airways during or after strenuous exercise, defined as a decline of 15% or more in FEV_1 after exercise; occurs in 40 to 80% of asthmatics.

exercise management—A profession involved in the application of exercise science and business knowledge and principles to the design, delivery, promotion and evaluation of physical activity programs for the widest possible audience.

exercise prescription and programming—Developing an exercise program for a client (or group of clients) designed to meets the client's health, fitness, performance, and other goals and needs.

exercise rehabilitation—The inclusion of exercise in a multifaceted program to help restore the patient's functional capacity and health.

extrinsic reward—A prize or incentive external to the individual and activity, for example, social recognition.

fitness assessment—Use of standardised tests to measure various components of physical fitness (refer to physical fitness).

flexibility—The ability of a specific joint to move through its full range of motion.

functional capacity—A general term referring to cardiorespiratory fitness and the ability to perform tasks of daily living.

gait—Walking pattern.

girth—The circumference value of a given site using a standard tape measure.

glucose tolerance—The ability of the body to maintain the blood glucose level within the recommended range of <6.1 mmol $\cdot$ L^{-1} (fasting).

glycaemic index (GI)—A measure of the magnitude of rise in blood glucose 2 h after ingestion of 50 g of a particular food relative to pure glucose.

glycogen—Polymer of multiple glucose molecules; the main storage form of glucose in the body, primarily in muscle and liver; provides a major substrate for high intensity exercise.

Healthy People 2000, 2010—A national strategy by the U.S. Departments of Health and Human Services and Education to improve the health of all Americans by encouraging cooperation between all government and non-government stakeholders to develop programs that support healthy lifestyles.

heart disease—Pathologies of the heart and coronary arteries, including heart failure.

heart rate reserve (HRR)—A method to calculate recommended exercise heart rate based on the difference between maximum heart rate and resting heart rate.

hemiplegia—Impaired neurological function and movement on one side of the body; occurs in disorders such as cerebral palsy or acquired brain injury.

herniation or **prolapse**—A herniated or "slipped" disk, a protrusion or tearing of the intervertebral disk causing compression of the spinal cord or nerve roots, resulting in back pain and sometimes disability.

high-density lipoprotein (HDL)—A category of cholesterol transported on proteins that has a protective effect on the development of atherosclerosis; high levels of HDL are associated with a reduced risk of developing coronary artery disease.

Hillary Commission for Sport, Fitness and Leisure—The government body that supports sport and active living in New Zealand by creating opportunities for its residents to be physically active through sport and other means.

hypoglycaemia—Low blood glucose level below 3.5 mmol $\cdot$ L^{-1}, which in the diabetic may result from the combined effect of insulin injection and exercise, both of which enhance glucose uptake by the tissues.

hypokinetic diseases—Chronic diseases associated with low levels of physical activity and movement.

individual anaerobic threshold (IAT)—An exercise intensity eliciting a blood lactate concentration of 4 mmol · L^{-1} in an incremental exercise test.

informed consent—A written document signed by the participant which notifies the participant of all procedures and potential risks of participation.

International Society for the Advancement of Kinanthropometry (ISAK)—The international organisation promoting scientific endeavours in the area of kinanthropometry, the quantitative measurement of human structure and function; founded in 1986.

intervention—Strategy or tool designed to help an individual or group achieve, usually a lifestyle habit, influenced by both external an dinternal stimuli.

intrinsic reward—A prize or incentive inherent to the individual and activity, for example, enjoyment.

iron-deficiency anaemia—Iron deficiency, characterised by clinically low concentrations of red blood cells, haemoglobin and serum ferritin (the body's storage form of iron).

isokinetic contraction—A dynamic muscular contraction with a constant speed of movement and variable resistance.

isolated exercise—An exercise movement using a single joint and muscle or muscle group, for example, a biceps curl.

isometric contraction—A muscular contraction against a fixed resistance with no change in muscle length.

isotonic contraction—A dynamic muscular contraction against a constant resistance.

job description—A summary of what an employee does in his or her work.

juvenile rheumatoid arthritis (JRA)—An autoimmune disorder in which substances produced by the body's immune system accumulate within the joints, causing inflammation and pain.

lactate threshold—A point during exercise of increasing intensity at which blood lactic acid levels begin to rise exponentially above resting levels.

lactate tolerance—The ability to continue exercising at a high intensity despite high muscle and blood lactic acid levels.

leadership—Influencing others' behaviour to accomplish group goals.

legislation—A statute or act derived by Parliament.

leisure-time physical activity (LTPA)—A common measure of participation in physical activity in large studies, usually by self-report using physical activity diaries or other types of surveys.

litigation—Conduct of legal proceedings by parties before a court.

low-density lipoprotein (LDL)—A category of cholesterol transported on proteins; most of the plasma cholesterol is transported as LDL, which may accelerate accumulation of lipoproteins on the artery wall; high levels of LDL are associated with an increased risk of coronary artery disease.

management—Administration (includes planning, organising, controlling) of resources (human, physical, financial, information) to achieve organisational goals.

market research—The process of gathering information for management to decide on a course of action.

marketing—Determining the needs and wants of potential clients and how to deliver the desired satisfaction.

maximum heart rate (HRmax)—The highest heart rate achieved during fatiguing exercise; can be estimated by 220 minus age, although there is considerable individual variation.

maximum oxygen uptake ($\dot{V}O_2$max)—Maximum capacity of the body to utilise oxygen during exercise; a good predictor, although not the best, of endurance exercise capacity; also known as aerobic power.

metabolic conditions—Impairments or disorders of the body system(s) used to convert nutrients to usable energy.

metabolic equivalent (MET)—A unit used to express the energy cost of physical activity, expressed as a multiple of resting metabolic rate; by definition, 1 MET = resting metabolic rate, or ~3.5 ml $O_2 \cdot kg^{-1} \cdot min^{-1}$ (e.g., 10 METs = energy cost of 10 times resting metabolic rate).

metabolic syndrome (syndrome X)—A clustering of risk factors for cardiovascular disease, including impaired glucose tolerance, obesity, hypertension and dyslipidaemia.

mission statement—The primary purpose of an organisation.

mortality—An epidemiological term to quantify death rate.

multiple sclerosis (MS)—An autoimmune neurological disease in which the body's immune cells breach the blood-brain barrier and attack myelin; the resulting demyelination of nerves disrupts smooth conduction along the neuron, causing disorders of movement and coordination.

muscle hypertrophy—Growth of a muscle or muscle group, generally as a result of resistance training; individual muscle fibres increase in diameter by adding new contractile and connective tissue proteins.

muscular dystrophy (MD)—An inherited disease in males causing progressive deterioration of muscle cells, muscle wasting, weakness and loss of muscle function.

muscular endurance—The ability of a muscle or muscle group to generate force repeatedly or continuously over time; an important component of sports requiring repetitive application of force, such as swimming, rowing or cycling.

muscular power—The rate at which a muscle or muscle group can develop force, defined as force per unit time; an important component of explosive movements such as sprinting, jumping and throwing.

muscular strength—The maximum force a muscle or muscle group can generate in a single maximal contraction or movement.

musculoskeletal exercise rehabilitation—Exercise programs designed for individuals with musculoskeletal disorders, such as arthritis, injury or low back pain, to help restore physical function and fitness and, if possible, prevent future injury.

negligence—Duty of care breached through a careless act or omission that results in damage.

negotiation—A process of resolving conflict by searching for a solution to a problem that is satisfactory for all parties involved.

nurturing—Genuine support, encouragement and development of another.

omission—Failure to act that may constitute an offence where duty of care exists.

organisation—A group of people working in a structured and coordinated way to achieve their goals.

organisational structure—The pattern of formal grouping of people and their tasks.

osteoarthritis (OA)—The most common form of arthritis in which joint inflammation is caused by structural changes and degradation of articular cartilage in the affected joints, often as a result of injury.

osteoporosis—A disorder of the skeleton characterised by low bone mass (or bone mineral density) and structural deterioration of bone, causing bone fragility and increased risk of fracture.

overtraining syndrome (OTS)—In athletes, a state of persistent fatigue, poor sport performance, mood state alterations and other symptoms resulting from prolonged periods of excessive training with inadequate rest and recovery.

overuse injuries—Exercise-induced repetitive microtrauma causing an inflammatory response, and possibly chronic inflammation, leading to structural changes in tissues such as bone, tendons, ligaments or joints.

oximetry—Measurement of arterial oxygen saturation.

paraplegia—Impaired neurological function and movement in the lower extremities resulting from injury to the spinal cord in the thoracic region (T2-T12); can be partial or complete.

Parkinson's disease (PD)—A progressive neurological condition involving the extrapyramidal system due to deficiency in the neurotransmitter dopamine that results in a variety of movement disorders such as tremor, akinesia (freezing during movement), muscle rigidity and dyskinesia (involuntary movements).

periodisation of training—A process of dividing an athlete's season into phases and planning a varied training program to optimise performance at certain times and to avoid overtraining.

personal trainer—An exercise professional who works with individual clients to develop and maintain an ongoing, individualised exercise program; the personal trainer may also exercise with the client.

Physical Activity Readiness Questionnaire (PAR-Q)—A seven-question pre-activity questionnaire for people aged 15 to 69 years.

physical activity—(According to the U.S. Surgeon General) Bodily movement produced by contraction of skeletal muscle that increases energy expenditure above the basal level.

physical fitness—Ability to perform physical tasks without undue fatigue; components include cardiorespiratory endurance, muscular strength and endurance, muscle flexibility, agility, balance and body composition.

planned behaviour—A psychological theory that explains behaviour change based on intention to change and perceived control.

planning—The process of deciding how to achieve an organisation's goals.

plyometrics—A type of power training used by speed and power athletes that includes exercises to pre-stretch the muscle group before each movement to enhance muscle force and power.

population attributable risk (PAR)—An epidemiological measure of the proportion of a given health outcome attributable to a risk factor in the population; includes both relative risk and the prevalence of that risk among the population.

post-exercise recovery period—The period after intense exercise (training or competition) when the body returns to a resting state. During recovery, the body restores resting levels of substrates (e.g., glycogen) and fluids (e.g., blood volume), and repairs injured tissue.

pre-activity screening—Use of questionnaires and/or health information to assess an individual's health risk factors to optimise safety and effectiveness of fitness assessment and physical activity prescription.

precontemplation—A stage of behaviour change during which the individual expresses no intention to change behaviour.

preparation—A stage of behaviour change during which the individual begins to change behaviour.

primary prevention—Interventions aimed at preventing the development of disease in healthy people or those without known disease.

principle of specificity—A principle stating that specific types of physical fitness (e.g., cardiorespiratory, muscular strength, flexibility) will optimally improve with specific types of training; the basis for prescribing exercise.

processes of change—Cognitive, affective and behavioural activities that may help an individual change behaviour.

profession (professional, professionalism)—Occupation requiring advanced knowledge in a specialised area; a professional is a practitioner of a particular profession; professionalism is an expected level of professional behaviour.

program evaluation—Systematic collection and reporting of information on the delivery of a client service.

progression—Changes to program intensity, duration or frequency (e.g., workload) to continue to improve a specific component of fitness.

promotional mix—Group of promotional tools including advertising, personal selling, sales promotions and publicity.

promotion—Communication to inform, persuade and influence potential clients.

proprioceptive neuromuscular facilitation (PNF)—A type of stretching exercise that involves movement after an isometric contraction; it is thought that an isometric contraction suppresses contractile activity of the muscle and enhances the range of the stretch.

pulmonary function tests—Physical tests used to assess lung capacity and airflow such as spirometry and breathing patterns.

quadriplegia—Impaired neurological function and movement in all four extremities resulting from injury to the spinal cord in the cervical or upper thoracic region (C1-8, T1); can be partial or complete.

quality of life (QOL)—A psychological construct to assess an individual's perception of his or her position in life; it is multidimensional, including facets of physical, psychological and social health.

rating of perceived exertion (RPE)—A participant's estimation of the level of effort undertaken during a specific physical activity; valid and reliable scales exist to help participants rate level of physical exertion (refer to figure 6.9).

relapse prevention—An approach used to help anticipate and cope with situations that may inhibit behaviour change.

relative risk (RR)—An epidemiological measure of the strength of relationship between a risk factor (e.g., physical inactivity) and the risk of disease (e.g., cardiovascular disease).

repetition maximum (RM)—The greatest amount of weight lifted in a specified number of repetitions; for example, a 1 RM is the greatest amount of weight lifted once, whereas a 3 RM is the greatest amount of weight lifted in three consecutive motions.

resistance training—Exercise training designed to enhance at least one component of muscular fitness (e.g., muscular strength, power or endurance), often but not always involving weightlifting.

respiratory exchange ratio (RER)—The ratio of expired carbon dioxide to consumed oxygen.

rheumatoid arthritis (RA)—An autoimmune disorder in which substances produced by the body's immune system accumulate within the joints, causing chronic inflammation of the synovial lining and tendons.

risk management—The process of identifying, evaluating and minimising risks that may lead to harm, together with the development of contingency plans and ongoing review of procedures.

risk stratification—Part of the health risk screening process to classify individuals by age and risk factors or symptoms to determine the appropriate type of fitness testing and degree of medical supervision needed before beginning an exercise program.

secondary prevention—Interventions aimed at preventing further disease progression, or restoring functional capacity, in those with documented disease.

self-efficacy—Confidence in one's ability to perform a specific behaviour.

service quality—The customer's perceived level of the provided service.

skinfold measurement—A measure of subcutaneous fat at a given site using specialised calipers.

social cognitive theory—A theory that a behaviour, such as physical activity, is strongly influenced by individual and environmental factors, and the ability to change depends on the individual's perception of his or her ability to control these factors and behaviour.

social marketing model—The application of business marketing techniques to social and health issues in an attempt to change health behaviour of a particular group or groups of people.

social norms—An individual's perception of positive and negative pressures from family, friends and cultural groups regarding a recommended behaviour change.

socio-economic status—A process of evaluating populations by the social environment and income.

spasticity (or hypertonicity)—Increased muscle tone; common in neurological disorders such as cerebral palsy or acquired brain injury; spastic muscles experience a nearly-continual state of contraction, reducing their function and range of motion around nearby joints.

Sports Medicine Australia (SMA)—A professional and community educational organisation in Australia made up of several professional groups with a common interest in sports medicine and sport science.

stakeholders—Individuals, groups or organisations directly involved in, or potentially affected by, a program, policy or law; the individual or group is said to have a "stake", or strong interest, in the outcome of the program or policy.

static balance—Control of postural sway during standing; is important for preventing falls especially in the elderly.

static stretch—A type of stretching exercise whereby the participant executes the exercise slowly to the point of mild discomfort and holds that position for a specificied length of time.

stress test—An exercise test (either maximal or submaximal) performed under controlled conditions with selected parameters monitored such as haemodynamics, electrocardiography and echocardiography.

stroke, or **cerebrovascular accident (CVA)**—Caused by vascular insufficiency to the brain as a result of thrombosis (blood clot), haemorrhage (bleeding) or embolism (clot moving through the circulation); often causes permanent loss of physical or cognitive function in the affected part of the brain.

SWOT analysis—A component of the marketing plan that identifies an organisation's strengths, weaknesses, opportunities and threats.

tapering—Practice by athletes of reducing training volume and possibly intensity for up to 3 weeks before a major competition.

total cholesterol—The measured amount of cholesterol in the bloodstream; cholesterol is an essential lipid, but elevated levels of total cholesterol indicate an increased risk of coronary artery disease; cholesterol is transported through the blood on proteins (lipoproteins), and it is beneficial to measure the different categories of lipoproteins, particularly high-density lipoprotein and low-density lipoprotein.

transtheoretical (or stages of change) model—A model theorising that behaviour change is a process of five stages based on the individual's motivational readiness to change. These stages range from precontemplation (not yet thinking about changing health behaviour) through to maintenance (maintaining long-term changes in health behaviour).

triglyceride—A fat transported in the blood on a lipoprotein (often chylomicrons and very low-density lipoproteins); elevated triglyceride levels are associated with an increased risk of coronary artery disease if accompanied by low HDL or elevated LDL levels.

U.S. Surgeon General's Report on Physical Activity and Health—A landmark report, published in 1996, that summarised research to date showing a strong relationship between moderate physical activity and health and that called for further promotion of a physically active lifestyle for all Americans.

Valsalva manoeuvre—Forced exhalation against a closed glottis, which causes increased intrathoracic pressure, thus reducing venous return and possibly leading to excessively elevated systolic and diastolic blood pressure.

waist to hip ratio (WHR)—The ratio of circumferences of the waist to hip; gives a simple, non-invasive indication of the degree of abdominal fat deposition.

REFERENCES

Active Australia. 1998. *Campaign news.* Sydney: The Better Health Centre.

American Association of Cardiovascular and Pulmonary Rehabilitation. 1995. *Guidelines for cardiac rehabilitation and secondary prevention programs,* 2nd ed. Champaign, IL: Human Kinetics.

American Association of Cardiovascular and Pulmonary Rehabilitation. 1999. *Guidelines for cardiac rehabilitation and secondary prevention programs,* 3rd ed. Champaign, IL: Human Kinetics.

American College of Obstetricians and Gynecologists. 1994. *Exercise during pregnancy and the postpartum period* (Technical Bulletin 189). Washington, DC: American College of Obstetricians and Gynecologists.

American College of Sports Medicine. 1978. The recommended quantity and quality of exercise for developing and maintaining fitness in healthy adults. *Medicine and Science in Sports and Exercise* 10: vii-x.

American College of Sports Medicine. 1990. The recommended quantity and quality of exercise for developing and maintaining cardiorespiratory and muscular fitness in healthy adults. *Medicine and Science in Sports and Exercise* 22: 265-74.

American College of Sports Medicine. 1998a. Exercise and physical activity for older adults. *Medicine and Science in Sports and Exercise* 30: 992-1008.

American College of Sports Medicine. 1998b. The recommended quantity and quality of exercise for developing and maintaining cardiorespiratory and muscular fitness, and flexibility in healthy adults. *Medicine and Science in Sports and Exercise* 30: 975-91.

American College of Sports Medicine. 2000. *ACSM's guidelines for exercise testing and prescription,* 6th ed. Philadelphia: Lippincott Williams & Wilkins.

Armstrong, T., Bauman, A., & Davies, J. 2000. *Physical activity patterns of Australian adults: Results of the 1999 National Physical Activity Survey.* Canberra: Australian Institute of Health and Welfare. See also [Online]. Available: http://www.aihw.gov.au/publications/health/papaa/papaa.pdf [21 May 2002].

Australian Institute of Health and Welfare. 2000. *National health priority areas.* [Online]. Available: http://www.aihw.gov.au/nhpa/index.html [21 May 2002].

Australian Sports Commission. 1999a. *Active women: National policy on women and girls in sport, recreation and physical activity 1999-2002.* Canberra: Australian Sports Commission.

Australian Sports Commission. 1999b. *How to include women and girls in sport, recreation and physical activity: Strategies and good practice.* Canberra: Australian Sports Commission.

Bailey, D.A., Faulkner, R.A., & McKay, H.A. 1996. Growth, physical activity and bone mineral acquisition. *Exercise and Sport Sciences Reviews* 24: 233-266.

Bandura, A. 1986. *Social foundations of thought and action: A social cognitive theory.* Englewood Cliffs, NJ: Prentice-Hall.

Blair, S.N., & Connelly, J. 1996. How much physical activity should we do? The case for moderate amounts and intensities of physical activity. *Research Quarterly for Exercise and Sport* 67 (2): 193-205.

Blair, S.N., Kampert, J.B., Kohl, H.W., Barlow, C.E., Macera, C.A., Paffenbarger, R.S., & Gibbons, L.W. 1996. Influences of cardiorespiratory fitness and other precursors on cardiovascular disease and all-cause mortality in men and women. *Journal of the American Medical Association* 276: 205-210.

Blair, S.N., Kohl, H.W. III, Barlow, C.E., Paffenbarger, R.S. Jr., Gibbons, L.W., & Macera, C.A. 1995. Changes in physical fitness and all-cause mortality: A prospective study of healthy and unhealthy men. *Journal of the American Medical Association* 273: 1093-1098.

Bolton, R. 1996. *People skills: How to assert yourself, listen to others, and resolve conflicts.* Brookvale, Australia: Simon Schuster.

Borg, G., 1998. *Borg's perceived exertion and pain scales.* Champaign, IL: Human Kinetics.

Brawley, L.R. 1993. The practicality of using social psychological theories for exercise and health research and intervention. *Journal of Applied Sport Psychology* 5: 99-115.

Brown, W.J., & Lee, C. 1994. Exercise and dietary modification with women of non-English speaking background: A pilot study with Polish-Australian women. *International Journal of Behavioral Medicine* 1: 195-203.

Brownson, R.C., Housemann, R.A., Brown, D.R., Jackson-Thompson, J., King, A.C., Malone, B.R., & Sallis, J.R. 2000. Promoting physical activity in rural communities: Walking trail access, use and effects. *American Journal of Preventive Medicine* 18: 235-241.

Bull, F.C., & Jamrozik, K. 1998. Advice on exercise from a family physician can help sedentary patients to become active. *American Journal of Preventive Medicine* 15 (2): 85-94.

Cameron, M., & MacDougall, C. 2000. *Crime prevention through sport and physical activity. Australian Institute of Criminology.* [Online]. Available: http://www.aic.gov.au/publications/tandi/tandi165.html [21 May 2002].

Canadian Society for Exercise Physiology. 1994. *PAR-Q and you.* Gloucester, ON: Canadian Society for Exercise Physiology.

Cardinal, B.J. 1997. Assessing the physical activity readiness of inactive older adults. *Adapted Physical Activity Quarterly* 14 (1): 65-73.

Cardinal, B.J., Esters, J., & Cardinal, M. 1996. Evaluation of the revised physical activity readiness questionnaire in older adults. *Medicine and Science in Sports and Exercise* 28 (4): 468-472.

Carter, N.D., Kannus, P., & Khan, K.M. 2001. Exercise in the prevention of falls in older people: A systematic literature review examining the rationale and the evidence. *Sports Medicine* 31: 427-438.

Clapp, J.F., & Little, K.D. 1995. Effects of recreational exercise on pregnancy weight gain and subcutaneous fat deposition. *Medicine and Science in Sports and Exercise* 27: 170-177.

Commonwealth (of Australia) Department of Health and Aged Care and Australian Sports Commission. 1999. *National physical activity guidelines for all Australians.* Active Australia. [Online]. Available: http://www.health.gov.au/pubhlth/publicat/document/physguide.pdf [21 May 2002].

Cordero, D.L., Sisto, S.A., Tapp, W.N., LaManca, J.J., Pareja, J.G., & Natelson, B.H. 1996. Decreased vagal power during treadmill walking in patients with chronic fatigue syndrome. *Clinical Autonomic Research* 6: 329-333.

Cox, D.L. 2000. *Occupational therapy and chronic fatigue syndrome.* London: Whurr.

Crouse, S.F., O'Brien, B.D., Grandjean, P.W., Lowe, R.C., Rohack, J.J., Green, J.W., & Tolson, H. 1997. Training intensity, blood lipids and apolipoproteins in men with high cholesterol. *Journal of Applied Physiology* 82: 270-277.

De Becker, P., Roeykens, J., Reynders, M., McGregor, N., & De Meileir, K. 2000. Exercise capacity in chronic fatigue syndrome. *Archives of Internal Medicine* 160: 3270-3277.

Dimeo, F., Fetscher, S., Lange, W., Mertelsmann, R., & Keul, J. 1997. Effects of aerobic exercise on the physical performance and incidence of treatment-related complications after high-dose chemotherapy. *Blood* 90: 3390-3394.

Dimeo, F., Tilmann, M.H.M., Bertz, H., Kanz, L., Mertelsmann, R., & Keul, J. 1997. Aerobic exercise in the rehabilitation of cancer patients after high dose chemotherapy and autologous peripheral stem cell transplantation. *Cancer* 79: 1717-1722.

Dishman, R.K. 1994a. Prescribing exercise intensity for healthy adults using perceived exertion. *Medicine and Science in Sports and Exercise* 26 (9): 1087-1094.

Dishman, R.K. 1994b. The measurement conundrum in exercise adherence research. *Medicine and Science in Sports and Exercise* 26 (11): 1382-1390.

Dishman, R.K., & Buckworth, J. 1996. Increasing physical activity: A quantitative synthesis. *Medicine and Science in Sports and Exercise* 28 (6): 706-719.

Dishman, R.K., Farquar, R.P., & Cureton, K.J. 1994. Responses to preferred intensities of exertion in men differing in activity levels. *Medicine and Science in Sports and Exercise* 26 (6): 783-790.

Dishman, R.K., Oldenberg, B., O'Neal, H., & Shephard, R.J. 1998. Worksite physical activity interventions. *American Journal of Preventive Medicine* 15: 344-361.

Dunn, A.L., Anderson, R.E., & Makicic, J.M. 1998. Lifestyle physical activity interventions: History, short- and long-term effects, and recommendations. *American Journal of Preventive Medicine* 15: 398-412.

Durnin, J., & Womersley, J. 1974. Body fat assessed from total body density and its estimation from skinfold thickness: Measurements on 481 men and women aged 16 to 72 years. *British Journal of Nutrition* 32: 77-97.

Epstein, L.H., Coleman, K.J., & Myers, M.D. 1996. Exercise in treating obesity in children and adolescents. *Medicine and Science in Sports and Exercise* 28: 428-435.

Eriksson, J., Tuominen, J., Valle, T., Sundberg, S., Sovijarvi, A., Lindholm, H., Tuomilehto, J., & Koivisto, V. 1998. Aerobic endurance exercise or circuit-type resistance training for individuals with impaired glucose tolerance? *Hormone and Metabolic Research* 30: 37-41.

Feigenbaum, M., & Pollock, M. 1997. Strength training, rationale for current guidelines for adult fitness programs. *The Physician and Sportsmedicine* 25 (2): 44-64.

Flynn, M.G., Carroll, K.K., Hall, H.L., Bushman, B.A., Brolinson, P.G., & Weideman, C.A. 1998. Cross training: Indices of training stress and performance. *Medicine and Science in Sports and Exercise* 30: 294-300.

Freeman, R., & Komaroff, A.L. 1997. Does the chronic fatigue syndrome involve the autonomic nervous system? *American Journal of Medicine* 102 (4): 357-364.

Gauvin, L., Spence, J.C., & Anderson, S. 1999. Exercise and psychological well-being in the adult population: Reality or wishful thinking? In J.M. Rippe (ed.), *Lifestyle medicine* (pp. 957-966). Malden, MA: Blackwell Science.

Gore, C.J., & Australian Sports Commission. (eds.). 2000. *Physiological tests for elite athletes.* Champaign, IL: Human Kinetics.

Gore, C.J., & Edwards, D.A. 1992. *Australian fitness norms: A manual for fitness assessors.* South Australia: The Health Development Foundation.

Halbert, J.A., Silagy, C.A., Finucane, P., Withers, R.T., Hamdorf, P.A., & Andrews, G.R. 1997. The effectivenss of exercise training in lowering blood pressure: A meta-analysis of randomized controlled trials of 4 weeks or longer. *Jounal of Human Hypertension* 11: 641-649.

Hardman, A.E. 1999. Accumulation of physical activity for health gains: What is the evidence? *British Journal of Sports Medicine* 33: 87-92.

Hicks, J.E. 1990. Exercise for cancer patients. In J.V. Basmajian & S.L. Wolf (eds.), *Therapeutic exercise* (pp. 351-367). Baltimore: Williams & Wilkins.

Hillary Commission for Sport, Fitness and Leisure Web site. Available: www.hillarysport.org.nz [21 May 2002].

Hooper, S.L., Mackinnon, L.T., & Ginn, E.M. 1998. Effects of three tapering techniques on the performance, forces and psychometric measures of competitive swimmers. *European Journal of Applied Physiology* 7: 258-263.

Hooper, S.L., Mackinnon, L.T., & Howard, A. 1999. Physiological and psychometric variables for monitoring recovery during tapering for major competition. *Medicine and Science in Sports and Exercise* 31: 1205-1210.

Houmard, J.A., Scott, B.K., Justice, C.L., & Chenier, T.C. 1994. The effects of taper on performance in distance runners. *Medicine and Science in Sports and Exercise* 26: 624-631.

Johnson, D., Perrault, H., Fournier, A., Leclerc, J.-M., Bigras, J.-L., & Davignon, A. 1997. Cardiovascular responses to dynamic submaximal exercise in children previously treated with anthracycline. *American Heart Journal* 133: 169-173.

King, A. 1994. Community and public health approaches to the promotion of physical activity. *Medicine and Science in Sports and Exercise* 26 (11): 1405-1412.

Lee, I., Hsieh, C., & Paffenbarger, R. 1995. Exercise intensity and longevity in men, the Harvard Alumni Health Study. *The Journal of the American Medical Association* 273 (15): 1179-1184.

Long, B.J., Calfas, K.J., Wooten, W., Sallis, J.F., Patrick, K., Goldstein, M., Marcus, B.H., Schwenk, T.L., Chenoweth, J., Carter, R., Torres, T., Palinkas, L.A., & Heath G. 1996. A multi-site field test of the acceptability of physical activity counseling in primary health care: Project PACE. *American Journal of Preventive Medicine* 12 (2): 73-81.

MacDougall, J.D., Wenger, H.A., & Green, H.J. 1991. *Physiological testing of the high-performance athlete.* Champaign, IL: Human Kinetics.

Maister, D.H. 1993. *Managing the professional service firm.* New York: Free Press.

Marcus, B.H. 1995. Exercise behaviour and strategies for intervention. *Research Quarterly for Exercise and Sport* 66 (4): 319-323.

Marcus, B.H., Banspach, S.W., Lefebvre, R.C., Rossi, J., Carleton, R., & Abrams, D. 1992. Using the stages of change model to increase the adoption of physical activity among community participants. *American Journal of Health Promotion* 6 (6): 424-430.

Marcus, B.H., Eaton, C.A., Rossi, J.S., & Harlow, L.L. 1994. Self-efficacy, decision-making, and stages of change: An integrative model of physical activity. *Journal of Applied Social Psychology* 24 (6): 489-508.

Marcus, B.H., Nigg, C.R., Riebe, D., & Forsyth, L.H. 2000. Interactive communication strategies: Implications for population-based physical-activity promotion. *American Journal of Preventive Medicine* 19: 121-126.

Marcus, B.H., Owen, N., Forsyth, L.H., Caavill, N.A., & Fridinger, F. 1998. Physical activity interventions using mass media, print media, and information technology. *American Journal of Preventive Medicine* 15: 362-378.

Marquez-Sterling, S., Perry, A.C., Kaplan, T.A., Halberstein, R.A., & Signorile, J.F. 2000. Physical and psychological changes with vigorous exercise in sedentary primigravidae. *Medicine and Science in Sports and Exercise* 32: 58-62.

Matthews, C.E., Heil, D.P., Freedson, P.S., & Pastides, H. 1999. Classification of cardiorespiratory fitness without exercise testing. *Medicine and Science in Sports and Exercise* 31 (3): 486-493.

McAuley, E., Talbot, H.M. & Martinez, S. 1999. Manipulating self-efficacy in the exercise environment in women: Influences on affective responses. *Health Psychology* 18 (3): 288-294.

McCarthy, J.P., Agre, J.C., Graf, B.K., Poziniak, M.A., & Vailas, A.C. 1995. Compatibility of adaptive responses with combining strength and endurance training. *Medicine and Science in Sports and Exercise* 27: 429-436.

McCully, K.K., Natelson, B.H., Iotti, S., Siston, S., & Leigh, J.S. 1996. Reduced oxidative muscle metabolism in chronic fatigue syndrome. *Muscle and Nerve* 19: 621-625.

McGill, S.M. 2001. Low back stability: From formal description to issues for performance and rehabilitation. *Exercise and Sport Sciences Reviews* 29: 26-31.

McKardle, W., Katch, F., & Katch, V. 1996. *Exercise physiology.* Baltimore: Williams & Wilkins.

Mensink, G., Heerstrass, D., Neppelenbroek, S., Schuit, A., & Bellach, B. 1997. Intensity, duration, and frequency of physical activity and coronary risk factors. *Medicine and Science in Sports and Exercise* 29 (9): 1192-1198.

Mock, V., Dow, K.H., Meares, C.J., Grimm, P.M., Dienemann, J.A., Haisfiled-Wolfe, M.E., Qutasol, W., Mitchell, S., Chakravarthy, A., & Gage, I. 1997. Effects of exercise on fatigue, physical functioning and emotional distress during radiation therapy for breast cancer. *Oncology Nursing Forum* 24: 991-1000.

Mujika, I., Goya, A., Padilla, S., Grijalba, A., Gorostiaga, E., & Ibancez, J. 2000. Physiological responses to a 6-d taper in middle-distance runners: Influence of training intensity and volume. *Medicine and Science in Sports and Exercise* 32: 511-517.

National Health Committee (New Zealand). 1998. *Active for life: A call for action. The health benefits of physical activity.* Hillary Commission for Sport, Fitness and Leisure. [Online]. Available: www.nhc.govt.nz/pub/activeforlife/index.htm [21 May 2002].

National Heart Foundation of Australia. 1998. *Recommendations for cardiac rehabilitation.* [Online]. Available: www.heartfoundation.com.au/prof/04_recom_rehab.html. [21 May 2002].

National Heart Foundation of Australia. 2000. *National Heart Foundation of Australia physical activity policy.* [Online]. Available: http://www.heartfoundation.com.au/prof/index_fr.html [21 May 2002].

New South Wales (Australia) Department of Health. 1999. *The Active Practice Project: A controlled trial of physical activity promotion in general practice.* [Online]. Available: http://www.health.nsw.gov.au/public-health/health-promotion/pdf/physicalact/active_prac/Active_prac.pdf [21 May 2002].

Nezu, K., Kushibe, K., Tojo, T., Takahama, M., & Kitamurra, S. 1998. Recovery and limitation of exercise capacity after lung resection for lung cancer. *Chest* 113: 1511-1516.

Nicklas, B.J., Katzel, L.I., Busby-Whitehead, J., & Goldberg, A.P. 1997. Increases in high-density lipoprotein cholesterol with endurance exercise training are blunted in obese compared with lean men. *Metabolism* 46: 556-561.

Norton, K., & Olds, T. 1996. *Anthropometrica.* Sydney: University of New South Wales Press.

Oldridge, N.B. 1997. Health-related quality of life and economic evaluation of cardiac rehabilitation. In A.S. Leon (ed.), *Physical activity and cardiovascular health: A national consensus* (pp. 183-190). Champaign, IL: Human Kinetics.

Olds, T., & Norton, K. 1999. *Pre-exercise health screening guide.* Champaign, IL: Human Kinetics.

Owens, S., Gutin, B., Allison, J., Riggs, S., Ferguson, M., Litaker, M., & Thompson, W. 1999. Effect of physical training on total and visceral fat in obese children. *Medicine and Science in Sports and Exercise* 31: 143-148.

Paffenbarger, R.S. Jr., Hyde, R.T., Alvin, M.A., Wing, A.L., & Hsieh, C.-C. 1986. Physical activity, all-cause mortality, and longevity in college alumni. *New England Journal of Medicine* 314: 605-613.

Pate, R. 1995. Physical activity and health: dose-response issues. *Research Quarterly for Exercise and Sport* 66 (4): 313-317.

Petajan, J.H., & White, A.T. 1999. Recommendations for physical activity in patients with multiple sclerosis. *Sports Medicine* 27: 179-191.

Prochaska, J.O., & DiClemente, C.C. 1983. Stages and processes of self-change in smoking: Towards an integrative model of change. *Journal of Consulting and Clinical Psychology* 51: 390-395.

Prochaska, J.O., DiClemente, C.C. & Norcross, J.C. 1992. In search of how people change: Applications to addictive behaviours. *American Psychologist* 47: 1102-1114.

Rall, L.C., Meydani, S.N., Kehayias, J.J., Dawson-Hughes, B., & Roubenoff, R. 1996. The effect of progressive resistance training in rheumatoid arthritis. *Arthritis and Rheumatism* 39: 415-426.

Rall, L.C., Rosen, C.J., Dolnikowski, G., Hartman, W.J., Lundgren, N., Abad, L.W., Dinarello, C.A., & Roubenoff, R. 1996. Protein metabolism in rheumatoid arthritis and aging: Effects of muscle strength training and tumor necrosis factor alpha. *Arthritis & Rheumatism* 39: 1115-1124.

Rall, L.C., Roubenoff, R., Cannon, J.G., Abad, L.W., Dinarello, C.A., & Meydani, S.N. 1996. Effects of progressive resistance training on immune response in aging and chronic inflammation. *Medicine and Science in Sports and Exercise* 28: 1356-1365.

Rankin, J.W. 1997. *Glycemic index and exercise metabolism.* Sports Science Exchange Article #64 [Online]. Available: http://www.gssiweb.com/bookstore/articleorderformsse.cfm [21 May 2002].

Reuter, I., Engelhardt, M., Stecker, K., & Baas, H. 1999. Therapeutic value of exercise training in Parkinson's disease. *Medicine and Science in Sports and Exercise* 31: 1544-1549.

Roberts, G. 1992. *Motivation in sport and exercise.* Champaign, IL: Human Kinetics.

Ross, R., Freeman, J.A., & Janssen, I. 2000. Exercise alone is an effective strategy for reducing obesity and related comordities. *Exercise and Sports Science Reviews* 28:165-170.

Rowbottom, D.G., Keast, D., Green, S., Kakulas, B., & Morton, A.R. 1998. The case history of an elite ultra-endurance cyclist who developed chronic fatigue syndrome. *Medicine and Science in Sports and Exercise* 30: 1345-1348.

Ryckman, R., Robbins, M., Thornton, B., & Cantrell, P. 1982. Development and validation of a physical self-efficacy scale. *Journal of Personality and Social Psychology* 42 (5): 891-900.

Sallis, J.F., Bauman, A., & Pratt, M. 1998. Environmental and policy interventions to promote physical activity. *American Journal of Preventive Medicine* 15: 379-397.

Sallis, J.F, & Owen, N. 1999. *Physical activity and behavioral medicine.* Thousand Oaks, CA: Sage.

Schell, J., & Leelarthaepin, B. 1994. *Physical fitness assessment in exercise and sport science,* 2nd ed. New South Wales: Leelar Biomediscience Services.

Sisto, S.A., LaManca, J., Cordero, D.L., Bergen, M.T., Ellis, S.P., Drastal, S., Boda, W.L., Tapp, W.N., & Natelson, B.H. 1996. Metabolic and cardiovascular effects of a progressive exercise test in patients with chronic fatigue syndrome. *American Journal of Medicine* 100: 634-640.

Skinner, J.S. 1993. *Exercise testing and exercise prescription for special cases.* Philadelphia: Lea & Febiger.

Spirduso, W.W. 1995. *Physical dimensions of aging.* Champaign, IL: Human Kinetics.

Sport and Recreation Ministers' Council (Australia). 1997. *Active Australia: A national participation framework.* Belconnen, ACT: Commonwealth of Australia. [Online]. Available: http://www.ausport.gov.au/pubcat/mainqry.asp?OrderingCode=11-002 [21 May 2002].

Sports Medicine Australia. 1994. *Participation of the pregnant athlete in contact and collision sports.* Canberra: Guideline One.

Stanley, R.K., Protas, E.J., & Jankovic, J. 1999. Exercise performance in those having Parkinson's disease and healthy normals. *Medicine and Science in Sports and Exercise* 31: 761-766.

Steadward, R. 1998. Musculoskeletal and neurological disabilities: Implications for fitness appraisal, programming, and counseling. *Canadian Journal of Applied Physiology* 23: 131-165.

Stephenson, J., Bauman, A., Armstrong, T., Smith, B., & Bellew, B. 2000. The costs of illness attributable to physical inactivity in Australia: A preliminary study. Canberra: Commonwealth Department of Health and Aged Care and the Australian Sports Commission. [Online]. Available: http://www.health.gov.au/pubhlth/publicat/document/phys_costofillness.pdf [21 May 2002].

Taafe, D.R., Duret, C., Wheeler, S., & Marcus, R. 1999. Once-weekly resistance exercise improves muscular strength and neuromuscular performance in older adults. *Journal of the American Geriatric Society* 47: 1208-1214.

Taafe, D.R., & Marcus, R. 2000. Musculoskeletal health and the older adult. *Journal of Rehabilitative Research* 37: 245-254.

Taylor, W.C., Baranowski, T., & Young, D.R. 1998. Physical activity interventions in low-income, ethnic minority, and populations with disability. *American Journal of Preventive Medicine* 15: 334-343.

Thomas, T., Ziogas, G., Smith, T., Zhang, Q., & Londeree, B. 1995. Physiological and perceived exertion responses to six modes of submaximal exercise. *Research Quarterly for Exercise and Sport* 66 (3): 239-246.

Thompson, P.D., Yurgalevitch, S.M., Flynn, M.M., Zmuda, J.M., Spannaus-Martin, D., Saritelli, A., Bausserman, L., & Herbert, P.N. 1997. Effect of prolonged exercise training without weight loss on high-density lipoprotein metabolism in overweight men. *Metabolism* 46 (2): 217-223.

Tolfrey, K., Campbell, I.G., & Batterham, A.M. 1998. Exercise training induced alterations in prepubertal children's lipid-lipoprotein profile. *Medicine and Science in Sports and Exercise* 30 (12): 1684-1692.

Trine, M.R. 1999. Physical activity and quality of life. In J.M. Rippe (ed.), *Lifestyle medicine* (pp. 989-998). Malden, MA: Blackwell Science.

Trost, S.G., Pater, R.R., Ward, D.S., Sauners, R., & Riner, W. 1999. Correlates of objectively measured physical activity in preadolescent youth. *American Journal of Preventive Medicine* 17: 120-126.

U.S. Department of Health and Human Services. 2000. *Healthy people 2000 and 2010.* U.S. Department of Health and Human Services. [Online]. Available: http://web.health.gov/healthypeople/ [21 May 2002].

U.S. Department of Health and Human Services, & Centers for Disease Control and Prevention. 1996. *Physical activity and health: A report of the Surgeon General.* Atlanta, GA: National Center for Chronic Disease Prevention and Health Promotion.

U.S. Department of Health and Human Services, & Department of Education. 2000. *Promoting better health for young people through physical activity and sports.* Chronic Disease Prevention. [Online]. Available: www.cdc.gov/nccdphp/dash/presphysactrpt/summary.htm [21 May 2002].

U.S. Department of Health and Human Services, Public Health Service, Centers for Disease Control and Prevention, National Center for Chronic Disease Prevention and Health Promotion, & Division of Nutrition and Physical Activity. 1999. *Promoting physical activity: A guide for community action.* Champaign, IL: Human Kinetics.

Van den Ende, C.H., Vlieland, T.P., Munneke, M., & Hazes, J.M. 1998. Dynamic exercise therapy in rheumatoid arthritis: A systematic review. *British Journal of Rheumatology* 37 (6): 677-687.

Van Der Weyden, M.B. 1999. The burden of disease and injury in Australia: Time for action. *Medical Journal of Australia* 171 (11-12): 581-582.

Wei, M., Kampert, J.B., Barlow, C.E., Naichaman, M.Z., Gibbons, L.W., Paffenbarger, P.S., & Blair, S.N. 1999. Relationship between low cardiorespiratory fitness and mortality in normal-weight, overweight and obese men. *Journal of the American Medical Association* 282: 1547-53.

Western Australia Department of Transport. 2000. TravelSmart. [Online]. Available: http://www.travelsmart.transport.wa.gov.au [21 May 2002].

Whittle, M.W. 1996. *Gait analysis.* Oxford: Butterworth-Heinemann.

Williams, P.T. 1996. High-density lipoprotein cholesterol and other risk factors for coronary heart disease in female runners. *New England Journal of Medicine* 334: 1298-1303.

Willis, J.D., & Campbell, L.F. 1992. *Exercise psychology.* Champaign, IL: Human Kinetics.

Wilson, G.J. 1994. Strength and power in sport. In J. Bloomfield, T.R. Ackland, & B.C. Elliott (eds.), *Applied anatomy and biomechanics in sport* (pp. 110-208). Melbourne: Blackwell Scientific.

Withers, R., Craig, N., Bourdon, P., & Norton, K. 1987. Relative body fat and anthropometric prediction of body density of male athletes. *European Journal of Applied Physiology* 56: 191-200.

Woolf-May, K., Kearney, E.M., Owen, A., Jones, D.W., Davison, C.R., & Bird, S.T. 1999. The efficacy of accumulated short bouts versus single daily bouts of brisk walking in improving aerobic fitness and blood lipid profiles. *Health Education Research* 14: 803-815.

World Health Organization. 1997. Health benefits of active living. Press release. WHO/19, 6 March 1997 [Online]. Available: http://www.who.int/archives/inf-pr-1997/en/pr97-19.html. See also *The untapped evident health, social benefits of active living.* [Online]. http://www.who.int/hpr/archive/active/benefits.html [21 May 2002]

SUGGESTED READINGS

Section 1

American College of Sports Medicine. 2000. *ACSM's guidelines for exercise testing and prescription,* 6th ed. Philadelphia: Lippincott Williams & Wilkins.

Bouchard, C. (ed.). 2001. Dose-response issues concerning physical activity and health: An evidence-based symposium. *Medicine and Science in Sports and Exercise* 33 (6 Suppl): S345-S640.

Centers for Disease Control and Prevention (U.S.), & National Center for Chronic Disease Prevention. 1999. *Promoting physical activity: A guide for community action.* Champaign, IL: Human Kinetics.

Grantham, W.C., Patton, R.W., York, T.D., & Winick, M.L. 1998. *Health fitness management: A comprehensive resource for managing and operating programs and facilities.* Champaign, IL: Human Kinetics.

Kriska, A.M., & Caspersen, C.J. (eds.). 1997. A collection of physical activity questionnaires for health-related research. *Medicine and Science in Sports and Exercise* 29 (6 Suppl): S1-S205.

Leon, A.S. (ed.). 1997. *Physical activity and cardiovascular health: A national consensus.* Champaign, IL: Human Kinetics.

Myers, A.M. 1999. *Program evaluation for exercise leaders.* Champaign, IL: Human Kinetics.

Rippe, J.M. (ed.). 1999. *Lifestyle medicine.* Malden, MA: Blackwell Scientific.

Sallis, J.F., & Owen, N. 1999. *Physical activity and behavioral medicine.* Thousand Oaks, CA: SAGE.

U.S. Department of Health and Human Services, & Centers for Disease Control and Prevention. 1996. *Physical activity and health: A report of the surgeon general.* Atlanta, GA: National Center for Chronic Disease Prevention and Health Promotion.

Section 2

Active Australia. 1998. *Campaign news.* Sydney: Better Health Centre.

American Association of Cardiovascular and Pulmonary Rehabilitation. 1999. *Guidelines for cardiac rehabilitation and secondary prevention programs,* 3rd ed. Champaign, IL: Human Kinetics.

American College of Sports Medicine. 1998. The recommended quantity and quality of exercise for developing and maintaining cardiorespiratory and muscular fitness, and flexibility in healthy adults. *Medicine and Science in Sports and Exercise* 30 (6): 975-991.

American College of Sports Medicine. 2000. *ACSM's guidelines for exercise testing and prescription,* 6th ed. Philadelphia: Lippincott Williams & Wilkins.

Armstrong, T., Bauman, A., & Davies, J. 2000. *Physical activity patterns of Australian adults: Results of the 1999 National Physical Activity Survey.* Canberra: Australian Institute of Health and Welfare.

Bandura, A. 1986. *Social foundations of thought and action: A social cognitive theory.* Englewood Cliffs, NJ: Prentice Hall.

Blair, S., & Connelly, J. 1996. How much physical activity should we do? The case for moderate amounts and intensities of physical activity. *Research Quarterly for Exercise and Sport* 67 (2): 193-205.

Cardinal, B.J. 1997. Assessing the physical activity readiness of inactive older adults. *Adapted Physical Activity Quarterly* 14 (1): 65-73.

Cardinal, B.J., Esters, J., & Cardinal, M. 1996. Evaluation of the revised physical activity readiness questionnaire in older adults. *Medicine and Science in Sports and Exercise* 28 (4): 468-472.

Dishman, R. 1994. Prescribing exercise intensity for healthy adults using perceived exertion. *Medicine and Science in Sports and Exercise* 26 (9): 1087-1094.

Dishman, R. 1994. The measurement conundrum in exercise adherence research. *Medicine and Science in Sports and Exercise* 26 (11): 1382-1390.

Fleck, S., & Kraemer, W. (eds.). 1997. *Designing resistance training programs.* Champaign, IL: Human Kinetics.

Goldberger, A.L. 1999. *Clinical electrocardiography,* 6th ed. St. Louis: Mosby.

Gore, C.J. 2000. *Physiological tests for elite athletes.* Champaign, IL: Human Kinetics.

Heyward, V.H. 1991. *Advanced fitness assessment and exercise prescription.* Champaign, IL: Human Kinetics.

Katula, J., McAuley, E., Mihalko, S., & Bane, S. 1998. Mirror, mirror on the wall: Exercise environment influences on self-efficacy. *Journal of Social Behaviour and Personality* 13 (2): 319-332.

King, A. 1994. Community and public health approaches to the promotion of physical activity. *Medicine and Science in Sports and Exercise* 26 (11): 1405-1412.

Lee, I., Hsieh, C., & Paffenbarger, R. 1995. Exercise intensity and longevity in men: The Harvard alumni health study. *Journal of the American Medical Association* 273 (15): 1179-1184.

MacDougall, J.D., Wenger, H.A., & Green, H.J. 1991. *Physiological testing of the high-performance athlete.* Champaign, IL: Human Kinetics.

Marcus, B.H. 1995. Exercise behaviour and strategies for intervention. *Research Quarterly for Exercise and Sport* 66 (4): 319-323.

Marcus, B.H., Banspach, S.W., & Lefebvre, R.C. 1992. Using the stages of change model to increase the adoption of physical activity among community participants. *American Journal of Health Promotion* 6 (6): 424-430.

Marcus, B.H., Simkin, L.R., Rossi, J.S., & Pinto, B.M. 1996. Longitudinal shifts in employees' stages and processes of exercise behaviour change. *American Journal of Health Promotion* 10 (3): 195-200.

McAuley, E., Katula, J., Mihalko, S., Blissmer, B., Duncan, T., Pena, M., & Dunn, E. 1999. Mode of physical activity and self-efficacy in older adults: A latent growth curve analysis. *Journal of Gerontology* 54B(5): 283-292.

McKardle, W., Katch, F., & Katch, V. 1996. *Exercise physiology.* Baltimore: Williams & Wilkins.

Mensink, G., Heerstrass, D., Neppelenbroek, S., Schuit, A., & Bellach, B. 1997. Intensity, duration, and frequency of physical activity and coronary risk factors. *Medicine and Science in Sports and Exercise* 29 (9): 1192-1198.

Norton, K., & Olds, T. 1996. *Anthropometrica.* Sydney: University of New South Wales Press.

Norton, K., Olds, T., Bowes, D., Van Ly, S., & Gore, C. 1998. Applying the Sports Medicine Australia pre-exercise screening procedures: Who will be excluded? *Journal of Science and Medicine in Sport* 1 (1): 38-51.

Olds, T., & Norton, K. 1999. *Pre-exercise health screening guide.* Champaign, IL: Human Kinetics.

Prochaska, J.O., & DiClemente, C.C. 1983. Stages and processes of self-change in smoking: Towards an integrative model of change. *Journal of Consulting and Clinical Psychology* 51: 390-395.

Prochaska, J.O., DiClemente, C.C., and Norcross, J.C. 1992. In search of how people change: Applications to addictive behaviours. *American Psychologist* 47: 1102-1114.

Roberts, G. 1992. *Motivation in sport and exercise.* Champaign, IL: Human Kinetics.

Rykman, R., Robbins, M., Thornton, B., & Cantrell, P. 1982. Development and validation of a physical self-efficacy scale. *Journal of Personality and Social Psychology* 42 (5): 891-900.

Schell, J., & Leelarthaepin, B. 1994. *Physical fitness assessment in exercise and sport science,* 2nd ed. New South Wales: Leelar Biomediscience Services.

Thomas, T., Ziogas, G., Smith, T., Zhang, Q., & Londeree, B. 1995. Physiological and perceived exertion responses to six modes of submaximal exercise. *Research Quarterly for Exercise and Sport* 66 (3): 239-246.

Whittle, M.W. 1996. *Gait analysis.* Oxford: Butterworth-Heinemann.

Section 3

Exercise Prescription for Individuals With Disease or Impairment

American Association of Cardiovascular and Pulmonary Rehabilitation. 1998. *Guidelines for pulmonary rehabilitation programs,* 2nd ed. Champaign, IL: Human Kinetics.

American Association of Cardiovascular and Pulmonary Rehabilitation. 1999. *Guidelines for cardiac rehabilitation and secondary prevention programs,* 3rd ed. Champaign, IL: Human Kinetics.

American College of Sports Medicine. 1997. *ACSM's exercise management for persons with chronic diseases and disabilities.* Champaign, IL: Human Kinetics.

American College of Sports Medicine. 1998. *ACSM's resource manual for guidelines for exercise testing and prescription,* 3rd ed. Baltimore: Williams & Wilkins.

American College of Sports Medicine. 2002. *ACSM's resources for clinical exercise physiology: Musculoskeletal, neuromuscular, neoplastic, immunologic, and hematologic conditions.* Baltimore: Lippincott Williams & Wilkins.

Bouchard, C. (ed.). 2000. *Physical activity and obesity.* Champaign, IL: Human Kinetics.

Carr, J.H, & Shepherd, R.B. 1998. *Neurological rehabilitation: Optimizing motor performance.* Oxford: Butterworth-Heinemann.

Courneya, K.S. 2001. Exercise interventions during cancer treatment: Biopsychosocial outcomes. *Exercise and Sport Sciences Reviews* 29: 60-64.

Cox, D.L. 2000. *Occupational therapy and chronic fatigue syndrome*. London: Whurr.

Durstine, J.L., Painter, P., Franklin, B.A., Morgan, D., Pitetti, K.H., & Roberts, S.O. 2000. Physical activity for the chronically ill and disabled. *Sports Medicine* 30: 207-219.

Fardy, P.S., Franklin, B.A., Porcari, J.P., & Verrill, D.E. 1998. *Training techniques in cardiac rehabilitation*. Champaign, IL: Human Kinetics.

Freidenreich, M., & Courneya, K.S. 1996. Exercise as rehabilitation for cancer patients. *Clinical Journal of Sports Medicine* 6: 237-244.

Frontera, W.R., Dawson, D.M., & Slovik, D.M. (eds.). 1999. *Exercise in rehabilitation medicine*. Champaign, IL: Human Kinetics.

Kell, R.T., Bell, G., & Quinney, A. 2001. Musculoskeletal fitness, health outcomes and quality of life. *Sports Medicine* 31: 863-873.

Khan, K., McKay, H., Kannus, P., Bennell, K., & Bailey, D. 2001. *Physical activity and bone health*. Champaign, IL: Human Kinetics.

Liemohn, W. 2000. *Exercise prescription and the back*. Sydney: McGraw-Hill.

Lockette, K.F., & Keyes, A.M. 1994. *Conditioning with physical disabilities*. Champaign, IL: Human Kinetics.

Lombard, T.N., & Lombard, D.N. 1999. Exercise management of the obese patient. In J.M. Rippe (ed.), *Lifestyle medicine* (pp. 1031-1040). Malden, MA: Blackwell Science.

Miller, P.D. 1995. *Fitness programming and physical disability*. Champaign, IL: Human Kinetics.

National Heart Foundation of Australia NSW Division. 1997. *How to plan a cardiac rehabilitation program*, 2nd ed. Sydney: National Heart Foundation of Australia NSW Division.

Ozer, M.N. 2000. *Management of persons with chronic neurologic illness*. Boston: Butterworth Heinemann.

Patarca-Montero, R. 2000. *Concise encyclopedia of chronic fatigue syndrome*. New York: Haworth Medical Press.

Shephard, R.J., & Bhambhani, Y. (eds.). 1998. Recommendations for fitness assessment, programming, and counselling of persons with a disability. *Canadian Journal of Applied Physiology* 23 (2) (Special Issue).

Exercise Prescription Through the Lifespan

American College of Sports Medicine. 1998. ACSM's position stand: Exercise and physical activity for older adults. *Medicine and Science in Sports and Exercise* 30 (6): 992-1008.

American College of Sports Medicine. 1998. *ACSM's resource manual for guidelines for exercise testing and prescription*, 3rd ed. Baltimore: Williams & Wilkins.

Cotton, R.T., Ekeroth, C.J., & Yancy, H. (eds.). 1998. *Exercise for older adults*. San Diego: American Council on Exercise; Champaign, IL: Human Kinetics.

Daley, M.J., & Spinks, W.L. 2000. Exercise, mobility and aging. *Sports Medicine* 29: 1-12.

Finch, C. (ed.). 2002. Pregnancy in sport. *Journal of Science and Medicine in Sport* 5: 9-57.

Forman, D.E., Pu, C.T., & Garber, C.E. 1999. Exercise counselling in the elderly. In J.M. Rippe (ed.), *Lifestyle medicine* (pp. 707-712). Malden, MA: Blackwell Science.

Goldberg, B. (ed.). 1995. *Sports and exercise for children with chronic health conditions*. Champaign, IL: Human Kinetics.

Hellerstein, S. 1999. Exercise and pregnancy. In J.M. Rippe (ed.), *Lifestyle medicine* (pp. 388-392). Malden, MA: Blackwell Science.

Hurley, B.F., & Roth, W.M. 2000. Strength training in the elderly: Effects on risk factors for age-related diseases. *Sports Medicine* 30: 249-268.

Jenkins, D., & Reaburn, P. 2000. *Guiding the young athlete*. St Leonards, NSW: Allen and Unwin.

Naughton, G., Farpour-Lambert, N.J., Carlson, J., Bradney, M., & Van Praagh, E. 2000. Physiological issues surrounding the performance of adolescent athletes. *Sports Medicine* 30: 309-325.

Rhodes, R.E., Martin, A.D., Taunton, J.E., Rhodes, E.C., Donnelly, M., & Elliot, J. 1999. Factors associated with exercise adherence among older adults. *Sports Medicine* 28: 397-411.

Rikli, R.E., & Jones, C.J. 2001. *Senior fitness test manual*. Champaign, IL: Human Kinetics.

Spirduso, W.W. 1995. *Physical dimensions of aging*. Champaign, IL: Human Kinetics.

Training Athletes

Baechle, T.R., & Earle, R.W. 2000. *Essentials of strength training and conditioning*, 2nd ed. Champaign, IL: Human Kinetics.

Brown, L.E., Ferrigno, V., & Santana, J.C. 2000. *Training for speed, agility, and quickness*. Champaign, IL: Human Kinetics.

Burke, L., & Deakin, V. 2000. *Clinical sports nutrition*, 2nd ed. Sydney: McGraw-Hill.

Foran, B. 2000. *High-performance sports conditioning*. Champaign, IL: Human Kinetics.

Gore, C.J. (ed.). 2000. *Physiological tests for elite athletes*. Champaign, IL: Human Kinetics.

Kreider, R.B., Fry, A.C., & O'Toole, M.L. (eds.). 1998. *Overtraining in sport*. Champaign, IL: Human Kinetics.

Reaburn, P., & Jenkins, D. (eds.). 1996. *Training for speed and endurance*. St Leonards, NSW: Allen and Unwin.

Sherman, S.M., & Lamb, D.R. (eds.). 1996. Fluid and energy replacement for physical activity. *Australian Journal of Nutrition and Dietetics* 53 (4 Suppl).

Wolinsky, I., & Driskell, J.A. (eds.). 2001. *Nutritional applications in exercise and sport*. Boca Raton, FL: CRC Press.

Section 4

Adair, J. 1988. *Effective leadership*. London: Pan Books.

Collins, J., & Porras, J. 1994. *Built to last: Successful habits of visionary companies*. New York: HarperCollins.

Coulthard, M., Howell, A., & Clarke, G. 1996. *Business planning: The key to success*. South Melbourne: Macmillan Education.

Covey, S.R. 1995. *The seven habits of highly effective people*. New York: Simon & Schuster.

Covey, S.R., & Merrill, A.R. 1994. *First things first*. New York: Simon & Schuster.

David, F.R. 1999. *Concepts of strategic management*. Upper Saddle River, NJ: Prentice Hall.

Davidson, P., & Griffin, R.W. 2000. *Management: Australia in a global context*. Brisbane: Wiley.

Davis, K.A. 1997. *Sport management: Successful private sector business strategies*. Madison, WI: Brown & Benchmark.

Fisher, R., & Ury, W. 1982. *Getting to yes*. London: Hutchinson.

Grantham, W.C., Patton, R.W., York, T.D., & Winick, M.L. 1998. *Health fitness management*. Champaign, IL: Human Kinetics.

Johnson, G., & Scholes, K. 1993. *Exploring corporate strategy*. New York: Prentice Hall.

Maister, D.H. 1993. *Managing the professional service firm*. New York: Free Press.

Maister, D.H. 1997. *True professionalism*. New York: Free Press.

Meredith, G.G. 1994. *Accounting and financial management for business decisions*. Sydney: McGraw-Hill.

Mohan, M.L. 1993. *Organisational communication and cultural vision: Approaches for analysis*. Albany, NY: SUNY Press.

Myers, A. 1999. *Program evaluation for exercise leaders*. Champaign, IL: Human Kinetics.

Parkhouse, B.L. 1996. *The management of sport: Its foundation and application*. St. Louis: Mosby.

Rossman, R.T. 1995. *Recreation programming: Designing leisure experiences*. Champaign, IL: Sagamore.

Sawyer, T., & Smith, O. 1999. *The management of clubs, recreation, and sport: Concepts and applications*. Champaign, IL: Sagamore.

Smith, M. 1991. *Analysing organisational behaviour*. London: Macmillan.

Ulrich, D., Zenger, J., & Smallwood, N. 1999 *Results-based leadership*. Boston: Harvard Business School Press.

Yukl, G. 1994. *Leadership in organizations*. Englewood, NJ: Prentice Hall.

INDEX

▪ ▪ ▪ ▪ ▪ ▪ ▪ ▪ ▪ ▪ ▪ ▪

Page numbers followed by *f* or *t* indicate pages with figures and tables.

ABOUT THE AUTHORS

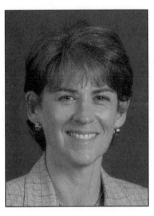

Laurel T. Mackinnon, PhD, is an associate professor at the University of Queensland at Brisbane, Australia. In 1992, Dr. Mackinnon authored *Exercise and Immunology*, the first book to explore the intriguing relationship between exercise and the immune system. She has received grant funding for projects related to overtraining and immune function in athletes.

Dr. Mackinnon is a fellow of Sports Medicine Australia and the American College of Sports Medicine. She is a former founding board member of the International Society of Exercise and Immunology (ISEI) and the Australian Association for Exercise and Sports Science. In 1997, she served as program chair for the international symposium of ISEI in Germany.

Dr. Mackinnon earned her PhD in exercise science at the University of Michigan. She previously held the position of research assistant professor at the University of New Mexico School of Medicine.

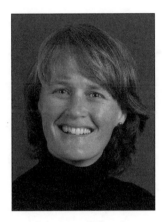

Carrie B. Ritchie, PhD, is a lecturer in clinical exercise science at the University of Queensland at Brisbane, Australia. Since 1993, she has lectured at the undergraduate and graduate levels in the areas of exercise prescription and programming for healthy populations and those requiring modifications and special considerations. Her research has focused on the design and implementation of physical activity options and adoption and maintenance of physical activity across various populations.

Dr. Ritchie is certified with the American College of Sports Medicine as a clinical exercise specialist. She earned her PhD in exercise physiology at the University of Queensland in 1996.

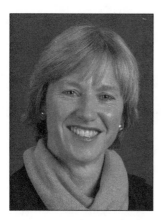

Sue L. Hooper, PhD, is director of the Centre for Physical Activity and Sport Education at the University of Queensland at Brisbane, Australia. She has more than 25 years of experience in exercise management, and she lectures at undergraduate and graduate levels in this field. She oversaw the management of 179 Olympic and Paralympic teams from 48 countries training and competing in Queensland before the 2000 Sydney Olympic Games. Dr. Hooper earned her PhD in exercise science at the University of Queensland in 1993.

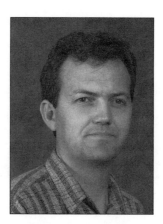

Peter J. Abernethy, PhD, is director of cardiovascular health programs for the National Heart Foundation (Queensland Division) at Brisbane, Australia. Prior to this he coordinated professional development and exercise management there for nine years at the University of Queensland. Dr. Abernethy has educated exercise management practitioners for 13 years.